Pediatric Anesthesia

Editors

VANESSA A. OLBRECHT
ALISON R. PERATE

ANESTHESIOLOGY CLINICS

www.anesthesiology.theclinics.com

Consulting Editor
LEE A. FLEISHER

September 2020 • Volume 38 • Number 3

ELSEVIER

1600 John F. Kennedy Boulevard • Suite 1800 • Philadelphia, Pennsylvania, 19103-2899

http://www.theclinics.com

ANESTHESIOLOGY CLINICS Volume 38, Number 3
September 2020 ISSN 1932-2275, ISBN-13: 978-0-323-76131-4

Editor: Joanna Collett
Developmental Editor: Kristen Helm

Anesthesiology Clinics (ISSN 1932-2275) is published quarterly by Elsevier Inc., 360 Park Avenue South, New York, NY 10010-1710. Months of issue are March, June, September, and December. Periodicals postage paid at New York, NY and at additional mailing offices. Subscription prices are $100.00 per year (US student/resident), $364.00 per year (US individuals), $446.00 per year (Canadian individuals), $728.00 per year (US institutions), $920.00 per year (Canadian institutions), $100.00 per year (Canadian student/resident), $225.00 per year (foreign student/resident), $474.00 per year (foreign individuals), and $920.00 per year (foreign institutions). To receive student and resident rate, orders must be accompanied by name of affiliated institution, date of term, and the *signature* of program/residency coordinator on institutions letterhead. Orders will be billed at individual rate until proof of status is received. Foreign air speed delivery is included in all *Clinics'* subscription prices. All prices are subject to change without notice. POSTMASTER: Send address changes to *Anesthesiology Clinics,* Elsevier Health Sciences Division, Subscription Customer Service, 3251 Riverport Lane, Maryland Heights, MO 63043. Customer Service (orders, claims, online, change of address): Elsevier Health Sciences Division, Subscription Customer Service, 3251 Riverport Lane, Maryland Heights, MO 63043. **Tel:1-800-654-2452 (U.S. and Canada); 314-447-8871 (outside U.S. and Canada). Fax: 314-447-8029. E-mail: journalscustomerservice-usa@elsevier.com (for print support); journalsonlinesupport-usa@elsevier.com (for online support)**.

Reprints. For copies of 100 or more of articles in this publication, please contact the Commercial Reprints Department, Elsevier Inc., 360 Park Avenue South, New York, NY 10010-1710. Tel.: 212-633-3874; Fax: 212-633-3820; E-mail: reprints@elsevier.com.

Anesthesiology Clinics, is also published in Spanish by McGraw-Hill Inter-americana Editores S. A., P.O. Box 5-237, 06500 Mexico D. F., Mexico.

Anesthesiology Clinics, is covered in *MEDLINE/PubMed (Index Medicus), Current Contents/Clinical Medicine, Excerpta Medica, ISI/BIOMED,* and *Chemical Abstracts.*

Contributors

CONSULTING EDITOR

LEE A. FLEISHER, MD, FACC, FAHA
Robert D. Dripps Professor and Chair of Anesthesiology and Critical Care, Professor of Medicine, Perelman School of Medicine, University of Pennsylvania, Philadelphia, Pennsylvania, USA

EDITORS

VANESSA A. OLBRECHT, MD, MBA
Associate Professor, Department of Anesthesia, Director of Quality Improvement and Accreditation for Procedural Sedation, Director of Anesthesia, Procedure Center, Associate Director of Research, Cincinnati Children's Hospital Medical Center, Cincinnati, Ohio, USA

ALISON R. PERATE, MD
Assistant Professor of Anesthesiology and Critical Care Medicine, Associate Director of Trauma, The Children's Hospital of Philadelphia, Perelman School of Medicine, University of Pennsylvania, Philadelphia, Pennsylvania, USA

AUTHORS

NIEKOO ABBASIAN, MD
Assistant Professor, Cincinnati Children's Hospital Medical Center, Cincinnati, Ohio, USA

ADAM C. ADLER, MS, MD, FAAP, FASE
Department of Anesthesiology, Perioperative and Pain Medicine, Texas Children's Hospital, Baylor College of Medicine, Houston, Texas, USA

ADITEE AMBARDEKAR, MD, MSEd
Associate Professor and Residency Program Director, Department of Anesthesiology and Pain Management, The University of Texas Southwestern Medical Center, Dallas, Texas, USA

KUMAR BELANI, MD
Professor, Department of Anesthesiology, University of Minnesota, Minneapolis, Minnesota, USA

TANNA J. BOYER, DO, MS
Associate Professor of Clinical Anesthesia, Director of Simulation, Department of Anesthesia, Indiana University School of Medicine, Indianapolis, Indiana, USA

ARVIND CHANDRAKANTAN, MD, MBA, FAAP, FASA
Department of Anesthesiology, Perioperative and Pain Medicine, Texas Children's Hospital, Baylor College of Medicine, Houston, Texas, USA

DEBNATH CHATTERJEE, MD, FAAP
Associate Professor of Anesthesiology, Children's Hospital Colorado, Anschutz Medical Campus, Director of Fetal Anesthesia, Colorado Fetal Care Center, Aurora, Colorado, USA

JOHN E. FIADJOE, MD
Associate Professor of Anesthesiology and Critical Care Medicine, The Children's Hospital of Philadelphia, Perelman School of Medicine, University of Pennsylvania, Philadelphia, Pennsylvania, USA

MICHAEL ANDREW FORD, DO
Clinical Anesthesia - 3 (PGY4) Resident, Department of Anesthesia, Indiana University School of Medicine, Indianapolis, Indiana, USA

ERICA GEE, MD
Clinical Fellow in Anesthesiology, Department of Anesthesia, Critical Care and Pain Medicine, Harvard Medical School, Massachusetts General Hospital, Boston, Massachusetts, USA

DIANE GORDON, MD
Associate Professor, Department of Anesthesiology, University of Colorado School of Medicine, Aurora, Colorado, USA

GRACE HSU, MD
Assistant Professor of Clinical Anesthesiology and Critical Care Medicine, The Children's Hospital of Philadelphia, Perelman School of Medicine, University of Pennsylvania, Philadelphia, Pennsylvania, USA

JI YEON JEMMA KANG, MD
Assistant Professor, Department of Anesthesia, University of Cincinnati College of Medicine, Cincinnati Children's Hospital Medical Center, Cincinnati, Ohio, USA

MEAGAN KING, MD
Department of Anesthesiology, Cincinnati Children's Hospital Medical Center, Cincinnati, Ohio, USA; Assistant Professor, Department of Anesthesiology, University of Minnesota, Minneapolis, Minnesota, USA

CHARLES DEAN KURTH, MD
John J. Downes MD Chair of Pediatric Anesthesiology and Critical Care Medicine, Anesthesiologist in Chief, Departments of Anesthesiology and Critical Care Medicine and Pediatrics, The Children's Hospital of Philadelphia, Perelman School of Medicine, University of Pennsylvania, Philadelphia, Pennsylvania, USA

MARY LANDRIGAN-OSSAR, MD, PhD
Senior Associate in Perioperative Anesthesia, Department of Anesthesiology, Critical Care and Pain Medicine, Boston Children's Hospital, Assistant Professor of Anaesthesia, Harvard Medical School, Boston, Massachusetts, USA

JOHANNA MEEHYUN LEE, MD
Clinical Fellow in Anesthesiology, Department of Anesthesia, Critical Care and Pain Medicine, Harvard Medical School, Massachusetts General Hospital, Boston, Massachusetts, USA

CHANG AMBER LIU, MD, MSc, FAAP
Assistant Professor, Department of Anaesthesia, Critical Care and Pain Medicine, Harvard Medical School, Massachusetts General Hospital, Boston, Massachusetts, USA

MARY ELLEN MCCANN, MD, MPH
Associate Professor of Anaesthesia, Department of Anesthesiology, Critical Care and Pain Medicine, Boston Children's Hospital, Harvard Medical School, Boston, Massachusetts, USA

SALLY A. MITCHELL, EdD, MMSc
Assistant Professor of Clinical Anesthesia, Vice Chair of Education, Statewide Assistant Clerkship Director, Department of Anesthesia, Indiana University School of Medicine, Indianapolis, Indiana, USA

ARUNA T. NATHAN, MD
Department of Anesthesia, Stanford University Medical Center, Stanford, California, USA

VANESSA A. OLBRECHT, MD, MBA
Associate Professor, Department of Anesthesia, Director of Quality Improvement and Accreditation for Procedural Sedation, Director of Anesthesia, Procedure Center, Associate Director of Research, Cincinnati Children's Hospital Medical Center, Cincinnati, Ohio, USA

ALISON R. PERATE, MD
Assistant Professor of Anesthesiology and Critical Care Medicine, Associate Director of Trauma, The Children's Hospital of Philadelphia, Perelman School of Medicine, University of Pennsylvania, Philadelphia, Pennsylvania, USA

NISHA PINTO, MD
Instructor of Anesthesiology, Department of Pediatric Anesthesiology, Ann & Robert H. Lurie Children's Hospital of Chicago, Feinberg School of Medicine, Northwestern University, Chicago, Illinois, USA

DAVID PRESTON, DO, MPH
Resident Physician, Department of Anesthesiology and Pain Management, The University of Texas Southwestern Medical Center, Dallas, Texas, USA

AMOD SAWARDEKAR, MD, MBA
Associate Professor of Anesthesiology, Department of Pediatric Anesthesiology, Ann & Robert H. Lurie Children's Hospital of Chicago, Feinberg School of Medicine, Northwestern University, Chicago, Illinois, USA

CHRISTOPHER TAN SETIAWAN, MD
Assistant Professor, Department of Anesthesiology and Pain Management, The University of Texas Southwestern Medical Center, Children's Medical Center, Dallas, Texas, USA

SULPICIO G. SORIANO, MD
Professor of Anaesthesia, Department of Anesthesiology, Critical Care and Pain Medicine, Boston Children's Hospital, Harvard Medical School, Boston, Massachusetts, USA

SANTHANAM SURESH, MD, MBA, FAAP
Anesthesiologist-in-Chief, Professor of Anesthesiology and Pediatrics, Department of Pediatric Anesthesiology, Ann & Robert H. Lurie Children's Hospital of Chicago, Feinberg School of Medicine, Northwestern University, Chicago, Illinois, USA

KHA M. TRAN, MD
Associate Professor of Clinical Anesthesiology and Critical Care Medicine, Perelman School of Medicine, University of Pennsylvania, Director of Fetal Anesthesia, Center for Fetal Diagnosis and Treatment, The Children's Hospital of Philadelphia, Philadelphia, Pennsylvania, USA

CHARLOTTE M. WALTER, MD
Assistant Professor, Cincinnati Children's Hospital Medical Center, Cincinnati, Ohio, USA

TING XU, MD
Departments of Anesthesiology, and Translational Neuroscience Center, West China Hospital, Sichuan University, The Research Units of West China (2018RU012) Chinese Academy of Medical Sciences, Chengdu, Sichuan, China; Department of Anesthesiology, Sichuan Academy of Medical Sciences & Sichuan Provincial People's Hospital, Chengdu, China

JIAN YE, MD
Assistant Professor of Clinical Anesthesia, Department of Anesthesia, Indiana University School of Medicine, Indianapolis, Indiana, USA

IAN YUAN, MD
Department of Anesthesiology and Critical Care Medicine, The Children's Hospital of Philadelphia, Perelman School of Medicine, University of Pennsylvania, Philadelphia, Pennsylvania, USA

Contents

> Children have unique characteristics that make them particularly vulnerable to perioperative adverse events. Skilled airway management is a cornerstone of high-quality anesthetic management. The use of hybrid airway techniques is a critical tool for the pediatric anesthesiologist. Point-of-care ultrasonography has an expanding role in airway management, from preoperative assessment of airway pathology and gastric contents to confirmation of tracheal intubation and identification of the cricothyroid membrane. The exciting fields of 3-dimensional printing, artificial intelligence, and machine learning are areas of innovation that will transform pediatric difficult airway management in years to come.

> There are compelling preclinical data that common general anesthetics cause increased neuroapoptosis in juvenile animals. Retrospective studies demonstrate that young children exposed to anesthesia have school difficulties, which could be caused by anesthetic neurotoxicity, perioperative hemodynamic and homeostatic instability, underlying morbidity, or the neuroinflammatory effects of surgical trauma. Unnecessary procedures should be avoided. Baseline measures of blood pressure are important in determining perioperative blood pressure goals. Inadvertent hypocapnia or moderate hypercapnia and hyperoxia or hypoxia should be avoided. Pediatric patients should be maintained in a normothermic, euglycemic state with neutral positioning. Improving outcomes of infants and children requires the collaboration of anesthesiologists, surgeons, pediatricians and neonatologists.

> Over the past few decades, there have been many advances in pediatric surgery, some using new devices (eg, VEPTR, MAGEC rods) and others

using less invasive approaches (eg, Nuss procedure, endoscopic cranial suture release, minimally invasive tethered cord release). Although many of these procedures were initially met with caution or skepticism, continued experience over the past few decades has shown that these procedures are safe and effective. This article reviews the anesthetic considerations for these conditions and procedures.

Disaster medicine refers to situations in which the need to care for patients outweighs the available resources. It is imperative for anesthesiologists to be involved at a leadership level in mass casualty/disaster preparedness planning. Mass casualty disaster plans should be clear, concise, and easy to follow. Terror events and natural disasters can differ significantly in anesthesia preparedness. Resiliency is an important aspect of the recovery phase that decreases psychological damage in the aftermath of a mass casualty event.

Management of the pediatric burn patient presents a variety of clinical challenges for the pediatric anesthesiologist. Despite the high incidence of burn injuries, standard management strategies are far from universal. The complex physiologic changes presented by burn injuries present airway management and resuscitation challenges and mandate careful consideration of adequate nutritional support. Long hospital stays with frequent operations and dressing changes necessitate creative approaches to anxiolysis and pain control. Underutilized modalities warranting further research include regional anesthesia and nonpharmacologic approaches, such as virtual reality. Further research and collaboration between burn centers are needed to standardize care for this population.

Children and adults with congenital heart disease undergoing noncardiac surgery are at higher risk of perioperative adverse events. Patients have significant comorbidities and syndromic associations that increase perioperative risk further. The complexity of congenital heart disease requires a thorough understanding of lesion-specific pathophysiology in order to provide safe care. Comprehensive multidisciplinary planning and the use of skilled and experienced teams achieve the best outcomes. The anesthesiologist is a perioperative physician charged with providing safe anesthesia care, instituting appropriate hemodynamic monitoring, and determining appropriate postoperative disposition on an individual basis.

This article discusses modernizing the education of pediatric anesthesiologists in the United States. First, the current education requirements to become an American Board of Anesthesiology certified pediatric anesthesiologist are detailed and then, through a historical lens, the development of the subspecialty is examined. Gaps and challenges in the current training system are identified and interventions for improvement discussed. Additionally, suggestions are made and questions posed on how to move from a time-based model towards a competency-based curriculum.

Nisha Pinto, Amod Sawardekar, and Santhanam Suresh

The scope of pediatric regional anesthesia is expanding, with increased safety and efficacy data over the past few years. As familiarity and expertise has developed with ultrasonography, regional anesthesia has played an important role in the management of acute pain in the postsurgical population.

Mary Landrigan-Ossar and Christopher Tan Setiawan

Anesthesia care performed outside the operating room is a growing area of pediatric anesthesia practice. The anesthesiology team expects to care for children in diverse locations, which include diagnostic and interventional radiology, gastroenterology and pulmonary endoscopy suites, radiation oncology sites, and the cardiac catheterization laboratory. To provide safe, high-quality care the anesthesiologist working in these environments must understand the unique environmental, logistical, and perioperative considerations and risks involved with each remote location. This 2-part review provides an overview of safety and system considerations in pediatric nonoperating room anesthesia before describing in more detail considerations for particular remote anesthetizing locations.

Christopher Tan Setiawan and Mary Landrigan-Ossar

Anesthesiology teams care for children in diverse locations, including diagnostic and interventional radiology, gastroenterology and pulmonary endoscopy suites, radiation oncology units, and cardiac catheterization laboratories. To provide safe, high-quality care, anesthesiologists working in these environments must understand the unique environmental and perioperative considerations and risks involved with each remote location and patient population. Once these variables are addressed, anesthesia and procedural teams can coordinate to ensure that patients and families receive the same high-quality care that they have come to expect in the operating room. This article also describes some of the considerations for anesthetic care in outfield locations.

Kha M. Tran and Debnath Chatterjee

Fetal anesthesia teams must understand the pathophysiology and rationale for the treatment of each disease process. Treatment can range from minimally invasive procedures to maternal laparotomy, hysterotomy, and major fetal surgery. Timing may be in early, mid-, or late gestation. Techniques continue to be refined, and the anesthetic plans must evolve to meet the needs of the procedures. Anesthetic plans range from moderate sedation to general anesthesia that includes monitoring of 2 patients simultaneously, fluid restriction, invasive blood pressure monitoring, vasopressor administration, and advanced medication choices to optimize fetal cardiac function.

The most common congenital anomalies are congenital heart defects, cleft lip and palate, Down syndrome, and neural tube defects. Anesthetic considerations for Down syndrome include cervical spine instability, history of congenital heart disease, risk of bradycardia, hematologic, endocrine, and behavioral considerations. Patients with cleft lip and palate can have associated syndromes, and the potential for underlying abnormalities should be investigated prior to their anesthetic. A major anesthetic consideration for neural tube defect surgery is positioning for intubation. Fetal surgery for myelomeningocele has been shown to reduce the need for ventriculoperitoneal shunting and improved motor outcomes.

The focus of this article is noncardiac surgery in the adult with congenital heart disease (CHD). The purpose is to provide the general and pediatric anesthesiologist with a basic overview of the most common congenital cardiac lesions, their long-term sequelae, and expected perioperative concerns during noncardiac surgery. Because of the very heterogeneous nature of CHD, it is difficult to make a single article a comprehensive guide for every lesion and its associated perioperative concerns. The authors hope to provide those who are not specifically trained in congenital cardiac anesthesia the basic principles and a greater understanding of each defect.

Trends in pediatric pain management are moving toward thinking beyond opioids. Regional anesthetic techniques, such as quadratus lumborum and erector spinae plane blocks, demonstrate efficacy and safety in pediatric populations. Extremity blocks with motor-sparing characteristics also are used. Adjuvants may be added to pediatric peripheral nerve blocks to increase duration of action and improve block efficacy. For medical management, pediatric pain management frequently uses nonopioid medications. These opioid-sparing medications and regional techniques are used to facilitate enhanced recovery after surgery in pediatric surgical patients. Virtual reality is a field where technology can aid in managing acute pain in pediatric patients.

Diane Gordon

Climate change will be the defining health crisis of the twenty-first century, and environmental health is directly linked with human health. The health sector should lead the sustainability effort by greening itself and reducing its ecological footprint to improve global health and the health of the planet. Anesthesiology has an oversized role in production of greenhouse gases and waste, and thus its impact on affecting change is also over-sized. Decreasing the waste of volatile anesthetic agents, medications, and anesthesia equipment is a powerful start to the many sustainability changes needed in health care.

Arvind Chandrakantan and Adam C. Adler

Pediatric obstructive sleep apnea affects a large number of children and has multiple end-organ sequelae. Although many of these have been demonstrated to be reversible, the effects on some of the organ systems, including the brain, have not shown easy reversibility. Progress in this area has been hampered by lack of a preclinical model to study the disease. Therefore, perioperative and sleep physicians are tasked with making a number of difficult decisions, including optimal surgical timing to prevent disease evolution, but also to keep the perioperative morbidity in a safe range for these patients.

Ian Yuan, Ting Xu, and Charles Dean Kurth

Sevoflurane and propofolebased anesthetics are dosed according to vital signs, movement, and expired sevoflurane concentrations, which do not assess the anesthetic state of the brain and, therefore, risk underdose and overdose. Electroencephalography (EEG) measures cortical brain activity and can assess hypnotic depth, a key component of the anesthetic state. Application of sevoflurane and propofol pharmacology along with EEG parameters can more precisely guide dosing to achieve the desired anesthetic state for an individual pediatric patient. This article reviews the principles underlying EEG use for sevoflurane and propofol dosing in pediatric anesthesia and offers case examples to illustrate their use in individual patients.

ANESTHESIOLOGY CLINICS

SERIES OF RELATED INTEREST

Pediatric Clinics

THE CLINICS ARE AVAILABLE ONLINE!
Access your subscription at:
www.theclinics.com

Foreword

Moving Beyond the Ordinary: Transcending Traditions in Pediatric Anesthesia

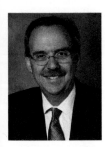

Lee A. Fleisher, MD
Consulting Editor

Surgical and procedural interventions in complex pediatric patients have evolved greatly over the years. Many of these patients undergo surgery at children's hospitals, but they could present in any hospital setting, and therefore, knowledge of their care is important for a large number of anesthesiologists. In addition, patients with congenital heart disease can survive into adulthood and require further interventions, and therefore, all anesthesiologists need to understand the care of the adult patient with congenital heart disease. In this issue of *Anesthesiology Clinics*, the editors have brought together a series of articles that cover a broad array of pediatric anesthesia topics that would be of interest to a wide variety of anesthesiologists.

This issue was edited by rising pediatric leaders from two of the preeminent pediatric hospitals in the United States. Vanessa A. Olbrecht, MD, MBA is an Associate Professor of Anesthesiology at Cincinnati Children's Hospital Medical Center and an outcomes researcher. She is also Director of Quality Improvement and Accreditation for Procedural Sedation. Alison R. Perate, MD is Assistant Professor of Anesthesiology at the University of Pennsylvania and The Children's Hospital of Philadelphia. She is also

Anesthesiology Clin 38 (2020) xiii–xiv
https://doi.org/10.1016/j.anclin.2020.07.002
1932-2275/20/© 2020 Published by Elsevier Inc.

Associate Director of the Trauma Center. Together they have assembled an amazing group of leaders in pediatric anesthesia to describe unique practices.

Lee A. Fleisher, MD
Perelman School of Medicine
University of Pennsylvania
3400 Spruce Street, Dulles 680
Philadelphia, PA 19104, USA

E-mail address:
Lee.Fleisher@uphs.upenn.edu

Preface

Moving Beyond the Ordinary: Transcending Traditions in Pediatric Anesthesia

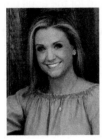
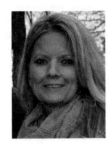

Vanessa A. Olbrecht, MD, MBA   Alison R. Perate, MD
Editors

Prior to the adoption of ether anesthesia in 1846, children undergoing procedures such as circumcisions or amputations did not receive anesthesia or analgesia. Pain was simply accepted as a necessary part of the surgical intervention. Despite the advances in the field of anesthesia over the next several decades, children were often misrepresented as "little adults." Even in the 1980s, the belief that infants did not require pain control prevailed. The advent of pediatric anesthesia and other advances in medical science and patient care have revolutionized pediatric surgery and improved the quality of care received by children.

The field of pediatric anesthesia emerged in the 1940s, when pediatric surgeons began performing complex operations on children. Since then, many innovations and new trends in pediatric anesthesia, such as the discovery of different anesthetic agents and airway management with tracheal intubation, have led to the continued evolution of modern pediatric anesthesia care. Because of increasingly complex procedures performed on children and the discovery of other successful therapies, many children with significant congenital abnormalities now live into adulthood, and the prevalence of these patients continues to rise. While pediatric anesthesiologists receive special training to care for these patients, non–pediatric anesthesia providers will increasingly face pediatric-based challenges in their practice.

This issue of *Anesthesiology Clinics* focuses on innovations and new trends in pediatric anesthesia and is intended to update anesthesia providers who care for children and adults with congenital disease. It also strives to highlight areas of unique innovation, such as advances in fetal surgery, optimization of education of the anesthesia provider, and how to be more ecologically friendly in our practice. We start with discussions about new techniques to care for pediatric patients with a difficult airway. We

Anesthesiology Clin 38 (2020) xv–xvi
https://doi.org/10.1016/j.anclin.2020.07.001
1932-2275/20/© 2020 Published by Elsevier Inc.

discuss neurologic implications of anesthetics, including current research on neuro-toxicity, a pressing question often asked of the anesthesia provider. We explore a se-ries of interesting topics in pediatric anesthesia, including anesthesia for innovative pediatric surgical procedures, mass casualty preparedness, anesthesia for pediatric burns, managing the child with complex congenital heart disease, and modernizing the education of the pediatric anesthesiologist. This issue also explores care for the pediatric patient outside of the operating room, including the use of regional analgesia and providing safe care to patients in remote locations. We discuss the emerging topic of fetal anesthesia and how to optimally provide care for the fetal patient, a hybrid of pediatric and obstetric anesthesia. Finally, we review how to care for the adult patient with complex congenital disease, address the increasingly common problem of obstructive sleep apnea, and address how we can use electroencephalogram to bet-ter tailor anesthesia therapy. We also include an article focusing on moving beyond opioids in the care of pediatric perioperative pain, a topic of great interest in light of the opioid epidemic as well as an article addressing environmental sustainability in the operating room to help reduce our impact on the planet.

While this issue of *Anesthesiology Clinics* is certainly not a comprehensive review of all new topics and trends in pediatric anesthesia, the authors provide interesting and thought-provoking discussions of many exciting innovations in our field. We sincerely thank the authors for sharing their considerable knowledge, expertise, and insights. We hope you enjoy their contributions as much as we have.

Vanessa A. Olbrecht, MD, MBA
Cincinnati Children's Hospital Medical Center
3333 Burnet Avenue, MLC 2001
Cincinnati, OH 45229, USA

Alison R. Perate, MD
The Children's Hospital of Philadelphia
3401 Civic Center Boulevard
Philadelphia, PA 19104, USA

E-mail addresses:
Vanessa.Olbrecht@cchmc.org (V.A. Olbrecht)
PerateA@email.chop.edu (A.R. Perate)

The Pediatric Difficult Airway: Updates and Innovations

Grace Hsu, MD*, John E. Fiadjoe, MD

KEYWORDS

- Pediatric difficult airway • Can't intubate can't oxygenate • Point-of-care-ultrasound
- Artificial intelligence • Machine learning • Three-dimensional printing

KEY POINTS

- Children are particularly vulnerable to adverse events during airway management.
- Understanding how to use hybrid techniques to manage the pediatric airway is critical for the pediatric anesthesiologist.
- Point-of-care ultrasonography, 3-dimensional printing, artificial intelligence, and machine learning are technologies that are bringing innovation to the management of the pediatric difficult airway.

INTRODUCTION

Skilled airway management is a cornerstone of high-quality anesthetic management. Respiratory complications remain a frequent cause of anesthetic-related complications in children due to their unique anatomy and physiology.[1] The infant or child with a difficult airway poses even greater challenges for clinicians. New technologies have improved the safety and management of pediatric difficult airways. The use of hybrid airway techniques, point-of-care ultrasonography (POCUS), novel ventilation devices, 3-dimensional (3-D) printing, artificial intelligence, and machine learning are transforming pediatric difficult airway management. This article summarizes the recent scientific literature, introduces novel airway devices and techniques, and highlights areas of innovation that are advancing pediatric difficult airway management forward.

UNIQUE CHARACTERISTICS OF THE PEDIATRIC AIRWAY

Children have anatomic characteristics that make airway management potentially challenging. They have a large occiput that naturally flexes the neck while they are lying supine, leading to upper airway obstruction and soft tissue compression. Their large occiput and more cephalad larynx make it challenging to align their oral,

Children's Hospital of Philadelphia, Perelman School of Medicine at the University of Pennsylvania, 3401 Civic Center Boulevard, Suite M905, Philadelphia, PA 19104, USA
* Corresponding author.
E-mail address: HsuG@email.chop.edu
Twitter: @Jef042 (J.E.F.)

Anesthesiology Clin 38 (2020) 459–475
https://doi.org/10.1016/j.anclin.2020.05.001
1932-2275/20/© 2020 Elsevier Inc. All rights reserved.

pharyngeal, and laryngeal axes during laryngoscopy. Their tongue and tonsils are proportionally larger than their oropharynx, leading to upper airway obstruction. The pediatric epiglottis is stiff, omega-shaped, and difficult to lift to obtain a view of the glottic opening. The cricoid cartilage is the narrowest point of the airway in an infant, increasing the risk of subglottic trauma with endotracheal tube (TT) placement. The trachea and lower airways are small in diameter, leading to exponential increases in airflow resistance when narrowed.

Children also have respiratory characteristics that predispose them to rapid oxygen desaturation during intubation. Their soft chest wall is compliant due to lack of ossification of the rib cage and is prone to collapse during tidal volume breathing under anesthesia, leading to atelectasis and loss of functional reserve capacity. Children consume more oxygen than do adults, leading to rapid oxygen desaturation during apnea. The infant's parasympathetic system is more fully developed than their sympathetic system, causing infants to respond to hypoxic stress with bradycardia and consequent cardiac arrest.

INCIDENCE AND PREDICTORS OF THE PEDIATRIC DIFFICULT AIRWAY

Challenges in airway management are categorized as occurring during mask ventilation, intubation, or supraglottic airway (SGA) placement. Patient characteristics help predict when one of these steps may be difficult. Congenital and acquired abnormalities of the head and neck often are associated with difficult airway management. The Committee on Nomenclature and Classification of Craniofacial Anomalies of the American Cleft Palate-Craniofacial Association has organized anomalies into 5 categories[2]: clefts, synostosis, hypoplasia, hyperplasia, and unclassified—with each of the categories associated with difficult airway management. Large cleft palates are associated with difficulty intubating. Craniosynostosis occurs when there is premature closure of 1 or more cranial sutures. Some of the most common craniosynostosis syndromes include Apert, Pfeiffer, Crouzon, Saethre-Chotzen, Carpenter, and Muenke syndromes and these syndromes are associated with difficult intubation. Examples of syndromes associated with craniofacial hypoplasia include Pierre Robin sequence and Goldenhar syndrome. Ease of intubation tends to improve with age in children with hypoplastic craniofacial dysmorphisms. Mucopolysaccharidoses, including Hunter and Hurler syndromes, and vascular malformations are hyperplastic anomalies associated with difficult airway management.

Difficult Mask Ventilation

The incidence of difficult bag-mask ventilation (DBMV) among healthy children in the 0 to 8-year age range is reported to be 6.6%.[3] This is much higher than the reported incidence of 1.5% of DBMV in adults.[4] Valois-Gomez and colleagues[3] studied a population of 484 children between the ages of 0 to 8 years undergoing elective surgery requiring bag-mask ventilation (BMV) and tracheal intubation. They defined DBMV as the occurrence of greater than or equal to 2 of the following events during BMV: application of continuous positive airway pressure of greater than or equal to 5 cm H_2O, required use of an oral/nasal airway, need for 2-person ventilation, desaturation less than 95%, and unanticipated need to increase fraction of inspired oxygen. Patient risk factors for DBMV were age less than 1 year and otolaryngology (ear, nose, and throat [ENT]) surgery.

Difficult Tracheal Intubation

Valois-Gomez and colleagues[3] determined the incidence of difficult tracheal intubation in children to be 1.2% and defined difficult tracheal intubation as the presence of greater than or equal to 2 of the following: Cormack-Lehane laryngoscopic view grade III or grade IV; greater than 3 attempts at intubation; intubation time greater than 5 minutes in total (sum of all attempts between the time the operator holds the laryngoscope until the TT passes the cords and the position is verified by auscultation and positive $EtCO_2$); and presence of desaturation less than 95%. The incidence of difficult intubation in children is similar to the incidence reported in adults of 1.8%.[5]

Heinrich and colleagues[6] found a similar incidence (1.35%) of difficult direct laryngoscopy (DL) in pediatric patients ages 0 to 18 years old. They analyzed a cohort of 11,219 pediatric patients undergoing anesthesia over a 5-year period and found patient age less than 1 year, American Society of Anesthesiologists physical status class III or IV, Mallampati score class III or IV, and low body mass index as risk factors associated with difficult DL. In the cohort, infants had the highest incidence of difficult DL (5%), followed by neonates (3.2%). The study also found that patients undergoing pediatric cardiac or oromaxillofacial surgery have a high incidence of difficult laryngoscopy—potentially explained by the finding that congenital heart defects often are associated with craniofacial dysmorphisms.

Difficult Supraglottic Airway Device Placement

SGAs, including laryngeal mask airways (LMAs), may be used as the primary airway device during general anesthesia or as a secondary technique during rescue and emergency airway management. SGAs are indicated for rescue ventilation in pediatric difficult airway algorithms when mask ventilation or tracheal intubation is difficult or impossible.[7] In a retrospective study of 11,910 anesthetic cases in pediatric patients less than 18 years old, Mathis and colleagues[8] identified that LMAs failed to rescue the airway in 0.86% of attempts. Risk factors for LMA failure were patient age less than 2 years old, ENT procedures, inpatient status, prolonged surgical duration, airway abnormalities, and room-to-room transport with an LMA in place.

COMPLICATIONS DURING PEDIATRIC DIFFICULT AIRWAY MANAGEMENT

A relatively high rate of severe critical events occurs during anesthetic management of children. The Anaesthesia Practice in Children Observational Trial (APRICOT), a prospective observational study of children less than 15 year old undergoing 31,127 anesthetic procedures across 261 hospitals in Europe, found that the incidence of perioperative severe critical events was 5.2%.[1] The incidence of respiratory critical events, including laryngospasm, bronchospasm, bronchial aspiration, and postanesthesia stridor, was 3.1%. Severe critical events occurred more often in children who were considered difficult to intubate. This finding was corroborated by a study from the Pediatric Difficult Intubation Collaborative. The group analyzed 1018 difficult pediatric tracheal intubation encounters across 13 children's hospitals and showed that 20% of pediatric patients with difficult intubations experienced perioperative complications, including cardiac arrest, hypoxemia, laryngospasm, and airway trauma[9]; 3% of these children had severe complications, including 1% having cardiac arrest. Children with unanticipated difficult airways had an even higher incidence of cardiac arrest, at a 3% rate. Complications during difficult tracheal intubation were associated with the following risk factors: weight less than 10 kg, short thyromental distance, multiple tracheal intubation attempts (>2), and persistent DL attempts ($\geq$3). Important takeaways from these studies are that the anesthetic management of a child less than 10 kg and with a short thyromental distance requires particular attention and preparation for a suspected difficult airway. Additionally, for children at risk of difficult tracheal intubation, each intubation attempt should be treated as a critical intervention and the number of DL and intubation attempts should be limited.

DEVICES AND TECHNIQUES FOR THE PEDIATRIC DIFFICULT AIRWAY
Oxygenation for the Pediatric Difficult Airway

Hypoxemia is one of the most common complications associated with pediatric difficult airway management.[9] In both adult and pediatric populations, oxygen delivery during tracheal intubation attempts reduce the incidence of hypoxemia.[10] Oxygen may be delivered during intubation while patients are kept spontaneously ventilating or while they are apneic.

Apneic oxygenation is a concept first described by Martin Holmdahl in 1956.[11] During apnea, oxygen is taken up from the alveoli due to the differential rate between alveolar oxygen absorption and carbon dioxide excretion, producing a mass flow of gas from the upper respiratory tract into the lungs. Apneic oxygenation may be delivered in a variety of ways, including via nasal cannula,[10] modified nasopharyngeal airway,[12] modified oral Ring-Adair-Elwyn (RAE) TT,[13] or heated humidified high-flow nasal cannula (HHHFNC) (**Fig. 1**).

HHHFNC is technique that originally was used in neonatology as a mode of respiratory support for premature infants, decreasing the need for tracheal intubation.[14] Cool dry gas delivered through nasal cannula at flows greater than 2 L/min quickly dry nasopharyngeal and oropharyngeal mucosa and is not well tolerated in young children.[15] HHHFNC heats gas to body temperature and humidifies it to greater than 99% relative humidity, allowing for comfortable delivery of gas flow rates matching or exceeding a patient's inspiratory flow rate. This technique is used during adult difficult

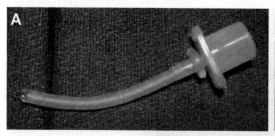
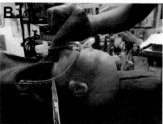
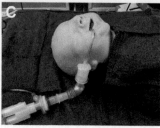

Fig. 1. (*A*) A modified nasopharyngeal airway for passive oxygenation. A TT 15-mm adapter taken from a TT of appropriate size for the patient is tunneled through the proximal end of the nasopharyngeal airway. (*B*) A modified oral RAE TT for passive oxygenation. Obtain an oral RAE TT of age-appropriate size for patient. Cut the distal TT so that the TT is equal lengths on both sides of the preformed bend. (*C*) A modified oral RAE TT for passive oxygenation. (*From [B, C]* Man JY, Fiadjoe JE, Hsu G. Technique utilizing a modified oral Ring-Adair-Elwyn tube to provide continuous oxygen and sevoflurane delivery during nasotracheal intubation in an infant with a difficult airway: a case report. *A A Pract* 2018;10:254-7, with permission.)

airway management to prolong the apneic time postinduction and is referred to as transnasal humidified rapid-insufflation (THRIVE).[16] THRIVE also has been described to be effective in delaying hypoxia in children during apnea after induction of anesthesia. Humphreys and colleagues[17] showed that children who received THRIVE doubled their time to desaturation to 92%. The flow rates used by Humphreys and colleagues are shown in **Table 1**. Anesthesiologists should consider delivering supplemental oxygen during difficult airway management of a child to reduce the risk of hypoxemia, using one of the numerous options available.

Videolaryngoscopy

Videolaryngoscopy (VL) allows the larynx to be visualized indirectly via a camera at the end of a laryngoscope blade. As opposed to DL, where the oral, pharyngeal, and laryngeal axes must be aligned to view the glottis, VL with a camera and video cable allows the operator to see around curves. An ever-increasing number of VL systems continue to be developed, including standard blades and hyperangulated options.

Standard blade videolaryngoscopes
Standard blade VLs have a similar shape and size to conventional Miller and Macintosh blades with the addition of a camera at the tip of the blade. The 2 main techniques for standard blade VL use are (1) traditional VL and (2) video-assisted DL. Video-assisted DL is a technique where the laryngoscopist performs DL and has the backup of the VL in the setting where DL is challenging. The application of this technique is increasingly popular in medical education. A trainee is able to perform DL with the VL, with an instructor looking on at the video screen, giving real-time feedback and coaching.[18,19] This technique has been useful particularly in teaching learners the intubation technique for neonates and infants, a population known to have a higher incidence of DBMV and difficult tracheal intubation and prone to rapid oxygen desaturation during airway management.

Hyperangulated videolaryngoscopes
There are several hyperangulated VLs available for use in children. Hyperangulated VLs cannot be used to perform standard DL because of the blade's acute angle, typically between 55° and 90°. A common problem with hyperangulated blades is a phenomenon called view-tube discrepancy, or when a good view of the glottis is obtained but there is difficulty advancing the TT into the trachea. The inherent angle of the blade, curvature of the styletted TT, and potentially challenging patient anatomy all contribute to this difficulty of advancing the TT into the trachea. Zhang and colleagues[20] conducted a prospective observational study of 225 GlideScope (Verathon; Bothell, Washington)-guided intubations in children less than 6 years of age and determined that 58% of attempts had technical difficulties, with the most common difficulty

Table 1	
Flow rates for children receiving heated humidified high-flow nasal cannula	
Weight	**Flow Rate**
0–15 kg	2 L/kg/min
15–30 kg	35 L/min
30–50 kg	40 L/min
>50 kg	50 L/min

Data from Humphreys S, Lee-Archer P, Reyne G, et al. Transnasal humidified rapid-insufflation ventilatory exchange (THRIVE) in children: a randomized controlled trial. *Br J Anaesth* 2017;118:232-8.

being "view-tube discrepancy." Technical difficulty was most likely to occur when the TT was advanced between the arytenoid cartilages just beyond the vocal cords. The TT often would catch on the arytenoid cartilage. Clockwise rotation of the TT was the most helpful maneuver to resolve this issue. The overall success rate of tracheal intubation with this technique was 98%, with first-attempt success rate of 80%.

Channeled VLs are a subset of hyperangulated VLs that have a guidance channel for a TT to be integrated into the blade of the scope. The potential benefit of channeled VLs is that when a view of the glottis is obtained, advancing the TT through the channel theoretically leads the tip of the tube through the glottic opening. Channeled devices, however, also have been associated with view-tube discrepancy. **Table 2** shows commonly used pediatric videolarygoscope systems.

Table 2
Commonly used pediatric laryngoscope systems

Manufacturer	Hyperangulated			Nonangulated		
	Neonatal/Infant	Pediatric	Teen	Neonatal/Infant	Pediatric	Teen
GlideScope[a] (Verathon)	+	+	+	Forthcoming	Forthcoming	+
C-MAC[b] (Karl Storz, El Segundo, California)	+/−	+	+	+	+	+
McGrath[c] (Medtronic, Minneapolis, Minnesota)	−	−	+	+	+	+
Airtraq[d] (Teleflex, Morrisville, North Carolina)	+	+	+	−	−	−
Truview PCD (Truphatek, Netanya, Israel)	+	+	+	−	−	−
UE Scope (UE Medical Devices, Newton, Massachusetts)	−	+	+	+	−	−
King Vision[d] (Ambu, Columbia, Maryland)	+	+	+	−	−	−

[a] Miller 0, 1, and 2 GlideScope VL blades are expected to become available in early 2020, in addition to existing Macintosh 3 and 4 blades.
[b] C-MAC pediatric hyperangulated blade (D-BLADE) may be used in infants, but it is less well suited for small or premature neonates. C-MAC nonangulated VLs are available in both Miller and Macintosh blades.
[c] McGrath nonangulated VLs are available in Macintosh blades.
[d] Airtraq and King Vision offer channeled hyperangulated VLs.
From Stein ML, Park RS, Kovatsis PG. Emerging trends, techniques, and equipment for airway management in pediatric patients. *Paediatr Anaesth* 2020;00:1-11, with permission.

Videolaryngoscopy with Fiberoptic Bronchoscopy

Hybrid techniques have become increasingly important in difficult airway management because no individual device has a perfect success rate. Hybrid techniques involve the simultaneous use of 2 different techniques, with the aim of capitalizing on the strengths of each device while overcoming their individual limitations. The combination technique of VL with flexible bronchoscopy is the technique where a flexible bronchoscope is used as a controllable and maneuverable stylet during VL. In this technique, the particular challenge of advancing a TT around the hyperangulated curve of a VL is overcome with fine motor control of the TT using the flexible bronchoscope. Another major advantage of this technique is that the clinician has 2 views of the tip of the TT: the flexible bronchoscopic view and the view of the TT with the VL. In addition, the challenges of using the flexible bronchoscope on its own with its narrow-angle view of the airway prone to distortion by oropharyngeal soft tissue are addressed by the videoscope creating space for the bronchoscope. This combined technique has been compared in the adult difficult airway population to GlideScope intubation alone and found to have a higher first-attempt intubation success rate (91% vs 67%) and faster tracheal intubation time (50 seconds vs 64 seconds).[21]

A downside of this combined technique is that it requires 2 skilled clinicians — 1 to operate the VL and the other to operate the flexible bronchoscope. The TT is preloaded onto the flexible bronchoscope. The videoscope then is placed into the oropharynx and the best view of the glottis is obtained. The videoscope is tilted slightly to the left of the oropharynx to provide a midline path for the flexible bronchoscope and TT. The flexible bronchoscope then is advanced toward the glottic opening and then into the trachea until a view of the carina is seen. The TT is advanced over the bronchoscope through the glottis under VL guidance, allowing the clinician to correct any TT obstacles at the cords under visualization. The final TT position is confirmed with the bronchoscope (**Fig. 2**).

In this combined technique, the flexible scope images may become difficult to see because of excessive lighting caused by having both VL and flexible scope lighting on simultaneously. Reducing the lighting of either the flexible bronchoscope or VL mitigates this problem. The bronchoscope never should be advanced blindly into the trachea, because airway trauma can occur. If the bronchoscope light is turned down during intubation, it should be turned back up as the scope tip passes through the vocal cords.

New systems with split screens have been developed by device manufacturers to allow for visualization of both the videoscope view and flexible bronchoscope view on the same screen.

Flexible Bronchoscopic Intubation via a Supraglottic Airway Device

Flexible bronchoscopic intubation can be performed through an SGA. This technique is useful particularly for pediatric patients with severe upper airway obstruction. One unique advantage of this technique is the ability to continue oxygenation, ventilation, anesthetic gas delivery, and gas sampling through the SGA during tracheal intubation.[22] The technique starts with preparation of the SGA and the TT. The 15-mm adapter is removed from the SGA and the TT is advanced two-thirds of the way down the shaft of the SGA. The TT cuff then is inflated to create a seal. A bronchoscope swivel adapter is attached to the end of the TT (**Fig. 3**). The prepared apparatus is placed into the oropharynx of the patient. The SGA position then is optimized and connected to the anesthesia circuit, allowing for continuous ventilation and delivery of oxygen and anesthetic gas. The flexible bronchoscope is inserted through the

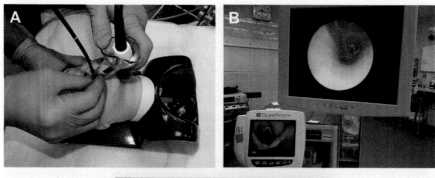

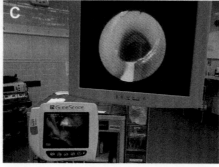

Fig. 2. (*A*) Proper positioning of a VL and flexible bronchoscope during a combined technique. (*B*) VL and flexible bronchoscopic views of the glottis. (*C*) Flexible bronchoscopic view of the carina, and simultaneous view of TT advancement under VL guidance. (*From* Olomu PN, Hsu G, Lockman JL. Hybrid approaches to the difficult pediatric airway. In: Jagannathan N, Fiadjoe JE, editors. *Management of the Difficult Pediatric Airway.* Cambridge: Cambridge University Press 2020. p.123, with permission. Used with permission, ©Verathon Inc.)

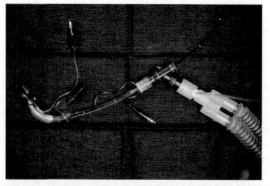

Fig. 3. SGA and TT apparatus. (*From* Olomu PN, Hsu G, Lockman JL. Hybrid approaches to the difficult pediatric airway. In: Jagannathan N, Fiadjoe JE, editors. *Management of the Difficult Pediatric Airway.* Cambridge: Cambridge University Press 2020. p.121, with permission.)

swivel adapter into the TT, past the SGA to the glottis, and finally into the trachea until a view of the carina is obtained. The TT cuff then is deflated and the tube is advanced into the trachea with the flexible scope as a guide. When the TT position has been confirmed, the SGA is removed—this is the only time during the procedure when ventilation must be briefly stopped.

Removal of the SGA over the TT is the highest-risk portion of this technique because the TT can be easily dislodged.[23] To remove the SGA from the oropharynx, disconnect the anesthesia circuit from the apparatus. Remove the TT 15-mm circuit adapter and place in a safe and easy-to-recover location. Stabilize the TT in place with laryngeal forceps, a disposable air-Q stabilizer rod, or a second uncuffed TT a half-size smaller tunneled into the proximal end of the intubated TT. Remove the SGA over the TT. Remove the stabilizing device, reinsert the 15 mm circuit adapter into the TT, reconnect the TT to the anesthesia circuit, and reinitiate positive pressure ventilation. Finally, reconfirm the TT position with flexible bronchoscopy via the bronchoscopic swivel adapter.

Ultrasonography for Airway Management

POCUS has become an important and transformative tool for clinical practice across multiple disciplines. It has unique characteristics of being a portable, noninvasive, and repeatable technique. POCUS has numerous applications in pediatric airway management, including in children with difficult airways. Some of the most useful airway applications of ultrasound are (1) choosing the correct TT size; (2) confirming correct TT placement; (3) identifying the cricothyroid membrane (CTM) and trachea prior to induction of anesthesia in a patient with suspected difficult airway; and (4) gastric ultrasound for qualitative and quantitative assessment of gastric contents prior to induction of anesthesia. There are many other proposed uses for ultrasonography in anesthesiology, including prediction of difficult laryngoscopy, assessment of obstructive sleep apnea, confirmation of SGA placement, and ruling out pneumothorax[24]; however, only a select number of applications are discussed.

Airway ultrasound

Ultrasonography can be used to identify subglottic stenosis. Knowing a patient's subglottic diameter can help a clinician choose the correct TT size to minimize trauma and subsequent edema. Ultrasound measurement of the subglottic diameter has been shown superior to age-based formulas in estimating the correct TT size in children.[25]

Tracheal intubation usually is confirmed with capnography or auscultation of lung fields. Capnography may be unreliable, however, in low cardiac output states, such as cardiac arrest, and auscultation has been shown to be surprisingly poor for detecting tracheal intubation, particularly in the neonatal population.[26] This is exacerbated when a patient is in severe bronchospasm. In these scenarios, the ability to confirm tracheal intubation via ultrasonography is a valuable tool. In successful tracheal intubation, only 1 air-mucosa interface is seen at the transverse view of the CTM. There also may be acoustic shadowing, known as the snowstorm sign, or a flutter behind the thyroid cartilage, when the TT passes through the glottis and touches the anterior tracheal wall. This is in contrast to when the TT enters the esophagus, and a double-trachea sign is seen (**Fig. 4**). This occurs because 2 air-mucosa interfaces are seen simultaneously: the trachea and the TT in the esophagus. Without a TT in the esophagus, the esophagus usually appears empty and flat without air in it. Ultrasound is able to confirm tracheal intubation with sensitivity and specificity of 98% and 98%, respectively.[27]

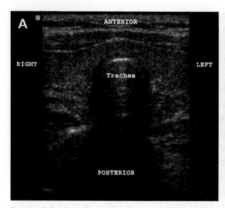
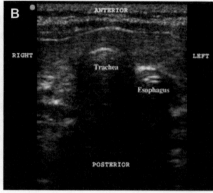

Fig. 4. (*A*) Ultrasonographic image of tracheal intubation. Only the shadowing posterior to the tracheal rings is visualized. The esophagus is not visualized. (*B*) Ultrasonographic image of esophageal intubation. Shadowing is seen posterior to the tracheal rings and in the left paratracheal space where the esophagus has been opened by the TT. (*From* Werner SL, Smith CE, Goldsetin JR, et al. Pilot study to evaluate the accuracy of ultrasonography in confirming endotracheal tube placement. *Ann Emerg Med* 2007;49:75-80, with permission.)

Emergency front-of-neck access (FONA) is a life-saving procedure in the "can't intubate, can't oxygenate" (CICO) scenario. Identification of the pediatric CTM by palpation alone, however, yields low success rates. Fennessy and colleagues[28] performed a study in which anesthesiologists evaluated 97 children and attempted to identify the CTM. Accuracy of identification of the CTM by palpation was 29.4% for children ages 37 weeks to less than 1 year, 28.6% for children 1 year old to 8 years old, and 38.2% for children 9 years old to 16 years old. In contrast, ultrasound can provide rapid and accurate identification of the CTM or midline trachea.[29] Ultrasound can be used to identify these structures preoperatively in the anticipated difficult airway or at point-of-care in the unanticipated emergency FONA scenario. The longitudinal (string-of-pearls) technique is described (**Fig. 5**):

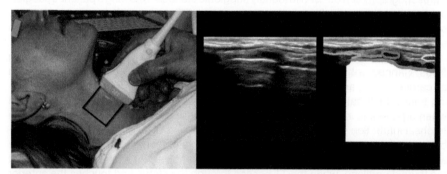

Fig. 5. CTM. (*Left*) The linear high-frequency transducer is placed in the midsagittal plane. (*Right*) The CTM (*orange*); thyroid cartilage (*green*); cricoid cartilage (*purple*); anterior part of tracheal rings (*dark blue*); tissue/air border (*light blue*); and isthmus of the thyroid gland (*yellow*). Below the tissue/air border are artifacts (*white*). (*From* Kristensen MS, Teoh WH, Graumann O, et al. Ultrasonography for clinical decision-making and intervention in airway management: from the mouth to the lungs and pleurae. *Insights Imaging* 2014;5:254-79, with permission.)

1. Stand at the right side of the patient and face the patient. Palpate the sternal bone and place the ultrasound probe transversely on the patient's neck cephalad to the suprasternal notch. The trachea is seen as a horseshoe-shaped, dark structure with a posterior white line.
2. Slide the transducer to the right side of the neck, so that the right border of the transducer is positioned over the midline trachea.
3. Keeping the right end of the transducer fixed on the midline trachea, rotate the transducer 90° clockwise, so the left end of the transducer is rotated into the sagittal plane. Several dark rings (string-of-pearls) are seen anterior to the white hyperechoic line. The dark rings are the anterior part of the tracheal rings.
4. Slide the transducer cephalad until the cricoid cartilage comes into view. The cricoid cartilage appears as a larger, elongated, anteriorly placed "pearl." Moving further cephalad, the thyroid cartilage is seen.
5. While holding the transducer still, a needle can be inserted midway between the caudal border of the thyroid cartilage and the cephalad border of the cricoid cartilage.
6. The transducer is removed. The needle marks the center of the CTM. This can be marked on the skin with a pen.

Gastric ultrasound

Gastric ultrasound can provide point-of-care information regarding gastric content quality (empty, clear fluid, or solid) and volume. Pulmonary aspiration of gastric contents is a serious complication with potentially devastating outcomes. Fasting guidelines are followed prior to nonurgent anesthesia induction. Although fasting guidelines are not applicable in surgical emergencies, ultrasound may help guide care in these circumstances. Algorithms have been proposed in adults to assess aspiration risk based on gastric ultrasonography.[30]

The application of gastric ultrasonography in the pediatric population also has been demonstrated. Quantitative gastric ultrasound assessment has been shown to correlate with gastric volume in children. Gagey and colleagues[31] performed a prospective cohort study of 34 infants undergoing pyloromyotomy. They quantitatively assessed the antrum of the stomach with ultrasound before and after aspiration of contents with a 10-French gastric tube (**Fig. 6**). They found a significant linear correlation between antral area measured in the right lateral decubitus (RLD) position and aspirated gastric volume, with a Pearson correlation coefficient of 0.83 (0.62–0.93; $P<.001$). Gagey and colleagues[32] also performed qualitative assessments of gastric contents in 143 children ages 2 months to 16 years presenting for urgent or emergency surgery. They used a 0 to 2 grading scale (0 = no gastric contents, 1 = clear fluid content in RLD only, and 2 = clear fluid content in both supine and RLD, suggesting high gastric volume or solid contents) to stratify the patients preoperatively. Based on the gastric ultrasound findings and clinical assessment, the anesthesiologist kept or modified their plan for anesthesia induction with either mask induction, intravenous induction, or modified rapid sequence. induction (RSI). After intubation, gastric contents were suctioned and defined as above risk threshold if there was presence of clear fluid greater than 0.8 mL/kg, thick fluid, or solid particulates. They found an improvement in the rate of appropriate anesthetic induction technique according to actual gastric contents after gastric ultrasound assessment versus after clinical assessment alone (85% vs 49%). They concluded that preoperative qualitative ultrasound assessment is a useful technique to guide choice of anesthetic induction in children presenting for urgent or emergent surgery. More studies are needed to assess the utility of

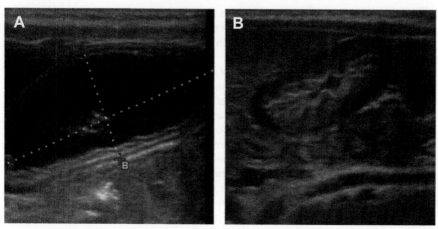

Fig. 6. Sonographic images of the antrum, (*A*) before and (*B*) after aspiration of the gastric contents through a nasogastric tube in an infant with pyloric stenosis. (*From* Gagey A-C, de Queiroz Siqueira M, Desgranges F-P, et al. Ultrasound assessment of the gastric contents for the guidance of the anaesthetic strategy in infants with hypertrophic pyloric stenosis: a prospective cohort study. *Br J Anaesth* 2016;116:649-54, with permission.)

gastric ultrasonography in pediatric patients and risk stratification of pulmonary aspiration under anesthesia.

Can't Intubate, Can't Oxygenate

Despite preparation, vigilance, and skill, the rare, life-threatening CICO emergency still may occur. In the CICO scenario, emergency FONA is indicated, with the goal of restoring oxygenation. FONA techniques are categorized based on the type of rescue airway used, including (1) scalpel and TT; (2) narrow-bore cannula (<4 mm); and (3) large-bore catheter (>4 mm). Examples of narrow-bore cannulas are the Emergency Transtracheal Airway Catheter (Cook Medical, Bloomington, Indiana) and nonsafety angiocatheters. Examples of large-bore catheters are emergency cricothyroidotomy sets and the Quicktrach (VBM Medical, Noblesville, Indiana). The best technique for emergency FONA in children has yet to be determined. As such, each institution must develop its own protocols and train with the equipment and techniques it has available.

The goal of emergency FONA is to provide a temporary route of oxygenation until a secure airway is established. A major concern with FONA with narrow-bore cannulas is that oxygenation through a cannula less than 4 mm provides little egress of air, increasing the risk of barotrauma and volutrauma. Patients in the CICO scenario typically suffer from significant upper airway obstruction that contributed to the emergency. Devices, such as Enk Oxygen Flow Modulator (Cook Medical) and Ventrain (Ventinova Medical, Eindhoven, The Netherlands), have been developed to decrease the risk of barotrauma during oxygenation and ventilation via a narrow-bore cannula.

Enk Oxygen Flow Modulator

The Enk Oxygen Flow Modulator is a transtracheal oxygenation device made up of a catheter with 5 finger holes connected to oxygen tubing. The catheter is connected to an oxygen source with a flow rate of approximately 1 L/(min) × years of age.[33] For example, a 6 year-old child would receive a flow rate of 6 L/min. All 5 of the holes are occluded and released intermittently using the thumb and index finger at a rate of approximately 100 cycles per minute. The chest is observed for slight outward and inward movement to confirm pulmonary inflation and exhalation. Flows above 15 L/min are potentially dangerous as the Enk Oxygen Flow Modulator fails to perform as an on-off device and delivers continuous high pressure to the lower airways. Flows less than 1 L/min risk no flow.

Ventrain
The Ventrain is another manual ventilation device designed for narrow-bore cannulas. It is the only ventilation device used during FONA that employs technology for active expiration by suction, via a Bernoulli effect, to decrease the risk of air-trapping and barotrauma. The active expiration technology shortens expiration time and thus increases achievable minute ventilation. There also is a connection for side-stream capnometry. This device has the unique ability for oxygenation, CO_2 removal, and capnometry. Ventrain currently is available only in Europe and New Zealand.

Three-Dimensional Printing and Difficult Airway Management

Scanning and printing in 3-D have allowed anesthesiologists to personalize a perioperative plan to individual patients to a degree of detail previously not possible. Patients with complex airway anatomy from radiation, previous surgery, or oncologic masses may pose significant challenges throughout the perioperative period. The innovation of 3-D reconstruction of images from computed tomography to print 3-D models of upper and lower airways is a new tool for clinicians to use in preoperative simulation—allowing for detailed planning of correct airway devices and sizes.[34] Another application of 3-D printing is the use of personalized prosthetics as airway adjuncts during intraoperative management. Fan and colleagues[35] demonstrated this application by using 3-D scanning, computer-aided design, and high-resolution 3-D printing to create a personalized facial prosthesis for a 73-year-old patient with significant right facial deformities after right mandibulectomy for alveolar carcinoma. The prosthesis helped to provide an anchoring platform for excellent mask seal.[35] Without the prosthesis, no mask seal was able to be obtained, rendering the patient DBMV. When the prosthesis was in place, however, positive-pressure ventilation was achieved, allowing for BMV prior to tracheal intubation. In pediatric difficult airway management, 3-D printing remains an area of opportunity for application.

Artificial Intelligence and Machine Learning in Pediatric Difficult Airway Management

Artificial intelligence and machine learning are rapidly growing fields that are being applied throughout health care to improve patient safety. Two examples of applications in health care include (1) predicting sepsis with streaming vital signs and (2) radiologic image-analysis and recognition of tumors. These tools also already have been utilized in adult difficult airway management and can have similar applications in pediatric difficult airway management.[36] Artificial intelligence uses complex algorithms and statistical models to analyze and interpret data, with limited or no direct human input. Artificial intelligence can solve complex problems that may be difficult or impossible for human intelligence alone to solve. Machine learning is a field of artificial intelligence that uncovers latent, nonlinear relationships in data and then creates predictive or prescriptive tools from the data. In contrast, traditional statistical methods focus on inference.

Machine learning has been used in the adult population to predict ease of intubation. Cuendet and colleagues[37] developed an automated face-analysis algorithm to detect morphologic traits associated with difficult intubation using a database of 970 patient photos and videos. The most discriminative structural facial features were selected by the machine learning algorithm. The positive predictive value of difficult intubation compared with an anesthesiologist's opinion was 77.9%. Connor and Segal[38] also developed a computer model that classified a patient as easy or difficult to intubate based on analysis of photographs of patients' faces. When the algorithm was tested against 80 male patients, it correctly classified 70 of 80 subjects as easy or challenging intubation. This was in contrast to more standard clinical assessments (Mallampati score and thyromental distance) that correctly classified only 47 of 80 subjects.[38] Machine learning is an exciting area of innovation in pediatric difficult airway management due to the ability of algorithms to improve exponentially as more data and images are collected.

Another area of innovation and application of machine learning for airway management is the ability to provide real-time guidance during airway procedures. Matava and colleagues[39] developed a machine learning algorithm that could classify vocal cords and tracheal airway anatomy in real time during VL and bronchoscopy. Using a data set of 775 VL and bronchoscopy videos for model training, their algorithm could identify the vocal cords and trachea with high sensitivity (0.87) and specificity (0.99).[39] The algorithm then labeled the airway anatomy on the VL screen for real-time clinical decision support during intubation. Technology like this may be used in medical education to teach trainees or clinicians learning to intubate. The real-time clinical decision support also may be applied to intubation of pediatric difficult airways for skilled practitioners.

Novel applications are being made in artificial intelligence and machine learning that can optimize the care of patients and will transform health care in the coming generation. The particular applications in difficult airway management are exciting, and one day may be life-saving. Children with difficult airways in particular will benefit from these advances.

SUMMARY

Children have unique characteristics that make them particularly vulnerable to perioperative adverse events. Skilled airway management is a cornerstone of high-quality anesthetic management. The use of hybrid airway techniques is a critical tool for the pediatric anesthesiologist. POCUS has an expanding role in airway management, from preoperative assessment of airway pathology and gastric contents to confirmation of tracheal intubation and identification of the CTM. The exciting fields of 3-D printing, artificial intelligence, and machine learning are areas of innovation that will transform pediatric difficult airway management in the years to come.

Clinics Care Points—Bulleted List of Evidence-Based Pearls and Pitfalls Relevant to the Point of Care

- Multiple tracheal intubation attempts (>2) and persistent DL attempts ($\geq$3) are associated with more anesthetic complications in children with difficult airways. Each tracheal intubation attempt should be treated as a critical intervention, and the number of DLs and tracheal intubation attempts should be limited.

- The delivery of supplemental oxygen should be considered during intubation attempts of the pediatric patient with a suspected difficult airway. Oxygenation can be performed via nasal cannula, modified nasopharyngeal airway, modified oral RAE TT, or THRIVE.

- The CICO scenario is rare but catastrophic. Continual practice of airway management techniques, meticulous preoperative planning, and clinical leadership for excellent team dynamics are necessary to minimize the potential for the CICO emergency.

DISCLOSURE

The authors have nothing to disclose.

REFERENCES

1. Habre W, Disma N, Virag K, et al. Incidence of severe critical events in paediatric anaesthesia (APRICOT): a prospective multicentre observational study in 261 hospitals in Europe. Lancet Respir Med 2017;5:412–25.
2. Whitaker LA, Pashayan H, Reichman J. A proposed new classification of craniofacial anomalies. Cleft Palate J 1981;18:161–76.
3. Valois-Gomez T, Oofuvong M, Auer G, et al. Incidence of difficult bag-mask ventilation in children: a prospective observational study. Paediatr Anaesth 2013;23: 920–6.
4. Kheterpal S, Han R, Tremper KK, et al. Incidence and predictors of difficult and impossible mask ventilation. Anesthesiology 2012;22:729–36.
5. Rose DK, Cohen MM. The airway: problems and predictors in 18,00 patients. Can J Anaesth 1994;41:372–83.
6. Heinrich S, Birkholz T, Ihmsen H, et al. Incidence and predictors of difficult laryngoscopy in 11,219 pediatric anesthesia procedures. Paediatr Anaesth 2012;22: 729–36.
7. Black AE, Flynn PE, Smith HL, et al. Development of a guideline for the management of the unanticipated difficult airway in pediatric practice. Paediatr Anaesth 2015;25:346–62.
8. Mathis MR, Haydar B, Taylor EL, et al. Failure of the laryngeal mask airway unique and classic in the pediatric surgical patient: a study of clinical predictors and outcomes. Anesthesiology 2013;119:1284–95.
9. Fiadjoe JE, Nishisaki A, Jagannathan N, et al. Airway management complications in children with difficult tracheal intubation from the Pediatric Difficult Intubation (PeDI) registry: a prospective cohort analysis. Lancet Respir Med 2016;4:37–48.
10. Bhagwan SD. Levitan's No Desat with nasal cannula for infants with pyloric stenosis requiring intubation. Paediatr Anaesth 2013;23:297–8.
11. Holmdahl MH. Pulmonary uptake of oxygen, acid-base metabolism, and circulation during prolonged apnea. Acta Chir Scand Suppl 1956;212:1–128.
12. Holm-Knudsen R, Eriksen K, Rasmussen L. Using a nasopharyngeal airway during fiberoptic intubation in small children with a difficult airway. Paediatr Anaesth 2005;15:839–45.
13. Man JY, Fiadjoe JE, Hsu G. Technique utilizing a modified oral Ring-Adair-Elwyn tube to provide continuous oxygen and sevoflurane delivery during nasotracheal intubation in an infant with a difficult airway: a case report. A A Pract 2018;10:254–7.
14. Hutchings FA, Hilliard TN, David PJ. Heated humidified high-flow nasal cannula therapy in children. Arch Dis Child 2015;100:571–5.
15. Milési C, Boubal M, Jacquot A, et al. High-flow nasal cannula: recommendations for daily practice in pediatrics. Ann Intensive Care 2014;4:29.
16. Patel A, Nouraei SA. Transnasal humidified rapid-Insufflation Ventilatory Exchange (THRIVE): a physiological method of increasing apnea time in patients with difficult airways. Anaesthesia 2015;70:323–9.
17. Humphreys S, Lee-Archer P, Reyne G, et al. Transnasal humidified rapid-insufflation ventilatory exchange (THRIVE) in children: a randomized controlled trial. Br J Anaesth 2017;118:232–8.
18. Weiss M, Schwarz U, Dillier CM, et al. Teaching and supervising tracheal intubation in paediatric patients using videolaryngoscopy. Paediatr Anaesth 2001;11:343–8.

19. O'Shea JE, Thio M, Kamlin CO, et al. Videolaryngoscopy to teach neonatal intubation: a randomized trial. Pediatrics 2015;135:912–9.
20. Zhang B, Gurnaney HG, Stricker PA, et al. A prospective observational study of technical difficulty with GlideScope-guided tracheal intubation in children. Anesth Analg 2018;127:467–71.
21. Mazzinari G, Rovira L, Henao L, et al. Effect of dynamic versus stylet-guided intubation on first-attempt success in difficult airways undergoing GlideScope laryngoscopy: a randomized controlled trial. Anesth Analg 2019;128:1264–71.
22. Kovatsis PG. Continuous ventilation during flexible fiberoptic-assisted intubation via supraglottic airways. Paediatr Anaesth 2016;26:457–8.
23. Galgon RE, Schroeder KM, Schmidt CS, et al. Fiberoptic-guided tracheal tube placement through the air-Q intubating laryngeal airway: a performance study in a manikin. J Anesth 2011;25:721–6.
24. Kristensen MS, Teoh WH, Graumann, et al. Ultrasonography for clinical decision-making and intervention in airway management: from the mouth to the lungs and pleurae. Insights Imaging 2014;5:253–79.
25. Shibasaki M, Nakajima Y, Ishii S, et al. Prediction of pediatric endotracheal tube size by ultrasonography. Anesthesiology 2010;113:819–24.
26. Roberts WA, Maniscalco WM, Cohen AR, et al. The use of capnography for recognition of esophageal intubation in the neonatal intensive care unit. Pediatr Pulmonol 1995;19:262–8.
27. Das SK, Choupoo NS, Haldar R, et al. Transtracheal ultrasound for verification of endotracheal tube placement: a systematic review and meta-analysis. Can J Anaesth 2015;62:413–23.
28. Fennessy P, Walsh B, Laffey JG, et al. Accuracy of pediatric cricothyroid membrane identification by digital palpation and implications for emergency front of neck access. Paediatr Anaesth 2020;30:69–77.
29. Kristensen MS, Teoh WH, Rudolph SS. Ultrasonographic identification of the cricothyroid membrane: best evidence, techniques, and clinical impact. Br J Anaesth 2016;117:i39–48.
30. Van de Putte P, Perlas A. Ultrasound assessment of gastric content and volume. Br J Anaesth 2014;113:12–22.
31. Gagey A-C, de Queiroz Siqueira M, Desgranges F-P, et al. Ultrasound assessment of the gastric contents for the guidance of the anaesthetic strategy in infants with hypertrophic pyloric stenosis: a prospective cohort study. Br J Anaesth 2016; 116:649–54.
32. Gagey A-C, de Queiroz Siqueira M, Monard C, et al. The effect of pre-operative gastric ultrasound examination on the choice of general anesthetic induction technique for non-elective paediatric surgery. A prospective cohort study. Anaesthesia 2018;73:304–12.
33. Baker PA, Brown AJ. Experimental adaptation of the Enk oxygen flow modulator for potential pediatric use. Paediatr Anaesth 2008;19:458–63.
34. Han B, Liu Y, Zhang X, et al. Three-dimensional printing as an aid to airway evaluation after tracheotomy in a patient with laryngeal carcinoma. BMC Anesthesiol 2016;16:6.
35. Fan S, Chan A, Au S, et al. Personalised anaesthesia: three-dimensional printing of facial prosthetic for facial deformity with difficult airway. Br J Anaesth 2018;121: 675–8.
36. Matava C, Pankiv, Ahumada L, et al. Artificial intelligence, machine learning and the pediatric airway. Paediatr Anaesth 2019;00:1–5.

37. Cuendet GL, Schoettker P, Yuce A, et al. Facial image analysis for fully automatic prediction of difficult endotracheal intubation. IEEE Trans Biomed Eng 2016;63: 328–39.
38. Connor CW, Segal S. Accurate classification of difficult intubation by computerized facial analysis. Anesth Analg 2011;112:84–93.
39. Matava C, Pankiv E, Raisbeck S, et al. A convolutional neural network for real time classification, identification, and labelling of vocal cord and tracheal using laryngoscopy and bronchoscopy video. J Med Syst 2020;44:44.

Is Anesthesia Bad for the Brain? Current Knowledge on the Impact of Anesthetics on the Developing Brain

Sulpicio G. Soriano, MD, Mary Ellen McCann, MD, MPH*

KEYWORDS

• Neurotoxicity • Hypotension • Pediatric anesthesia • Neurocognition

KEY POINTS

• There are compelling preclinical data that commonly used general anesthetics cause neuroapoptosis in juvenile animals in vitro and in vivo.

• Many but not all retrospective clinical studies in children demonstrate an association between anesthesia exposure at a young age and later neurocognitive difficulties.

• The only prospective randomized trial to date did not find an association between general anesthesia exposure in early infancy for inguinal hernia repair and neurocognitive difficulties.

• However, this study did not address the effects of prolonged anesthetic exposure during early childhood. Perioperative factors such blood pressure, arterial carbon dioxide tension, temperature, glycemic state, arterial oxygen saturation, and positioning are modifiable during anesthesia and, if abnormal, can lead to possible brain injury.

Concerns about long-term anesthetic-induced neurotoxicity have permeated the pediatric anesthesia community since landmark laboratory reports demonstrated neurodegeneration as well as behavioral deficits in juvenile animals exposed to general anesthetics and sedatives.[1,2] These preclinical findings led the US Food and Drug Administration in 2016 to issue a safety warning as well as change the labeling of general anesthetics and sedatives to reflect these concerns. The safety warning states that "repeated or lengthy use of general anesthetic and sedation drugs during surgeries or procedures in children younger than 3 years or in pregnant women during their third trimester may affect the development of children's brains." Regulatory bodies and medical societies in other countries have declined to issue specific warnings about the safety of general anesthetic exposure in young children, reflecting the

Department of Anesthesiology, Critical Care and Pain Medicine, Boston Children's Hospital, Harvard Medical School, 300 Longwood Avenue, Boston, MA 02115, USA
* Corresponding author.
E-mail address: mary.mccann@childrens.harvard.edu

Anesthesiology Clin 38 (2020) 477–492
https://doi.org/10.1016/j.anclin.2020.05.007
1932-2275/20/© 2020 Elsevier Inc. All rights reserved.
anesthesiology.theclinics.com

lack of compelling evidence that general anesthetic exposure at a young age leads to clinically relevant anesthetic-induced neurotoxicity.

Measuring the impact of general anesthesia on children undergoing procedures is difficult owing the many confounding factors. These confounders include the underlying pathology of the child which leads to the need for anesthesia for diagnostic tests and procedures as well as the neuroinflammatory effects of surgery. This neuroinflammation has been associated with postoperative neurocognitive deficits in older adults. There has been only a single randomized prospective trial published examining the effects of general anesthesia compared with regional anesthesia for hernia repair on young infants. Difficulty enrolling patients in a control group has limited the ability to conduct more research.[3,4] There is an ongoing international randomized controlled trial known as the TREX trial comparing sevoflurane alone with low-dose sevoflurane, remifentanil and dexmedetomidine for procedures lasting longer than 2 hours.[5]

One of the concerning negative effects of general anesthesia is neurotoxicity leading to cognitive dysfunction. However, other factors such as environmental factors and genetic background have a significant impact on neurodevelopment and are beyond the control of the clinician during a perioperative encounter.[6,7] In addition, the impact of surgery and anesthesia can provoke homeostatic variability and instability that can lead to brain injury. Factors that can contribute to this instability include alterations in blood pressure, $Paco_2$, blood glucose levels, temperature, Pao_2, and head positioning during procedures. In this review, we discuss the preclinical as well as clinical data available about the neurotoxic effects of general anesthesia on the developing brain as well as clinical data linking abnormal homeostasis perioperatively or in the intensive care unit with abnormal neurologic development.

PRECLINICAL DATA

The quest for determining whether commonly used general anesthetics in pediatrics causes long-term harm began about 20 years ago with reports that infant mice exposed to general anesthesia had increased neuronal apoptotic cell death and long-term behavioral and cognitive deficits. Apoptotic cell death is a normal developmental process whereby an organism rids itself of unnecessary cells.[8] Both in vitro and in vivo studies have shown that very young animals exposed to either GABA agonists (eg, volatile anesthetics, benzodiazepines, barbiturates and propofol) as well as N-methyl-D-aspartate (NMDA) antagonists (nitrous oxide and ketamine) develop abnormally high levels of neuronal apoptosis.[9] The vast majority of the animal studies have been on very young murine species who show an increased susceptibility to neuroapoptosis at postnatal day 7 of life. Slightly older murine species (postnatal days of life 14–20) exposed to these same general anesthetics develop increased but abnormal dendritic growth.[10,11] The clinical significance of this abnormal dendritic formation is unknown, but some human psychiatric and neurologic disorders such as autism spectrum disorder and schizophrenia are associated with abnormal dendritic formation and synaptogenesis.[12] Although most of these studies have been performed in rats and mice, there is also a convincing body of evidence that rhesus monkeys have increased neuroapoptosis when exposed to anesthetic drugs as fetuses or within the first 5 days of life.[13,14]

Anesthetic-induced neuroapoptosis has been found throughout the central nervous system and regional changes occur at different time points during development.[15] Exposure to general anesthetics also affects neuronal generation by causing abnormal neurogenesis in rats and mice. Glial cell formation is decreased and maturation is delayed by general anesthetic exposure.[16]

Laboratory animals such as rats, mice, guinea pigs, and rhesus monkeys exposed to anesthetic drugs in the neonatal period develop impairments in learning, memory, attention, emotional behavior, psychomotor speed, concept formation, motivation, emotional behaviors, and motor function.[17] Studies in rhesus monkey have shown that exposure to general anesthesia during infancy leads to animals with heightened emotional reactivity to perceived threats such as contact with strangers, as well as overall increased anxiety.[18] In addition, exposure to general anesthesia may lead to late findings in monkeys. Repeated exposure to general anesthetics in rhesus monkeys can lead to visual memory deficits that become apparent only after the first year of life.[19]

One of the possible mechanisms is that neuronal cells during exposure to general anesthesia are deprived of stimulating input and thus deprived of trophic support. This trophic or growth support is necessary for neurogenesis, synaptogenesis, and other context-sensitive modulation necessary for neuronal plasticity. This trophic factor dysregulation leads vulnerable cells toward an apoptotic pathway. General anesthetics can also cause mitochondrial dysfunction in immature animals, which can stress neuronal cells.[20] Aberrant cell cycle entry, where neurons abnormally enter the mitotic cell cycle and perish, is another mechanism observed with exposure to NMDA receptor antagonists.[21] Volatile anesthetics induce excitotoxicity and seizures by binding to immature GABA receptors and activating the cotransporter protein NKCC1, leading to chloride influx and neuronal depolarization.[22] With maturity, this protein is replaced by KCC2, which actively transports chloride out of the cellular membrane causing inhibition of depolarization.[23] In humans, this protein receptor starts to switch around 15 weeks after birth, but is not complete until 1 year of age. KCC2 expression determines the developmental stage-dependent impact of propofol anesthesia on the brain growth spurt.[24] Seizures can occur as well as increased neuroapoptosis in neonatal rats exposed to sevoflurane.[23] This neurotoxicity has been successfully mitigated with pretreatment with bumetanide, which blocks the NKCC1 channels. In addition, epigenetic modulation of transcription can be altered by general anesthetics, which can impede neurodevelopment.[25]

In addition to bumetanide, there have been several other nonspecific medications, which have been shown to ameliorate the effects of general anesthesia in animal models. These drugs include estradiol, erythropoietin, melatonin, L-carnitine, lithium, xenon, and dexmedetomidine. Currently, dexmedetomidine is the only medication commonly used as a sedative or adjunctive anesthetic in pediatric medicine that has been shown to mitigate anesthetic-induced developmental neurotoxicity Dexmedetomidine has been found in animal studies to mitigate the effects of isoflurane in rodent models, but high doses of dexmedetomidine in these same models induces a modest increase in neuroapoptosis.[26,27]

Although the preclinical animal data are compelling, a meta-analysis of more than 400 preclinical reports found no clear exposure duration threshold below which no injury or subsequent cognitive abnormalities followed. This meta-analysis did not clearly identify a specific age beyond which anesthetic exposure did not cause any structural or functional abnormalities.[28] The majority of animal studies that demonstrated increased histologic and behavioral derangements involve exposures of 4 hours or more, which has been associated with severe physiologic changes that can trigger neurodegenerative processes.[29,30] It is also important to note that several animals studies have compared general anesthetic exposures with no exposures in groups of young animals who were in either controlled or enhanced environments.[31,32] The effects of enhanced environments (cages with wheels and other toys) to a very large degree mitigated the neurotoxic effects of general anesthesia in rodent models.

Translating the findings of the preclinical studies to young children is problematic. The sensory and social deprivation seen in the rodent experimental paradigms, which use controlled environments (sterile cage, solitary confinement), is not a natural environment and thus calls into question the validity of developmental studies on rodents in such environments. It is also unknown whether the prolonged neurodevelopment of human beings as well as the generally enriched environments that children live in compared with other species may allow for restoration of function of any damage caused by general anesthetic. It is also unknown which neurodevelopmental domains would be affected in humans compared with animals.

CLINICAL STUDIES

There are many human studies that show an association between anesthetic exposure at a young age and later learning or behavioral difficulties. In contrast, there are also many studies that show no such associations. The outcome measures used include comprehensive neurocognitive testing, parental reports of school and medical issues, behavioral or medical diagnoses in large databases often derived from billing codes, or school reports of academic performance or readiness.[33] The age of exposure has also varied in these reports ranging from infancy to about 5 years of age.[34] Another difficulty encountered is that some of the neurocognitive domains such as executive function and some social emotional skills are not reliably tested in humans until early adolescence. Finally, it is important to consider the type of studies that have been reported. The vast majority have been retrospective in nature, although there have been some ambidirectional trials in which a retrospective cohort is developed and then prospectively evaluated and a single randomized control trial. In this review, we highlight some of the important trials that address the effects of anesthesia on neurodevelopment.

Retrospective Trials

One of the first studies published about this topic was in 2009 was from the Mayo Clinic.[35] Because of the stability of the population of Olmsted County, Minnesota, a wealth of information is known about school age children, including their health and school records. The first retrospective birth cohort study of children born between 1976 and 1982 found that more than 1 exposure to general anesthesia before the age of 4 years was associated with almost double the cumulative risk of a school referral for a learning difficulty. A single exposure was not associated with an increased risk. This study was criticized because the children mostly received halothane (an anesthetic generally not used anymore) and intraoperative pulse oximetry was not yet available. A similar cohort was developed examining a later birth cohort born between 1996 and 2000 who were exposed to contemporary anesthetics and monitoring in children less than 3 years of age.[36] Again, the findings were that a single exposure to general anesthesia did not confer an increased risk of school difficulties, but further exposures did.

The Western Australia Pregnancy (Raine) cohort, which was originally developed as randomized controlled trial to test the effects of fetal ultrasound examination on birth outcomes, has become one of the largest prospective cohorts of pregnancy and childhood.[37] Extensive secondary analysis has been done on this cohort looking at the effects of early anesthetic exposure and neurocognitive outcomes. From the original cohort of 2868 children, 148 children were anesthetized before the age of 3 years.[38] When tested at age 10 years, the exposed children were found to have increased risks of language deficits and overall intelligence, even after a single exposure. Further studies were done on this cohort using latent class analysis, in which the authors defined 4 classes of neurodevelopmental outcomes: normal or nearly normal testing, language and cognitive deficits, behavioral deficits, and global deficits.[39] They found that only language and cognitive deficits were associated with exposure to general anesthesia before the age of 3 years.

There have been 2 large database studies from Canada looking at school readiness using the Early Developmental Instrument, a 104-component questionnaire encompassing 5 developmental domains to assess developmental skills.[40,41] Both studies found a modest increase in risk for early developmental vulnerability for single anesthetic exposures in children, but only when the exposure was between the ages of 2 and 4 years. Exposure before the age of 2 did not confer any increased risk. A large Swedish cohort of more than 2 million individuals born between 1973 and 1993 found a modest decrease in overall IQ after single or multiple exposures to general anesthesia before the age of 4 years in military recruits who were tested at age 18 years.[42]

At least 2 retrospective studies used siblings as a control group to attempt to control for inherited traits, socioeconomic, and cultural factors. One of the studies published in 2009 examined the neurocognitive and academic outcomes of identical twins in the Netherlands from the National Twin Registry.[43] The authors examined general anesthetic exposure before the ages of 3 and 12 years. This study found that anesthetic exposure was a risk factor for poorer academic outcomes, but in discordant twin pairs of whom one was exposed and the other nonexposed, the academic outcomes were identical. The authors concluded that it was unlikely that general anesthesia exposure per se was a cause of poor academic outcomes. Another sibling study using the cohort developed in Ontario, Canada, found that there was no increased risk of developmental vulnerabilities in siblings exposed to general anesthesia compared with nonexposed siblings.[44]

Ambidirectional cohort studies
The Pediatric Anesthesia & NeuroDevelopment Assessment (PANDA) study tested the neurocognitive outcomes of 105 sibling pairs who were born within 36 months of each other and in which one of the siblings was exposed to general anesthesia for inguinal herniorrhaphy.[45] There were no meaningful differences in IQ, the primary outcome in this cohort, who were tested between ages 8 and 15 years. There were also no differences in mean scores between sibling pairs in memory/learning, motor/processing speed, visuospatial function, attention, executive function, language, or behavior. This trial highlights the difficulties in doing ambidirectional trials. Almost 10,000 sibling pairs were screened for this study, but only 105 sibling pairs were enrolled.

The Mayo Anesthesia Safety in Kids (MASK) study enrolled a total of 997 children: 411 were unexposed, 380 were singly exposed, and 206 were exposed more than once before the age of 3 years to determine whether anesthetic exposure was related to poor neurocognitive outcomes.[46] The children were propensity matched and underwent neuropsychologic testing between ages 8 to 12 years or 15 to 20 years. There were no significant differences found in the primary outcome measure, the full-scale IQ as determined by the Wechsler Abbreviated Scale of Intelligence. For secondary outcomes, children who had multiple anesthetic exposures were at higher risk for decreased processing speed and fine motor abilities.[47] Parental reports of the exposed children revealed an increased risk of difficulties with executive function as well as reading for children with both single and multiple exposures. The children of this cohort were also tested by the operant test battery, in which subjects operate a lever to complete a task and are rewarded with a small treat for task completion.[48] This type of testing has been done with nonhuman primates exposed to ketamine in early infancy who demonstrated deficits in motivation as well as deficits in accuracy of task performance and response speed.[13] The operant test battery did not detect a difference between the control and exposed groups in the MASK cohort.

Randomized, Controlled Trials

The General Anesthesia versus Spinal Anesthesia (GAS) trial, a prospective randomized controlled equivalence trial, compared the neurocognitive outcomes of infants less than 60 weeks postmenstrual age who were exposed to either sevoflurane general anesthesia or bupivacaine regional anesthesia for inguinal hernia repair. An interim analysis done at age 2 and using the Bayley III developmental test found no differences between the 2 groups.[3] The full-scale IQ using the Wechsler Primary and Preschool Scales of Intelligence was performed at age 5 years and also found no differences between the 2 groups.[4] The data was analyzed on a per-protocol and intention-to-treat basis. Criticisms of this trial include the medium length of exposure (55 minutes), mostly male enrollees (>80%), and the time of general anesthetic exposure was during a relatively narrow time during development.[49]

The TREX trial is currently prospectively enrolling subjects in the United States, Australia, New Zealand, and Great Britain. In this trial, patients are randomized to receive either standard dose sevoflurane as an aesthetic agent or low-dose sevoflurane, remifentanil, and dexmedetomidine for procedures expected to last longer than 2 hours in children less than 2 years of age. Neurocognitive testing is being done at age 3 years.[5]

PERIOPERATIVE FACTORS ASSOCIATED WITH ADVERSE PATHOPHYSIOLOGY IN PEDIATRIC PATIENTS

There are many factors that may lead to neurologic injury in susceptible patients undergoing procedures. Some of these factors may not be easily modifiable, such as the effects of neuroinflammation or abnormal circulatory patterns owing to congenital heart disease, but many factors are modifiable. Altered cerebral circulation can occur from high intrathoracic pressure or head positioning, leading to decreased cerebral venous drainage. Hypercapnia or hypocapnia cause cerebral arterial vasodilation or vasoconstriction. Low blood pressure can lead to inadequate cerebral perfusion pressure. Metabolic cellular insufficiency can result from inadequate metabolic fuel (hypoglycemia or hypoxia) or from unmet metabolic demand such as occurs with pain, stress, fever, or seizures. Neurotoxic mediators produced from hypoxic or ischemic neurons, as well as free radicals produced during periods of hyperoxia, can promote brain injury.

It is important to recognize that there may be some children who may be at higher risk for perioperative brain injury. There are many illnesses and conditions that put pediatric patients at risk for neuronal injury perioperatively. We discuss a few of these conditions to elucidate the manner in which a pediatric patient's underlying preoperative state may influence the anesthesiologist on methods to optimize the conduct of the general anesthetic.

Premature infants are at high risk for perinatal brain injury for many reasons, and the effects of intraoperative instability may increase this risk. These infants are born with much lower levels of neuroprotective hormones such as increased placental levels of estrogen, progesterone, and oxytocin, which increase during the third trimester of development and peak around 40-weeks of gestation. Levels of progesterone and estrogen increase 100-fold during the last trimester of fetal development. Estrogen acts as an antioxidant; promotes growth of dendrites, axons, and synapses; promotes the expression of neurotrophic factors; and acts as an antiapoptotic agent. Progesterone decreases postischemic inflammation and induces the production of brain-derived neurotrophic factor. Oxytocin in fetal rats promotes an excitatory to inhibition switch in GABA actions, further protecting the developing brain.

Premature infants are at risk for ventricular intravascular hemorrhage because of the immature and fragile nature of the choroid plexuses in the lateral cerebral ventricles. Alterations in cerebral perfusion can lead to rupture of these delicate blood vessels, which ultimately lead to a loss of white matter if there is intracerebral parenchymal hemorrhage or hydrocephalus if there is obstruction to cerebral spinal fluid flow. The time of maximum vulnerability for this injury is the first 72 hours of life, when the infant is transitioning from fetal circulation to extrauterine circulation, but the first 10 days of life is a time of heightened risk for this type of injury.

Premature infants are also at extremely high risk for leukomalacia or white matter injury and the majority of infants born before 30-weeks of gestation demonstrate some white matter injury.[50] There are several important factors that lead to this heightened risk. The arterial vascular supply to the brain is immature in premature infants, leading to a vulnerability to white matter injury in the end zones of the deep penetrating arteries and in the watershed areas between the deep and short penetrating arterial end zones. In addition, the estimated cerebral blood flow through the white matter is about one-tenth of that seen in that of the overall adult brain, suggesting that the premature brain has a narrower safety margin in terms of adequate cerebral blood flow compared with the mature adult brain.[51,52] The precursor oligodendrocytes or glial cells are at risk for both necrotic and apoptotic cell death in premature infants.[53] These cells are exquisitely sensitive to the effects of oxygen free radicals, which are produced during conditions of ischemia, hypoxia, or hyperoxia.

Former premature infants or infants that are greater than 37 weeks postmenstrual age but who were born prematurely may also be a high-risk group because of ongoing and recent brain injury and neuroinflammation. Diseases of prematurity such as necrotizing enterocolitis or sepsis can lead to an inflammatory state.[50] This state puts the infants at risk for perioperative injury in at least 2 ways. The ongoing inflammatory state can lead to baseline hypertension, which may or may not be recognized preoperatively, as well as lead to neuroinflammation.

Another group of susceptible neonates include those born with complex congenital cardiac disease.[54] The fetal cerebral circulation of these infants is abnormal, which leads to a delay in maturation of the brain. It is estimated that the delay in maturation for an infant born at term is about 4 weeks putting these infants at high risk for brain injury, especially white matter injury.

There are also many neurologic conditions that put the developing brain at risk during general anesthesia, including poorly controlled seizure disorders, traumatic brain injury, anatomic brain abnormalities, and tumors. Careful collaboration with the patient's care team including neurologists, neonatologists, and pediatric and intensive care specialists is needed to craft an anesthetic plan to optimize the brain health of these pediatric patients.

Modifiable Factors

Blood pressure

Blood pressure goals during anesthesia should be defined before the initiation of general anesthesia, especially in vulnerable patient populations. There is no generally accepted definition of hypotension in pediatric practice. Many pediatricians consider a blood pressure below the 10th percentile for age in a child that is clinically ill or distressed as hypotension. In addition, there is no absolute agreement on the best method to improve blood pressure in pediatric patients who are hypotensive. Many algorithms include fluid boluses of 10 to 20 mL/kg followed by the initiation of vasoactive agents.[55] The maximal allowable decrease in blood pressure during anesthesia to maintain cerebral perfusion in pediatrics is even less well-defined, but there are a few studies that can guide practice. Many practitioners strive to keep the blood pressure above the lower limit of cerebral autoregulation, because there is less risk of inadvertent ischemia. Although there are some research methods that can approximate the lower limit of autoregulation in infancy and childhood using Doppler technology and near infrared spectroscopy, for most pediatric anesthesia cases using these methods is not feasible. These methods have demonstrated that every patient has their own individual autoregulatory curve, which can change depending on their physiologic status. The lower limit of autoregulation in children from age 6 months to 14 years was found to be approximately 60 mm Hg and did not vary with age using Doppler technology.[56] The baseline mean arterial pressure (MAP) for infants is lower than that for older children, indicating that infants have less autoregulatory reserve. The maximal allowable decrease in MAP in infants less than 6 months of age compared with older children undergoing sevoflurane anesthesia with end-tidal CO_2 levels controlled was found to be 20% in the young infants versus 40% in the older infants and children.[57] Another study found that, in infants less than 6 months of age undergoing similar anesthesia, there was adequate cerebral blood flow and oxygenation at a MAP of 45 mm Hg but when the MAPs were less than 35 mm Hg, there was both decreased cerebral blood flow and decreased cerebral oxygenation.[58] A root cause analysis of a very small series of infants less than 4 kg in weight undergoing 2 to 3 hours of general anesthesia who developed postoperative seizures and evidence of cerebral ischemic hypoperfusion injury in MRI and computed tomography imaging determined that mean MAPs between 32 and 38 mm Hg were a contributing cause.[59]

Hypocapnia or hypercapnia

There is a linear relationship between the tissue partial pressure of arterial carbon dioxide and cerebral blood flow as estimated by the tissue oxygen index using near infrared spectroscopy values over a large range in neonates.[60] In children, the cerebral blood flow decreases by up to 3% for every 1 mm Hg decrease in the tissue partial pressure of arterial carbon dioxide.[61] Mechanical ventilation to hypocapnic levels can independently decrease cerebral perfusion to ischemic ranges in critically ill children with preserved autoregulation. Many of the studies examining the effects of hypocapnia have been done in neonates who have sustained a hypoxic ischemic birth injury. A large multicenter trial examining hypothermia as a treatment for neonatal encephalopathy found that both the minimum $Paco_2$ value as well as the cumulative exposure to $Paco_2$ were risk factors for death and disability.[62] The incidence of PVL is also increased in preterm infants who have had known hypocapnia of less than 35 mm Hg.[63]

Mild hypercapnia may be beneficial to some neonates requiring ventilatory support. In a small randomized trial of extreme premature infants, it was found that mild hypocapnia ($Paco_2$ of 45–55 mm Hg) led to fewer days requiring respiratory support.[64] Patients with congenital diaphragmatic hernia also have been shown to benefit from mild hypercapnia versus normcapnia with decreased mortality rates.[65] However, moderate hypercapnia ($Paco_2$ of >55 mm Hg) has not been beneficial over normocapnia or mild hypercapnia in very premature infants.[66,67]

Hypoxia or hyperoxia

Hypoxic ischemic injury is the most common cause of death and disability in the neonate.[68] The disabilities incurred include persistent motor, sensory, and cognitive impairment. Every effort should be made to ensure that there is adequate oxygen delivery to the brain to meet metabolic demand.

Hyperoxia can increase the risk of retinopathy of prematurity, chronic lung disease, and brain injury in premature infants.[69–71] The generally accepted target goal for blood oxygen saturation levels in premature infants to minimize these risks is between 90% and 94%.[72] Term and older infants are at less risk for retinopathy of prematurity, so many practitioners aim for an oxygen saturation of greater than 95%.[72] Regional anesthesia in young infants carries less of a risk of either hyperoxia or hypoxia compared with general anesthesia.[73] Oxygen free radicals generated from hyperoxia can lead to both necrotic and apoptotic neuronal cell death. Oxidative stress is particularly harmful to neonates because the scavenging systems that detoxify reactive oxygen species are poorly developed in neonates.[69]

Glucose homeostasis

Metabolic requirements decrease during general anesthesia for infants and older children but because the energy requirements of neonates is up to 6 times greater per body weight than adults, they may be at risk for intraoperative hypoglycemia.[74] The risk of hypoglycemia is greatest during the first hours of life before the first feeding with almost 5% of normal neonates having a glucose concentration of 28 mg/dL or less.[75] Then, after the first feeding, the glucose typically increases to near adult levels in the range of 70 to 100 mg/dL.

A single low blood glucose measurement in the first few hours of life does not put the infant at risk for long-term neurologic deficits.[76–78] However, prolonged mild (glucose levels between 47–70 mg/dL) to moderate (glucose levels between 35–47 mg/dL) hypoglycemia is associated with long-term neurocognitive consequences. Infants with measured glucose levels of less than 47 mg/dL on 5 or more days had 3.5 times the incidence of cerebral palsy.[79] Studies looking at the effects of mild hypotension and mild hypoglycemia in nonhuman primates found that the risks of neurocognitive injury is similar to the effects of moderate hypotension alone.[80]

Temperature

The risks of hypothermia in pediatric patients during surgery are significant. In premature infants, the risks are high because of their greater surface to body mass proportion, low subcutaneous fat and keratin content, immature thermoregulatory mechanisms, and limited glycogen and brown adipose tissue stores. Radiant, conductive, and evaporative losses are most predominant in infants in the operating room. The risks to infants who are hypothermic on admission to the neonatal intensive care unit are great, with a multicenter prospective cohort study of almost 2000 premature infants finding that more than 50% of them were hypothermic on admission; hypothermia in this population was associated with an increased risk of death.[81]

Keeping infants euthermic in the operating room is difficult and usually requires active warming measures. A quality improvement project found that raising the room temperature to 29.4°C when the infants were undraped, using warmed fluids, warming blankets and/or thermal mattresses, and keeping the transport incubator warm decreased the risk of hypothermia upon arrival to the neonatal intensive care unit by almost 4-fold.[82]

Hyperthermia increases the patient's metabolic rate and increases the risk of ischemic injury. Term neonates with hypoxic ischemic encephalopathy who were hyperthermic had worse neurocognitive outcomes compared with normothermic infants in the National Institute of Child Health and Human Development Neonatal Research Network randomized trial.[83]

Positioning

The importance of intraoperative positioning is unclear. Often, because the endotracheal tube of a small neonate is prone to instability, pediatric anesthesiologists prefer to position the infant's head in a lateral position. However, this position may not be optimal for brain health because this position can lead to obstruction to venous drainage. There is a correlation between lateral head rotation and decreased cerebral oxygen index as measured by near infrared spectroscopy and an increase in cerebral blood volume in very low birth weight infants.[84,85] Intracranial pressures are lowest in infants positioned with their heads midline with the head of the bed raised 30°. However, a Cochrane meta-analysis studying the effects of neutral head position and head elevation did not find a decreased incidence of intravascular hemorrhage or an improvement in cerebral oxygenation.[86] Further research on this topic is needed. However, if feasible, maintaining the patient's head in a neutral position may decrease the chance of venous outflow obstruction.

Parental counseling The best approach to parents and pediatric care providers who are concerned about anesthetic-induced neurotoxicity is to be cognizant and

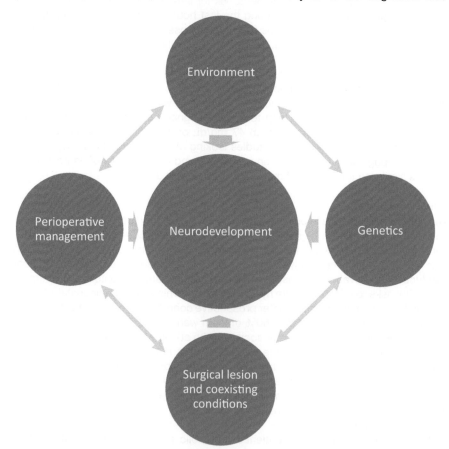

Fig. 1. Neurodevelopmental framework in pediatric surgical patients encompasses complex interplay between genetics, environment (socioeconomic status and education), perioperative factors (prolonged surgery and hospitalization and anesthetic management) and the surgical lesion and coexisting disease processes.

conversant about the available pediatric anesthesia literature on this topic. There is little to no evidence for anesthetic neurotoxicity in prospective human studies in children exposed to short to moderate length general anesthetics. The median length of general anesthetics in children less than 18 years of age is less than 1 hour.[49] It is also important to reassure parents that every effort will be made to ensure that their child will be stable throughout the general anesthetic and the surgeon and anesthesiologist will strive to minimize the length of exposure. Many of the procedures that are done in young children are also very important for their neurodevelopment, such as strabismus surgery to ensure binocular vison and ear surgery to ensure adequate hearing. Parents and providers should be informed that there is ongoing research examining the effects of anesthetic exposures lasting longer than 2 hours.

SUMMARY

Several factors have an impact on neurodevelopment in pediatric surgical patients. These factors include the genetics and environment in addition to the surgical lesion and the perioperative management of the patient (**Fig. 1**). Pediatric anesthesiologists and intensivists are tasked to minimize the risk of brain injury throughout the perioperative period. This effort requires close attention and understanding of the patient's underlying medical condition and working closely with their entire medical team to optimize care. Unnecessary procedures and imaging studies should be avoided to limit exposure to potentially toxic general anesthetics. Baseline measures of blood pressure are important in determining perioperative blood pressure goals. Inadvertent hypocapnia or moderate hypercapnia as well as hyperoxia or hypoxia should be avoided in all patients. Pediatric patients should be maintained in a normothermic, euglycemic state with neutral positioning unless there are good reasons to deviate from these goals. Most of all, the task of improving the developmental outcomes of infants and children requires collaboration between anesthesiologists, surgeons, pediatricians, and neonatologists.

DISCLOSURE

The authors have nothing to disclose.

REFERENCES

1. Ikonomidou C, Bosch F, Miksa M, et al. Blockade of NMDA receptors and apoptotic neurodegeneration in the developing brain. Science 1999;283:70–4.
2. Jevtovic-Todorovic V, Hartman RE, Izumi Y, et al. Early exposure to common anesthetic agents causes widespread neurodegeneration in the developing rat brain and persistent learning deficits. J Neurosci 2003;23:876–82.
3. Davidson AJ, Disma N, de Graaff JC, et al. Neurodevelopmental outcome at 2 years of age after general anaesthesia and awake-regional anaesthesia in infancy (GAS): an international multicentre, randomised controlled trial. Lancet 2016;387:239–50.
4. McCann ME, de Graaff J, Dorris L, et al, Davidson AJ for the GAS Consortium. Neurodevelopmental outcome at 5 years of age after general anaesthesia or awake-regional anaesthesia in infancy (GAS): an international, multicentre, randomised, controlled equivalence trial. Lancet 2019;393:664–77.
5. Szmuk P, Andropoulos D, McGowan F, et al. An open label pilot study of a dexmedetomidine-remifentanil-caudal anesthetic for infant lower abdominal/lower extremity surgery: the T REX pilot study. Paediatr Anaesth 2019;29:59–67.

6. Homsy J, Zaidi S, Shen Y, et al. De novo mutations in congenital heart disease with neurodevelopmental and other congenital anomalies. Science 2015;350: 1262–6.

7. Miguel PM, Pereira LO, Silveira PP, et al. Early environmental influences on the development of children's brain structure and function. Dev Med Child Neurol 2019;61:1127–33.

8. Buss RR, Sun W, Oppenheim RW. Adaptive roles of programmed cell death during nervous system development. Annu Rev Neurosci 2006;29:1–35.

9. Vutskits L. General anesthesia: a gateway to modulate synapse formation and neural plasticity? Anesth Analg 2012;115:1174–82.

10. De Roo M, Klauser P, Briner A, et al. Anesthetics rapidly promote synaptogenesis during a critical period of brain development. PLoS One 2009;4:e7043.

11. Briner A, De Roo M, Dayer A, et al. Volatile anesthetics rapidly increase dendritic spine density in the rat medial prefrontal cortex during synaptogenesis. Anesthesiology 2010;112:546–56.

12. Penzes P, Cahill ME, Jones KA, et al. Dendritic spine pathology in neuropsychiatric disorders. Nat Neurosci 2011;14:285–93.

13. Paule MG, Li M, Allen RR, et al. Ketamine anesthesia during the first week of life can cause long-lasting cognitive deficits in rhesus monkeys. Neurotoxicol Teratol 2011;33:220–30.

14. Talpos JC, Chelonis JJ, Li M, et al. Early life exposure to extended general anesthesia with isoflurane and nitrous oxide reduces responsivity on a cognitive test battery in the nonhuman primate. Neurotoxicology 2019;70:80–90.

15. Deng M, Hofacer RD, Jiang C, et al. Brain regional vulnerability to anaesthesia-induced neuroapoptosis shifts with age at exposure and extends into adulthood for some regions. Br J Anaesth 2014;113:443–51.

16. Brambrink AM, Back SA, Riddle A, et al. Isoflurane-induced apoptosis of oligodendrocytes in the neonatal primate brain. Ann Neurol 2012;72:525–35.

17. Jevtovic-Todorovic V. Exposure of developing brain to general anesthesia: what is the animal evidence? Anesthesiology 2018;128:832–9.

18. Raper J, Alvarado MC, Murphy KL, et al. Multiple anesthetic exposure in infant monkeys alters emotional reactivity to an acute stressor. Anesthesiology 2015; 123:1084–92.

19. Alvarado MC, Murphy KL, Baxter MG. Visual recognition memory is impaired in rhesus monkeys repeatedly exposed to sevoflurane in infancy. Br J Anaesth 2017;119:517–23.

20. Boscolo A, Starr JA, Sanchez V, et al. The abolishment of anesthesia-induced cognitive impairment by timely protection of mitochondria in the developing rat brain: the importance of free oxygen radicals and mitochondrial integrity. Neurobiol Dis 2012;45:1031–41.

21. Soriano SG, Liu Q, Li J, et al. Ketamine activates cell cycle signaling and apoptosis in the neonatal rat brain. Anesthesiology 2010;112:1155–63.

22. Ben-Ari Y. Excitatory actions of GABA during development: the nature of the nurture. Nat Rev Neurosci 2002;3:728–39.

23. Edwards DA, Shah HP, Cao W, et al. Bumetanide alleviates epileptogenic and neurotoxic effects of sevoflurane in neonatal rat brain. Anesthesiology 2010; 112:567–75.

24. Puskarjov M, Fiumelli H, Briner A, et al. K-Cl Cotransporter 2-mediated Cl- Extrusion Determines Developmental Stage-dependent Impact of Propofol Anesthesia on Dendritic Spines. Anesthesiology 2017;126:855–67.

25. Dalla Massara L, Osuru HP, Oklopcic A, et al. General anesthesia causes epigenetic histone modulation of c-fos and brain-derived neurotrophic factor, Target genes important for neuronal development in the immature rat hippocampus. Anesthesiology 2016;124:1311–27.
26. Sanders RD, Xu J, Shu Y, et al. Dexmedetomidine attenuates isoflurane-induced neurocognitive impairment in neonatal rats. Anesthesiology 2009;110:1077–85.
27. Liu JR, Yuki K, Baek C, et al. Dexmedetomidine-induced neuroapoptosis is dependent on its cumulative dose. Anesth Analg 2016;123:1008–17.
28. Lin EP, Lee JR, Lee CS, et al. Do anesthetics harm the developing human brain? An integrative analysis of animal and human studies. Neurotoxicol Teratol 2017; 60:117–28.
29. Johnson SC, Pan A, Sun GX, et al. Relevance of experimental paradigms of anesthesia induced neurotoxicity in the mouse. PLoS One 2019;14:e0213543.
30. Loepke AW, McCann JC, Kurth CD, et al. The physiologic effects of isoflurane anesthesia in neonatal mice. Anesth Analg 2006;102:75–80.
31. Zheng H, Dong Y, Xu Z, et al. Sevoflurane anesthesia in pregnant mice induces neurotoxicity in fetal and offspring mice. Anesthesiology 2013;118:516–26.
32. Shih J, May LD, Gonzalez HE, et al. Delayed environmental enrichment reverses sevoflurane-induced memory impairment in rats. Anesthesiology 2012;116: 586–602.
33. Davidson AJ, Sun LS. Clinical evidence for any effect of anesthesia on the developing brain. Anesthesiology 2018;128:840–53.
34. McCann ME, Soriano SG. Does general anesthesia affect neurodevelopment in infants and children? BMJ 2019;367:l6459.
35. Wilder RT, Flick RP, Sprung J, et al. Early exposure to anesthesia and learning disabilities in a population-based birth cohort. Anesthesiology 2009;110: 796–804.
36. Hu D, Flick RP, Zaccariello MJ, et al. Association between exposure of young children to procedures requiring general anesthesia and learning and behavioral outcomes in a population-based birth cohort. Anesthesiology 2017;127:227–40.
37. Straker L, Mountain J, Jacques A, et al. Cohort profile: the Western Australian pregnancy cohort (Raine) study-Generation 2. Int J Epidemiol 2017;46: 1384–1385j.
38. Ing C, DiMaggio C, Whitehouse A, et al. Long-term differences in language and cognitive function after childhood exposure to anesthesia. Pediatrics 2012;130: e476–85.
39. Ing C, Wall MM, DiMaggio CJ, et al. Latent class analysis of neurodevelopmental deficit after exposure to anesthesia in early childhood. J Neurosurg Anesthesiol 2017;29:264–73.
40. Graham MR, Brownell M, Chateau DG, et al. Neurodevelopmental assessment in kindergarten in children exposed to general anesthesia before the age of 4 years: a retrospective matched cohort study. Anesthesiology 2016;125:667–77.
41. O'Leary JD, Janus M, Duku E, et al. A population-based study evaluating the association between surgery in early life and child development at primary school entry. Anesthesiology 2016;125:272–9.
42. Glatz P, Sandin RH, Pedersen NL, et al. Association of anesthesia and surgery during childhood with long-term academic performance. JAMA Pediatr 2017; 171:e163470.
43. Bartels M, Althoff RR, Boomsma DI. Anesthesia and cognitive performance in children: no evidence for a causal relationship. Twin Res Hum Genet 2009;12: 246–53.

44. O'Leary JD, Janus M, Duku E, et al. Influence of surgical procedures and general anesthesia on child development before primary school entry among matched sibling pairs. JAMA Pediatr 2019;173:29–36.

45. Sun LS, Li G, Miller TL, et al. Association between a single general anesthesia exposure before age 36 months and neurocognitive outcomes in later childhood. JAMA 2016;315:2312–20.

46. Warner DO, Zaccariello MJ, Katusic SK, et al. Neuropsychological and behavioral outcomes after exposure of young children to procedures requiring general anesthesia: the Mayo Anesthesia Safety in Kids (MASK) study. Anesthesiology 2018; 129(1):89–105.

47. Zaccariello MJ, Frank RD, Lee M, et al. Patterns of neuropsychological changes after general anaesthesia in young children: secondary analysis of the Mayo Anesthesia Safety in Kids study. Br J Anaesth 2019;122:671–81.

48. Warner DO, Chelonis JJ, Paule MG, et al. Performance on the Operant Test Battery in young children exposed to procedures requiring general anaesthesia: the MASK study. Br J Anaesth 2019;122:470–9.

49. Bartels DD, McCann ME, Davidson AJ, et al. Estimating pediatric general anesthesia exposure: quantifying duration and risk. Paediatr Anaesth 2018;28:520–7.

50. McCann ME, Lee JK, Inder T. Beyond anesthesia toxicity: anesthetic considerations to lessen the risk of neonatal neurological injury. Anesth Analg 2019;129: 1354–64.

51. Altman DI, Powers WJ, Perlman JM, et al. Cerebral blood flow requirement for brain viability in newborn infants is lower than in adults. Ann Neurol 1988;24: 218–26.

52. Fan AP, Jahanian H, Holdsworth SJ, et al. Comparison of cerebral blood flow measurement with [15O]-water positron emission tomography and arterial spin labeling magnetic resonance imaging: a systematic review. J Cereb Blood Flow Metab 2016;36:842–61.

53. Volpe JJ. Perinatal brain injury: from pathogenesis to neuroprotection. Ment Retard Dev Disabil Res Rev 2001;7:56–64.

54. DiNardo JA. Should what we know about neurobehavioral development, complex congenital heart disease, and brain maturation affect the timing of corrective cardiac surgery? Paediatr Anaesth 2011;21:781–6.

55. Dasgupta SJ, Gill AB. Hypotension in the very low birthweight infant: the old, the new, and the uncertain. Arch Dis Child Fetal Neonatal Ed 2003;88:F450–4.

56. Vavilala MS, Lee LA, Lam AM. The lower limit of cerebral autoregulation in children during sevoflurane anesthesia. J Neurosurg Anesthesiol 2003;15:307–12.

57. Rhondali O, Mahr A, Simonin-Lansiaux S, et al. Impact of sevoflurane anesthesia on cerebral blood flow in children younger than 2 years. Paediatr Anaesth 2013; 23(10):946–51.

58. Rhondali O, Pouyau A, Mahr A, et al. Sevoflurane anesthesia and brain perfusion. Paediatr Anaesth 2015;25:180–5.

59. McCann ME, Schouten ANJ, Dobija N, et al. Infantile postoperative encephalopathy after general anesthesia: perioperative factors as a cause for concern. Pediatrics 2014;133:e751–7.

60. Vanderhaegen J, Naulaers G, Vanhole C, et al. The effect of changes in tPCO2 on the fractional tissue oxygen extraction–as measured by near-infrared spectroscopy–in neonates during the first days of life. Eur J Paediatr Neurol 2009;13: 128–34.

61. Ashwal S, Stringer W, Tomasi L, et al. Cerebral blood flow and carbon dioxide reactivity in children with bacterial meningitis. J Pediatr 1990;117:523–30.

62. Pappas A, Shankaran S, Laptook AR, et al. Hypocarbia and adverse outcome in neonatal hypoxic-ischemic encephalopathy. J Pediatr 2011;158:752–758 e1.
63. Fabres J, Carlo WA, Phillips V, et al. Both extremes of arterial carbon dioxide pressure and the magnitude of fluctuations in arterial carbon dioxide pressure are associated with severe intraventricular hemorrhage in preterm infants. Pediatrics 2007;119:299–305.
64. Mariani G, Cifuentes J, Carlo WA. Randomized trial of permissive hypercapnia in preterm infants. Pediatrics 1999;104:1082–8.
65. Guidry CA, Hranjec T, Rodgers BM, et al. Permissive hypercapnia in the management of congenital diaphragmatic hernia: our institutional experience. J Am Coll Surg 2012;214:640–5, 647.e1.
66. Thome UH, Genzel-Boroviczeny O, Bohnhorst B, et al. Neurodevelopmental outcomes of extremely low birthweight infants randomised to different PCO2 targets: the PHELBI follow-up study. Arch Dis Child Fetal Neonatal Ed 2017;102:F376–82.
67. Thome UH, Genzel-Boroviczeny O, Bohnhorst B, et al. Permissive hypercapnia in extremely low birthweight infants (PHELBI): a randomised controlled multicentre trial. Lancet Respir Med 2015;3:534–43.
68. Millar LJ, Shi L, Hoerder-Suabedissen A, et al. Neonatal hypoxia ischaemia: mechanisms, models, and therapeutic challenges. Front Cell Neurosci 2017; 11:78.
69. Noh EJ, Kim YH, Cho MK, et al. Comparison of oxidative stress markers in umbilical cord blood after vaginal and cesarean delivery. Obstet Gynecol Sci 2014;57: 109–14.
70. Felderhoff-Mueser U, Bittigau P, Sifringer M, et al. Oxygen causes cell death in the developing brain. Neurobiol Dis 2004;17:273–82.
71. Kaindl AM, Sifringer M, Zabel C, et al. Acute and long-term proteome changes induced by oxidative stress in the developing brain. Cell Death Differ 2006;13: 1097–109.
72. Schmidt B, Whyte RK, Asztalos EV, et al. Canadian Oxygen Trial G: effects of targeting higher vs lower arterial oxygen saturations on death or disability in extremely preterm infants: a randomized clinical trial. JAMA 2013;309:2111–20.
73. McCann ME, Withington DE, Arnup SJ, et al. Consortium GAS: differences in blood pressure in infants after general anesthesia compared to awake regional anesthesia (GAS Study-A Prospective Randomized Trial). Anesth Analg 2017; 125:837–45.
74. Jain V, Chen M, Menon R. Disorders of carbohydrate metabolism. In: Gleason C, Devaskar S, editors. Avery's diseases of the newborn. 9th edition. Philadelphia: Elsevier Health Sciences; 2012. p. 1320–30.
75. Alkalay AL, Sarnat HB, Flores-Sarnat L, et al. Population meta-analysis of low plasma glucose thresholds in full-term normal newborns. Am J Perinatol 2006; 23:115–9.
76. McKinlay CJ, Alsweiler JM, Ansell JM, et al. Neonatal glycemia and neurodevelopmental outcomes at 2 years. N Engl J Med 2015;373:1507–18.
77. Simmons R, Stanley C. Neonatal hypoglycemia studies–is there a sweet story of success yet? N Engl J Med 2015;373:1567–9.
78. Tin W, Brunskill G, Kelly T, et al. 15-year follow-up of recurrent "hypoglycemia" in preterm infants. Pediatrics 2012;130:e1497–503.
79. Lucas A, Morley R, Cole TJ. Adverse neurodevelopmental outcome of moderate neonatal hypoglycaemia. BMJ 1988;297:1304–8.
80. Inder T. How low can I go? The impact of hypoglycemia on the immature brain. Pediatrics 2008;122:440–1.

81. de Almeida MF, Guinsburg R, Sancho GA, et al, Brazilian Network on Neonatal Research. Hypothermia and early neonatal mortality in preterm infants. J Pediatr 2014;164:271–5.e1.

82. Witt L, Dennhardt N, Eich C, et al. Prevention of intraoperative hypothermia in neonates and infants: results of a prospective multicenter observational study with a new forced-air warming system with increased warm air flow. Paediatr Anaesth 2013;23:469–74.

83. Laptook A, Tyson J, Shankaran S, et al. Elevated temperature after hypoxic-ischemic encephalopathy: risk factor for adverse outcomes. Pediatrics 2008; 122:491–9.

84. Elser HE, Holditch-Davis D, Levy J, et al. The effects of environmental noise and infant position on cerebral oxygenation. Adv Neonatal Care 2012;12(Suppl 5): S18–27.

85. Eichler F, Ipsiroglu O, Arif T, et al. Position dependent changes of cerebral blood flow velocities in premature infants. Eur J Pediatr 2001;160:633–9.

86. Romantsik O, Calevo MG, Bruschettini M. Head midline position for preventing the occurrence or extension of germinal matrix-intraventricular hemorrhage in preterm infants. Cochrane Database Syst Rev 2017;(7):CD012362.

Anesthesia for Innovative Pediatric Surgical Procedures

Johanna Meehyun Lee, MD, Erica Gee, MD,
Chang Amber Liu, MD, MSc*

KEYWORDS

- Pectus excavatum • Nuss procedure • Thoracic insufficiency syndrome
- Vertical expandable prosthetic titanium rib (VEPTR) • Craniosynostosis
- Endoscopic cranial suture release • Tethered cord syndrome
- Minimally invasive tethered cord release

KEY POINTS

1. The Nuss procedure is a minimally invasive approach to pectus excavatum repair. Anesthetic considerations include the potential for massive blood loss, injury to the heart, and arrhythmias, as well as significant postoperative pain, which can be treated with multimodal analgesia including regional techniques.

2. Vertical expandable prosthetic titanium ribs (VEPTR) can be used to treat children with thoracic insufficiency syndrome, and in contrast to spine fusion, allow for stabilization and continued growth of the spine. Patients who were dependent on tracheostomy and mechanical ventilation preoperatively may need continued mechanical ventilation and ICU admission for the immediate postoperative period before their ventilation begins to improve from the surgical intervention.

3. Endoscopic repair of craniosynostosis, when compared with open repair, decreases blood loss and transfusion, operative time, length of stay, and perioperative complications, including venous air embolism and transfusion-related complications. However, because of the young age and small size of patients undergoing this procedure, it is important to have blood available and transfuse preemptively.

4. New minimally invasive approaches to tethered cord release seem to be associated with reductions in postoperative pain, blood loss, and hospital stays. Although patients with tethered cord syndrome are typically otherwise healthy, preoperative evaluation should include an assessment of any other associated conditions, including anal atresia, cardiac anomalies, tracheoesophageal fistula, renal anomalies, and limb malformations.

Department of Anesthesia, Critical Care and Pain Medicine, Harvard Medical School, Massachusetts General Hospital, 55 Fruit Street, GRB 444, Boston, MA 02114, USA
* Corresponding author.
E-mail address: cliu19@partners.org

Anesthesiology Clin 38 (2020) 493–508
https://doi.org/10.1016/j.anclin.2020.06.004   anesthesiology.theclinics.com
1932-2275/20/© 2020 Elsevier Inc. All rights reserved.

INTRODUCTION

Over the past few decades, there have been numerous advances in pediatric surgery. This article focuses on anesthesia for innovative pediatric surgical procedures, namely the Nuss procedure for pectus excavatum repair, vertical expandable prosthetic titanium rib (VEPTR) for thoracic insufficiency syndrome, endoscopic cranial suture release for craniosynostosis, and minimally invasive tethered cord surgery for tethered cord syndrome.

THE NUSS PROCEDURE
Pectus Excavatum

Pectus excavatum is one of the most common congenital anomalies in the United States. It is the most common chest wall deformity in children, with an incidence of approximately 1:1000.[1] There is a male predominance, with an incidence of 1:400 in male children.[2] In pectus excavatum, the lower sternum is commonly depressed posteriorly relative to the upper sternum and costal cartilages, creating a concave chest wall deformity.[1] The etiology is unknown, but hypotheses include an intrinsic abnormality of the costal cartilage or overgrowth of the cartilages.[1,3]

Although usually present at birth, pectus excavatum is often diagnosed in early childhood or adolescence.[1] There has been a misconception that pectus excavatum is solely a cosmetic defect, which can delay correction of this condition until adulthood.[1] Clinically, patients can have a variety of symptoms that typically worsen with age.[1] The most common symptoms are dyspnea with exertion and loss of endurance, but also include chest pain, palpitations, and dizziness.[1] Associated conditions include mitral valve prolapse, cardiac dysrhythmias, and connective tissue disorders.[1,3]

Evaluation

The workup for pectus excavatum typically includes a computed tomography (CT) scan of the chest and may include echocardiography and pulmonary function tests (PFTs).[1–3] The severity of symptoms often does not correlate with the severity of the chest wall deformity.[1]

The Haller Index, a measure typically calculated on a CT scan, is the most commonly used objective measure of the degree of the defect in pectus excavatum.[2] To calculate this metric, the widest transverse diameter of the inner chest is divided by the distance between the posterior sternum and anterior spine.[1,2] A Haller Index of greater than 3.25 is generally thought to be an indicator of moderate to severe deformity and is an indication for surgery.[1] Of note, this number was initially determined by comparing a small group of patients with pectus excavatum who underwent repair with healthy controls, and was not subsequently validated with further studies.[2] The accuracy of the Haller Index can be limited with variations in thoracic shape, particularly with wide or narrow chests, and asymmetry.[2] A retrospective review in a series of patients who underwent repairs did not show a correlation between the Haller Index and operative time, postoperative bar infection, or length of hospitalization.[4] Nonetheless, at this time, this index is still the most commonly used index to quantify the severity of pectus excavatum.

Because the depressed portion of the sternum can result in compression of the anterior structures of the heart, namely the right atrium and right ventricle, an echocardiogram is useful for evaluation of cardiac anatomy and function.[1] Other features on echocardiogram to note include mitral valve prolapse, and if present, should include evaluation of the aortic root and valve in patients thought to have connective tissue disease.[1] An electrocardiogram (ECG) can identify any cardiac dysrhythmias that may result from this chest wall deformity.[1]

Static and exercise PFTs can be used to characterize the effect on lung mechanics.[1] PFTs may show features of both restrictive disease and mild obstructive disease.[1] Less commonly, cardiopulmonary exercise testing can be used to further assess the physiologic changes that are a result of the pectus excavatum and may suggest whether surgical repair could be beneficial.[1]

Surgical Approach

Indications for surgery can be found in **Box 1**.[1,3] Generally, modifications of 1 of 2 surgical approaches are used in the repair of pectus excavatum: the open approach described by Ravitch in 1949,[5] and the minimally invasive approach first described by Nuss in 1998.[6] In the open Ravitch procedure, deformed cartilage is resected, and a metal strut can be placed to support the sternum.[1] This strut is left in place for 6 months to 1 year before it is removed.[1] In contrast, in the minimally invasive Nuss procedure, 1 or 2 substernal concave bars are placed transthoracically posterior to the sternum, then rotated into a convex position, displacing the sternum outward.[1] This bar is left in place for approximately 2 years, allowing the sternum and chest wall to remodel, and then removed.[1] Thoracoscopy can also be used for better visualization of the heart and surrounding structures, to decrease the risk of cardiac injury during the insertion of the substernal bars.[1,7]

Over the past few decades, the Nuss procedure has become the standard approach in many centers because of its minimally invasive approach, with short operating time and good long-term cosmetic results.[3,8–10] However, disadvantages include longer hospitalization, severe postoperative pain, and the risk of hemorrhage due to cardiac or vascular injury as a result of the blind approach.[3,7]

Anesthetic Considerations

Preoperative
Preoperative evaluation must include a detailed assessment of the patient's cardiopulmonary function, as pectus excavatum can cause significant physiologic anomalies. In particular, chest CT, ECG, and if available, echocardiogram and PFTs should be reviewed. In addition, preoperative counseling about the operation and expectations for the postoperative period, including education on postoperative pain management strategies, have been shown to improve outcomes, increase patient and family satisfaction, and decrease length of hospitalization.[11]

Intraoperative
This procedure is performed under general anesthesia with an endotracheal tube. Although the procedure typically has minimal blood loss, there is a potential for

---

Box 1
Indications for surgical repair of pectus excavatum

- Symptoms (eg, dyspnea on exertion, exercise intolerance, chest pain)

- Haller Index greater than 3.25

- Abnormal pulmonary function tests

- Compression of right atrium or right ventricle on echocardiogram

Data from Jaroszewski D, Notrica D, McMahon L, Steidley DE, Deschamps C. Current management of pectus excavatum: A review and update of therapy and treatment recommendations. J Am Board Fam Med 2010;23:230-239; and Mavi J, Moore DL. Anesthesia and analgesia for pectus excavatum surgery. Anesthesiology Clin 2014;32:175-184.

massive blood loss due to the proximity to the heart and major vessels.[3] As such, depending on the patient's history and underlying conditions, it may be helpful to consider large-bore intravenous (IV) access, an arterial line, and type and screen with blood available in the event of significant blood loss.[3]

Although complications associated with the Nuss procedure are uncommon, there are a few complications to be aware of. Although rare, cardiac injury at the time of bar placement (or removal) is the most serious complication.[3,10] This risk can be mitigated by using thoracoscopy to guide placement of the bars.[3,10] Within the NSQIP-P 2012–2015 database, cardiothoracic injury occurred in 0.1% of cases.[12] This risk is highest in patients who have had prior cardiac surgery; as such, for these patients, there should be a cardiac surgeon, cardiac bypass circuit and perfusionist, and surgical instruments for open heart surgery available in the event of cardiac injury.[10]

Complications associated with the minimally invasive repair of pectus excavatum
During mediastinal dissection and insufflation of the chest, the patient should be monitored closely for possible arrhythmias that can occur due to irritation of the structures around the heart.[3] These arrhythmias can include frequent premature atrial and ventricular contractions, bradycardia, or even asystole. As such, preparation should include atropine, glycopyrrolate, ephedrine, and epinephrine.

After the bars are placed, the iatrogenic bilateral pneumothoraces should be mitigated using suctioning of the pleural spaces.[10] Chest tubes are not typically required, but may be necessary in certain scenarios, including the following: if residual CO_2 cannot be adequately removed from the pleural space, if there is intraoperative lung trauma, or if there is potential air leakage from the entry sites of the bars.[10] Nitrous oxide should be avoided, as it can cause significant expansion of these iatrogenic pneumothoraces.[11] Deep extubation or the use of opioid medications, or other medications like lidocaine or dexmedetomidine, may be helpful to avoid coughing or straining at the time of extubation.[3]

Postoperative
Pectus excavatum repair is one of the most painful surgeries performed in the pediatric population. As such, postoperative pain management has been a point of extensive research over the past several years, and studies have shown that multimodal analgesia is the most effective.[3] Although there is no unified consensus on the best approach at this time, there are many techniques that can be used for effective postoperative analgesia aside from opioids, including regional techniques and nonopioid adjuncts.[11] A thoracic epidural, placed at T5-T6 or T6-T7, is often used for pain control intraoperatively and postoperatively, but alternatives include bilateral paravertebral catheters or erector spinae plane blocks or catheters, which have a lower risk of hypotension but require more expertise.[11,13–15] Surgical interventions for pain control include intraoperative catheter placement into either the subpleural or subcutaneous space, and cryoablation of intercostal nerves at the level of the incision and 1 or 2 levels above and below the incision (**Fig. 1**).[11] In the perioperative period, the preceding measures are often supplemented with other adjuncts, including a patient-controlled anesthesia (PCA) or intermittent opioids, acetaminophen (Tylenol), diazepam (Valium), methocarbamol, ketorolac (Toradol), ketamine, methadone, dexamethasone, and clonidine.[3,11]

Key Points

- Preoperative evaluation should include a detailed assessment of the patient's cardiopulmonary function, including the chest CT scan, ECG, and, if available, echocardiogram and PFTs.

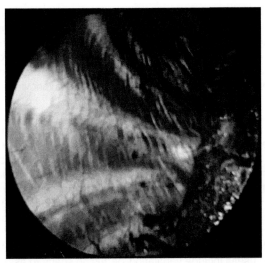

Fig. 1. Cryoablation of intercostal nerves during the Nuss procedure. This photograph shows the view via thoracoscopy after cryoablation of the intercostal nerves, as a regional technique for perioperative pain management.

- Although the procedure typically has minimal blood loss, there is a potential for massive blood loss due to the proximity to the heart and major vessels. As such, the patient should have an active type and screen, adequate IV access, and, if indicated, arterial line.
- Serious complications of the Nuss procedure include injury to the heart and cardiac arrhythmias. If a patient has had prior cardiac surgery, a cardiac surgeon, cardiac bypass circuit, and perfusionist should be available, because of the elevated risk of cardiac injury during this procedure.
- As the Nuss bar is advanced through the mediastinum, arrhythmias such as frequent premature atrial and ventricular contractions, bradycardia, or even asystole can occur due to irritation of the heart and surrounding structures.
- Although the Nuss procedure is minimally invasive, it is a very painful procedure, and multimodal analgesia should be used for postoperative pain management. This can include a combination of regional anesthesia (epidural, paravertebral, or erector spinae catheters), cryoablation, and other adjuncts like acetaminophen, diazepam, methocarbamol, ketorolac, ketamine, methadone, dexamethasone, and clonidine.

VERTICAL EXPANDABLE PROSTHETIC TITANIUM RIB
Thoracic Insufficiency Syndrome

Thoracic insufficiency syndrome encompasses congenital or acquired chest wall defects, spinal deformities, neuromuscular dysfunction, or other anatomic disorders of the thorax that can lead to restrictive lung disease.[16,17] Conditions that can lead to thoracic insufficiency syndrome include Jeune syndrome, Jarcho-Levin syndrome, connective tissue disorders, spina bifida, spinal muscular atrophy, scoliosis, and many others.[17] Children diagnosed with these syndromes can be extremely debilitated with chronic contractures and restrictive lung disease.[17,18]

The diagnosis of this syndrome relies on symptoms, signs, and radiography.[16,17] Symptoms include limited exercise tolerance, recurrent lower respiratory tract infections, and pulmonary hypertension, and signs can include tachypnea at rest, nocturnal hypercarbia and hypoxemia.[17] In early-onset scoliosis, the natural history of the disease leads to decreased life expectancy, with increased mortality rates of 2 times normal by age 40 and 3 times normal by age 60, largely due to respiratory failure or cardiovascular disease.[17] Early diagnosis and treatment is important in preventing or mitigating progression to significant thoracic insufficiency.

Evaluation

Although there is no standardized protocol for evaluating children with thoracic insufficiency syndrome, various imaging studies can provide an estimate of severity and can also be used for serial assessments of lung volume or pulmonary function.[17,18] Anteroposterior and lateral radiographs of the spine are used to measure the height of the thoracic spine and the Cobb angle, which is the maximal angle between the superior and inferior endplates of the terminal vertebrae of the spinal curvature.[17,19] The Cobb angle is often measured serially to assess for changes over time.[19] CT scans of the chest and lumbar spine can give a more accurate assessment of lung volume, particularly in children younger than 3 years if PFTs cannot be obtained.[17] Other studies that can be useful include ventilation-perfusion scans to assess for and quantify relative ventilation and perfusion in the right versus left lung, echocardiograms if there is a suspicion for early cor pulmonale, and MRI of the spine to assess for any spinal cord abnormalities.[17]

Surgical Approach

When limitation of respiratory function or normal lung growth due to thoracic insufficiency syndrome is progressive, surgical treatment can be pursued.[17] VEPTR can also be used for congenital scoliosis that does not respond to bracing.[17,18] Historically, early-onset scoliosis was treated with early spine fusion with immobilization, but many of these patients had poor pulmonary function, with loss of thoracic height from the spine fusion and decreased lung volumes.[17] As such, in younger children, this approach has largely been replaced by the use of various devices, including the growing rods, VEPTR, MAGnetic expansion control (MAGEC) rods, and bracing.[17]

Although studies are still being conducted to evaluate the efficacy of these newer growth-sparing interventions, evidence suggests that VEPTR insertion may improve respiratory function, allowing for the weaning of respiratory support in patients requiring mechanical ventilation or preventing the need for respiratory support in patients not currently requiring ventilation or supplemental oxygenation, and decrease mortality.[17]

Vertical Expandable Prosthetic Titanium Rib

The VEPTR was approved by the Food and Drug Administration (FDA) in 2004 as a humanitarian use device to treat children with thoracic insufficiency syndrome.[17,18] The VEPTR device is a construct that attaches to the ribs and, once placed, can be progressively expanded, allowing for continued growth of the spine while stabilizing it.[18] These are typically anchored to another rib, the spine, or pelvis.[18] The particular surgical approach using these devices is guided by the type of volume depletion deformity (VDD).[17,20]

In VDD Type I, characterized by absent ribs and early-onset scoliosis, the approach is a thoracotomy on the side without ribs, intraoperative correction of scoliosis by distraction, then stabilization using VEPTR devices.[17,20] In VDD Type II (the most common type), which is characterized by fused ribs and early-onset scoliosis, the surgical approach involves creating an opening wedge thoracostomy (thoracotomy on the side with fused ribs, followed by transverse rib osteotomy and distraction of the edges of the ribs), and stabilization of the expanded thorax using VEPTR devices.[17,18,20] In VDD Type IIIa, characterized by a short thorax (eg, Jarcho-Levin syndrome), a staged bilateral procedure is performed, using opening wedge thoracostomies and insertion of rib-to-rib VEPTR.[17] In VDD Type IIIb, characterized by a narrow thorax (eg, Jeune syndrome, infantile scoliosis with windswept deformity), staged bilateral dynamic segmental expansion thoracoplasties are performed, with rib osteotomies to mobilize the chest wall and insertion of a curved VEPTR to stabilize the chest wall.[18,20]

MAGnetic Expansion Control Rods

The MAGEC rods, approved by the FDA in 2014, use a magnetic expansion mechanism that can be activated by an external set of magnets.[17] As a result, the MAGEC rods do not require multiple expansion surgeries and can be lengthened more frequently without the need for general anesthesia.[17]

Anesthetic Considerations

Preoperative
Preoperative evaluation should include a comprehensive review of the available imaging studies, including radiographs, CT scans, PFTs, and echocardiograms, as well as assessment of comorbidities.[17] In the setting of an acute upper or lower respiratory infection, the surgery should be postponed until the infection is resolved or treated due to risk of prolonged intubation in the setting of baseline respiratory compromise.[17] Children presenting for VEPTR surgery can often have corrected or uncorrected congenital cardiac anomalies as part of their syndrome.

Intraoperative
The procedure is typically performed under general endotracheal anesthesia with prone positioning for posterior approaches or lateral decubitus positioning for anterior approaches, with standard monitors and an arterial line.[21] Phenylephrine can be used to increase mean arterial pressure (MAP) to improve spinal cord perfusion during the case, particularly if there are any changes noted on neuromonitoring. Although uncommon, there can be significant blood loss with these procedures; large-bore IV access and an active type and screen should be available.[21] In addition, antifibrinolytics like tranexamic acid or aminocaproic acid are commonly used to prevent or control significant blood loss, though their use is institution-dependent. Placement of a central line can be considered for patients with poor cardiac function or for patients with challenging intravenous access, particularly in those with chronic contractures.

During prone positioning, care must be taken to avoid mechanical compression, which can increase intrathoracic and pulmonary pressures. This can exacerbate difficulty with ventilation due to restrictive lung disease and can lead to acute right to left shunting in children with residual intracardiac defects. Patients with preexisting cardiac dysfunction, such as patients with Duchenne muscular dystrophy or Friedreich ataxia who have progressive cardiomyopathy, may not tolerate the prone position due to increased thoracic pressures causing a reduction in stroke volume and cardiac index.[22]

Somatosensory evoked potentials (SSEPs) and motor evoked potentials (MEPs) should be used to monitor for neurologic complications secondary to spinal cord damage from mechanical distraction or ischemia.[21] Anesthetic techniques that allow for effective SSEP and MEP monitoring include total intravenous anesthesia (TIVA) or a minimum alveolar concentration (MAC) of less than 1 with an inhaled anesthetic and nitrous oxide.[21] Neuromuscular blockade should also be avoided after intubation, and the use of succinylcholine for intubation should be considered. A neurologic examination is done at the end of the case by assessing for purposeful movement of all 4 extremities, and care should be taken that the patient is not overly sedated after extubation at the end of the case to be able to follow commands.[21] Rarely, intraoperative wake-up tests may need to be performed if neuromonitoring signals are poor or unreliable intraoperatively. Poor baseline signals can occur in children who are minimally mobile due to their preexisting conditions.

Postoperative

In patients who were preoperatively dependent on tracheostomy and mechanical ventilation due to severe thoracic insufficiency, most will require continued mechanical ventilation and admission to the intensive care unit (ICU) for the immediate postoperative period before their ventilation status begins to improve from surgical intervention.[21] Pain management is challenging in this population because of the extensive nature of the surgery. However, epidural analgesia is technically difficult because of the challenging anatomy with scoliosis and increased incidence of spinal cord abnormalities, although an epidural catheter placed under direct vision at the end of surgery has been shown to be effective.[21,23] Continuous opioid infusions, PCA or nurse-controlled analgesia (NCA), along with other adjuncts like nonsteroidal antiinflammatory drugs, can be used for pain management.[21,23]

Key Points

- Preoperative evaluation of thoracic insufficiency syndrome should include a review of the available imaging studies, including radiographs, CT scans, PFTs, and echocardiograms, as well as a thorough assessment of underlying comorbidities.
- If the patient has an acute upper or lower respiratory infection, surgery should be postponed until the infection is resolved or treated.
- The VEPTR and MAGEC rods are new FDA-approved devices that can be used in the treatment of thoracic insufficiency syndrome. Particularly in young patients, these devices provide an alternative to early spine fusion by providing stabilization and continued growth of the spine.
- During prone positioning of the patient, it is important to avoid chest wall compression, which can exacerbate difficulty with ventilation and can also lead to acute right to left shunting in children with intracardiac defects.
- SSEPs and MEPs should be used for neuromonitoring, and the anesthetic maintenance should be tailored to allow for neuromonitoring and a crisp wake-up test as necessary.
- Patients may need mechanical ventilation and ICU admission postoperatively if they were dependent on tracheostomy and mechanical ventilation preoperatively. Pain management will likely involve the use of opioids via continuous infusion, PCA, or NCA, in addition to other analgesic medications.

ENDOSCOPIC CRANIAL SUTURE RELEASE
Craniosynostosis

In normal development, infants have rapid brain growth over the first year of life, pushing apart the cranial sutures, which are growth plates that deposit new bone and allow for expansion of the brain and skull.[24,25] In craniosynostosis, one or more of the cranial sutures fuse prematurely, causing localized or global growth delay of the skull.[24,25] Craniosynostosis can be isolated or associated with various syndromes.[25] Most cases of craniosynostosis are nonsyndromic, but the cases of syndromic craniosynostosis can be very complex and challenging to manage.[25] This is because nonsyndromic craniosynostosis usually involves a single suture, whereas syndromic craniosynostosis can involve multiple sutures and other cranial vault bony abnormalities. Associated syndromes include Crouzon syndrome, Apert syndrome, Pfeiffer syndrome, Saethre-Chotzen syndrome, and Muenke syndrome. Children with these syndromes have various clinical features, particularly craniofacial anomalies that can make airway management difficult.[25] Nonsyndromic craniosynostosis is classified by the cranial suture affected: sagittal, metopic, coronal (bilateral or unilateral), or lamboid.

Of note, in children with complex craniosynostosis, approximately 50% may have intracranial hypertension, whereas in simple synostosis, approximately 15% may have intracranial hypertension.[25,26] Symptoms of elevated intracranial pressure (ICP) can be nonspecific in children and include poor feeding, failure to thrive, headaches, and developmental delay.[25]

Surgical Approach

Historically, in the late 1800s and mid-1900s, suturectomies or strip craniectomies were performed for the treatment of craniosynostosis, but were limited by early refusion at the craniectomy sites.[18,21] In the 1970s, a new, more invasive technique was introduced that involved the removal of large segments of bone, remodeling of the bone, and stabilization of the bone in a more anatomic position.[18,21] Although this led to more predictable outcomes, there was significant morbidity due to blood loss, lengthy operations, and prolonged hospitalizations.[18,21] Traditionally, open cranial vault surgeries for the correction of craniosynostosis are performed from 6 to 12 months of age.[21]

The use of endoscopic techniques for craniosynostosis has been documented in the literature since the 1990s; however, it is often considered to be an innovative procedure, despite its well established safety and efficacy.[24] In endoscopic surgery, the goal is to remove the fused portion of the bone, followed by the use of orthotic therapy (ie, with a helmet) to guide brain and skull growth to recreate normal anatomy.[24,27] Access requires 1 to 2 small incisions perpendicular to the fused suture, followed by the creation of burr holes over the suture.[24,28] An endoscope is used for dissection of the dura off of the suture, and a strip of fused bone is removed from the affected suture.[24,28]

In contrast to open vault surgeries, endoscopic repair of craniosynostosis should be undertaken in infants younger than 6 months, as the procedure relies on brain and skull growth following the procedure for correction.[24] If undertaken in children older than 6 months, there are expandable devices that can be used (springs, distractors) to drive skull growth in a defined direction, but this technique requires a second procedure to remove this device.[24,27] Research has shown that the endoscopic approach decreases blood loss and transfusion, operative time, length of stay, and perioperative complications including venous air embolism and transfusion-related complications,[29,30] in addition to improved patient and family experience and cosmetic outcomes.[24]

Anesthetic Considerations

Preoperative
It is important to assess these patients for any underlying or associated medical conditions, birth history (specifically history of prematurity and any oxygen requirements), evidence of elevated ICP, and potential for a difficult airway.[26,28] Of note, the risk of postoperative apnea increases with history of prematurity and anemia.[28]

In syndromic craniosynostosis, anatomic anomalies can make mask ventilation and/ or intubation challenging, and advanced airway techniques should be available.[28] Premedication is typically not necessary because of the young age of the patients, and should be avoided because of the risk of adversely affecting the post-operative wake-up test.[28]

Intraoperative

This procedure is typically performed under general endotracheal anesthesia with standard monitors and 2 IVs.[27] Although arterial lines are routine for open vault surgeries, invasive blood pressure monitoring is typically reserved for patients with significant comorbidities for endoscopic suture release.[28] After intubation, the endotracheal tube (ETT) can be displaced during neck flexion or extension, and the ETT position should be reconfirmed after all position changes.[26]

Positioning depends on the cranial suture affected: supine positioning for metopic or coronal suture repair, and prone positioning for sagittal or lamboidal suture repair.[28] The prone position increases the risk of venous air embolism, and, as such, patients can be monitored using precordial Doppler ultrasound.[28] However, the risk of venous air embolism is dramatically reduced with endoscopic repair (8%) when compared with open repair (up to 82.6%), and central venous catheters are typically not necessary.[28] However, brisk bleeding and subsequent reduced venous pressures leading to increased risk for venous air embolism can occur quickly due to surrounding large venous sinuses regardless of endoscopic or open repair. Other uncommon complications include intraoperative dural tear.[28] With the potential for intracranial hypertension in these patients, measures to avoid increased ICP should be used, including avoidance of hypercapnia, hypoxemia.[26]

There remains a potential for bleeding with the endoscopic approach, though less than the risk with an open approach.[28–30] Risk factors for blood loss and the need for transfusion include weight less than 6 kg, syndromic craniosynostosis, sagittal suture involvement, and the experience of the team.[28] It is recommended that packed red blood cells be available in the operating room.[24] Due to the young age and small size of children undergoing craniosynostosis repair, blood loss can be rapid because cardiac output to the brain is much higher in this age group. In some institutions, blood transfusion starts concomitantly with scalp incision to avoid inadvertent hypovolemia, which can occur quickly and insidiously in a small child.

Postoperative

With endoscopic repair, patients can typically be extubated in the operating room, and if there are no other complications or comorbidities, can be monitored on the floor postoperatively.[24] Patients can often be discharged on postoperative day 1.[24] As with any other surgical approach to craniosynostosis, there is a risk for refusion of the suture, whether fusion of the suture that was operated on or pan-synostosis.[24] As a result, all craniosynostosis repair patients should be serially followed with head circumference measurement and imaging as needed, until at least 6 years of age.[24]

Key Points

- Craniosynostosis can be associated with a myriad of syndromes, including Crouzon syndrome, Apert syndrome, and Pfeiffer syndrome, that may be characterized by various craniofacial anomalies that can make airway management challenging and may require advanced airway techniques.
- Although open repair was typically undertaken between 6 and 12 months of age, endoscopic repair of craniosynostosis is performed at a younger age (<6 months). The procedure is followed by orthotic therapy (ie, helmet) to guide

brain and skull growth and recreate normal anatomy. Expandable devices (springs, distractors) can be used to actively drive skull growth in a defined direction if this procedure is undertaken in children >6 months of age.

- Compared with open repair, endoscopic repair of craniosynostosis decreases blood loss and transfusion, operative time, length of stay, and perioperative complications including venous air embolism and transfusion-related complications. However, due to the young age and small size of patients undergoing this procedure, it is important to have blood available and transfuse preemptively.
- Brisk bleeding and subsequent reduced venous pressures leading to increased risk for venous air embolism can occur quickly due to surrounding large venous sinuses regardless of endoscopic or open repair.
- Otherwise healthy patients can typically be extubated in the operating room and be monitored on the neurosurgical floor overnight, before being discharged on postoperative day 1.

MINIMALLY INVASIVE TETHERED CORD RELEASE
Tethered Cord Syndrome

A tethered spinal cord is characterized by the tethering of the lumbosacral spinal cord to inelastic structures caudally, causing a stretching and traction effect on the spinal cord.[31] In tethered cord syndrome (TCS), this tension on the cord can cause symptoms, including back pain, leg pain, motor or sensory deficits in the lower extremities, diminished deep tendon reflexes, bladder dysfunction, incontinence, or scoliosis.[31–33] Tethered cord is also often associated with other physical signs, including sacral dimples or hair tufts.[31,32] Of note, although most patients with tethered cord are otherwise healthy, spinal cord abnormalities can often be associated with other anatomic anomalies (eg, VACTERL syndrome), and additional evaluation may be indicated.[34,35] Evaluation of TCS involves MRI of the spinal cord.[32] Although ultrasound can be used as an initial approach, an MRI is indicated if TCS is suspected.[32]

TCS can be classified into 3 categories.[31,32] Category 1 TCS includes patients with symptoms that are correlated with the stretch-induced injury to the caudal spinal cord.[31,32] Causes of category 1 TCS include caudal myelomeningocele (MMC), small lipomyelomeningocele (LMMC), and an inelastic filum terminale.[31,32] Category 2 TCS includes patients with similar symptoms that may not be fully attributed to the stretch-induced dysfunction, and may be due to injury resulting from local compression and ischemia from dorsal anomalies (eg, MMC, large LMMC).[31,32] As such, symptoms may be only partially relieved or not relieved at all after detethering of the cord in these patients.[31,32] Category 3 TCS includes patients with extensive neurologic deficits typically due to damage to the thoracic or high lumbar spinal cord.[31,32] Category 3 TCS is not true TCS in the sense that the deficits are not correlated with stretch-induced effects on the caudal spinal cord but rather are a result of irreversible neurologic deficits, which in some cases can be due to a lack of functional neurons or replacement of neuronal tissue with fat tissue.[31,32] This categorization of TCS is useful because surgical release of the tethered cord can only be beneficial in categories 1 and 2.[31,32]

Although tethered cord release is recommended in patients who are symptomatic, particularly in those with neurologic or urologic deficits, there is no consensus on surgery in the asymptomatic patient with an incidental finding on MRI.[35] Although every operation has its risks, prophylactic surgical intervention may be useful even in asymptomatic patients at risk for TCS, because neurologic and urologic symptoms may not be completely resolved by surgery once they develop.[35] Furthermore, early intervention appears to improve outcomes in patients with TCS.[35]

Surgical Approach

The current standard of care for the management of TCS is open tethered cord release (TCR) via 1-level lumbar laminectomy.[35,36] Minimally invasive surgery has become increasingly widespread due to shorter operative times and fewer complications.[36] Although most reported minimally invasive TCR procedures to date have been performed in adult patients, there have been reports of minimally invasive approaches for TCR release in children.[36,37]

The approaches described in these studies were specifically for tight filum terminale, not for more complex causes of TCS (eg, tumors, MMC).[36,37] As these minimally invasive approaches are still under development, the approaches were all slightly different, involving lumbar hemilaminectomy with endoscopic sectioning of the filum terminale,[33] microscopic tubular approach to laminotomy and sectioning of the filum,[36] and microscopic interlaminar approach that does not involve laminectomy or laminotomy with sectioning of the filum.[37] However, all of these minimally invasive approaches, though with small sample sizes, suggested reductions in postoperative pain, blood loss, and hospital stays.[33,36,37] In particular, there was a suggested likelihood of reduction in retethering with these strategies due to the minimization of injury and inflammation to the subarachnoid space.[36,37]

Anesthetic Considerations

Preoperative
Children with TCS, although typically otherwise healthy, may have other associated congenital conditions, including vertebral defects, anal atresia, cardiovascular anomalies, tracheoesophageal fistula, renal anomalies, and limb malformations (VACTERL syndrome).[34,38] A preoperative assessment of neurologic deficits and any history of prior spine surgery is essential.[34] It is also often important to prepare for a latex-free operating room environment as TCS, especially history of MMC, is associated with latex sensitivity.[38]

Intraoperative
TCR is performed under general endotracheal anesthesia in the prone position.[34,38] For otherwise uncomplicated TCR in patients with tight filum terminale, there is minimal estimated blood loss, and even less in minimally invasive approaches.[36,37] Careful attention to positioning and control of blood pressure is important to maintain spinal perfusion pressure (SCPP).[38]

Intraoperative neuromonitoring with SSEP and MEP are used to monitor neurophysiological function during tethered cord release.[39] As a result, neuromuscular blockade should be avoided after intubation and inhaled anesthetic agents should be minimized or avoided to ensure accurate neuromonitoring.[34] Intraoperative direct stimulation of the nerve roots is also used to monitor responses in the bilateral lower extremities and anal sphincter throughout the surgery.[36] Stimulation of the filum, in contrast, does not produce any response; this is used to distinguish and confirm the tethering structure before sectioning of the filum.[36] After dural closure, the surgeon will typically perform or ask for a Valsalva maneuver to ensure there is no dural leak of cerebrospinal fluid (CSF).[35]

Postoperative
Tethered cord release has a relatively safe risk profile, with the most common complications being wound infections, wound dehiscence, and CSF leak.[35] Unfortunately, there is also a risk of re-tethering and recurrence of TCS after tethered cord release, and long-term follow-up is recommended.[35,36]

The most common cause of reoperation after tethered cord release is CSF leak.[35] In the past, patients were required to remain flat for several days to avoid CSF leak,[34] but more recent evidence suggests that for simple TCR, 24 hours of postoperative recumbency may result in similar rates of CSF leak as longer periods.[40]

For minimally invasive approaches, postsurgical pain is thought to be lower than for open approaches, particularly when laminectomy or laminotomy is not required.[36,37] In simple TCR for tight filum terminale, perioperative pain can be managed with acetaminophen, opioids as needed, and, depending on institutional policies, ketorolac.[36,40] Epidural catheters are not typically used.[40]

Key Points

- Tethered cord can be associated with other congenital anomalies, including anal atresia, cardiac anomalies, tracheoesophageal fistula, renal anomalies, and limb malformations. However, typically patients with tethered cord are otherwise healthy.
- Tethered cord can be associated with latex sensitivity, and as such, the gloves and equipment used in the operating room should be latex-free.
- Minimally invasive approaches to TCR seem to be associated with reductions in postoperative pain, blood loss, and hospital stays.
- Intraoperative monitoring with SSEP, MEP, and intraoperative direct stimulation of the nerve roots is used to monitor neurophysiologic function throughout surgery. As a result, neuromuscular blockade should be avoided after intubation and inhaled anesthetic agents should be minimized or avoided to ensure accurate neuromonitoring.
- The most common cause of reoperation after tethered cord release is CSF leak.

Discussion

There have been many advances in pediatric surgery over the past few decades, with some advances using new devices (eg, VEPTR, MAGEC rods) and others using less invasive approaches (eg, Nuss procedure, endoscopic cranial suture release, minimally invasive TCR). Although many of these procedures were initially met with caution or skepticism, continued experience over the past few decades has shown that these procedures are safe and effective.

Clinics Care Points

- Although the Nuss procedure is minimally invasive, it is a very painful procedure, and multimodal analgesia should be used for postoperative pain management. This can include a combination of regional anesthesia (epidural vs paravertebral), cryoablation, and other adjuncts like acetaminophen, diazepam, ketorolac, ketamine, and methadone.

- The VEPTR and MAGEC rods are new FDA-approved devices that can be used in the treatment of thoracic insufficiency syndrome, and have been used with good effect. Particularly in young patients, these devices provide an alternative to early spine fusion by providing stabilization and continued growth of the spine. If the patient has an acute upper or lower respiratory infection, surgery should be postponed until the infection is resolved or treated.

- Craniosynostosis can be associated with a myriad of syndromes, including Crouzon syndrome, Apert syndrome, and Pfeiffer syndrome, that may be characterized by various craniofacial anomalies that can make airway management challenging and may require advanced airway techniques. Compared with open repair, endoscopic repair of craniosynostosis decreases blood loss and transfusion, operative time, length of stay, and perioperative complications, including venous air embolism and transfusion-related complications. However, because of the young age and small size of patients undergoing this procedure, it is important to have blood available and transfuse preemptively.

- TCS can be associated with other congenital anomalies, including anal atresia, cardiac anomalies, tracheoesophageal fistula, renal anomalies, and limb malformations. New minimally invasive approaches to TCR seem to be associated with reductions in postoperative pain, blood loss, and hospital stays. Due to the need for intraoperative neuromonitoring during these procedures, neuromuscular blockade should be avoided after intubation and inhaled anesthetic agents should be minimized or avoided.

DISCLOSURE

The authors have no disclosures.

REFERENCES

1. Jaroszewski D, Notrica D, McMahon L, et al. Current management of pectus excavatum: a review and update of therapy and treatment recommendations. J Am Board Fam Med 2010;23:230–9.
2. Sujka JA, St. Peter SD. Quantification of pectus excavatum: anatomic indices. Semin Pediatr Surg 2018;27:122–6.
3. Mavi J, Moore DL. Anesthesia and analgesia for pectus excavatum surgery. Anesthesiol Clin 2014;32:175–84.
4. Mortellaro VE, Iqbal CW, Fike FB, et al. The predictive value of Haller index in patients undergoing pectus bar repair for pectus excavatum. J Surg Res 2011;170: 104–6.
5. Ravitch MM. The operative treatment of pectus excavatum. Ann Surg 1949;129: 429–44.
6. Nuss D, Kelly RE Jr, Croitoru DP, et al. A 10-year review of a minimally invasive technique for the correction of pectus excavatum. J Pediatr Surg 1998;33: 545–52.
7. Frawley G, Frawley J, Crameri J. A review of anesthetic techniques and outcomes following minimally invasive repair of pectus excavatum (Nuss procedure). Paediatr Anaesth 2016;11:1082–90.
8. Nuss D. Minimally invasive surgical repair of pectus excavatum. Semin Pediatr Surg 2008;56:283–6.
9. Kelly RE, Goretsky MJ, Obermeyer R, et al. Twenty-one years of experience with minimally invasive repair of pectus excavatum by the Nuss procedure in 1215 patients. Ann Surg 2010;252:1072–81.
10. Goretsky MJ, McGuire MM. Complications associated with the minimally invasive repair of pectus excavatum. Semin Pediatr Surg 2018;27:151–5.
11. Singhal NR, Jerman JD. A review of anesthetic considerations and postoperative pain control after the Nuss procedure. Semin Pediatr Surg 2018;27:156–60.
12. Tetteh O, Rhee DS, Boss E, et al. Minimally invasive repair of pectus excavatum: analysis of the NSQIP database and the use of thoracoscopy. J Pediatr Surg 2018;53(6):1230–3.
13. Yoshizaki M, Murata H, Ogami-Takamura K, et al. Bilateral erector spinae plane block using a programmed intermittent bolus technique for pain management after Nuss procedure. J Clin Anesth 2019;57:51–2.
14. Bryskin RB, Robie DK, Mansfield FM, et al. Introduction of a novel ultrasound-guided extrathoracic sub-paraspinal block for control of perioperative pain in Nuss procedure patients. J Pediatr Surg 2017;52(3):484–91.

15. Nardiello MA, Herlitz M. Bilateral single shot erector spinae plane block for pectus excavatum and pectus carinatum surgery in 2 pediatric patients. Rev Esp Anestesiol Reanim 2018;65(9):530–3.
16. Hines RL, Marschall K. Pediatric diseases. In: Hines RL, Marschall K, editors. Handbook for Stoelting's anesthesia and co-existing disease. 4th edition. Philadelphia: Elsevier; 2013. p. 364–97.
17. Mayer O, Campbell R, Cahill P, et al. Thoracic insufficiency syndrome. Curr Probl Pediatr Adolesc Health Care 2016;46:72–97.
18. Parnell SE, Effmann EL, Song K, et al. Vertical expandable prosthetic titanium rib (VEPTR): a review of indications, normal radiographic appearance and complications. Pediatr Radiol 2015;45:606–16.
19. Malfair D, Flemming AK, Dvorak MF, et al. Radiographic evaluation of scoliosis: review. AJR Am J Roentgenol 2010;194:S8–22.
20. Campbell RM Jr, Smith MD. Thoracic insufficiency syndrome and exotic scoliosis. J Bone Joint Surg Am 2007;89(Suppl 1):108–22.
21. McCann ME, Brustowicz RM, Holzman RS. The musculoskeletal system and orthopedic surgery. In: Holzman RS, Mancuso TJ, Polaner DM, editors. A practical approach to pediatric anesthesia. 2nd edition. Philadelphia: Wolters Kluwer; 2016. p. 562–613.
22. Kwee MM, Ho Y, Rozen WM. The prone position during surgery and its complications: a systematic review and evidence-based guidelines. Int Surg 2015;100:292–303.
23. Cunliffe M. Bone and joint surgery: anesthetic considerations and postoperative management. In: Anderson B, Bissonnette B, editors. Pediatric anesthesia: basic principles, stage of the art, future. Shelton (CT): People's Medical Publishing House-USA; 2011. p. 1527–50.
24. Proctor MR. Endoscopic craniosynostosis repair. Transl Pediatr 2014;3:247–58.
25. Peters DA, Forrest CR. Craniofacial malformations: surgical considerations. In: Anderson B, Bissonnette B, editors. Pediatric anesthesia: basic principles, stage of the art, future. Shelton (CT): People's Medical Publishing House-USA; 2011. p. 1891–919.
26. Levin MF. Craniofacial malformations: anesthetic considerations. In: Anderson B, Bissonnette B, editors. Pediatric anesthesia: basic principles, stage of the art, future. Shelton (CT): People's Medical Publishing House-USA; 2011. p. 1920–33.
27. Proctor MR. Endoscopic cranial suture release for the treatment of craniosynostosis – is it the future? J Craniofac Surg 2012;23:225–8.
28. Nelson JH, Menser CC, Reddy SK. Endoscopic craniosynostosis repair. Int Anesthesiol Clin 2019;57:61–71.
29. Goyal A, Lu VM, Yolcu YU, et al. Endoscopic versus open approach in craniosynostosis repair: a systematic review and meta-analysis of perioperative outcomes. Childs Nerv Syst 2018;34:1627–37.
30. Riordan CP, Zurakowski D, Meier PM, et al. Minimally invasive endoscopic surgery for infantile craniosynostosis: a longitudinal cohort study. J Pediatr 2020;216:142–9.
31. Yamada S, Won DJ, Pezeshkpour G, et al. Pathophysiology of tethered cord syndrome and similar complex disorders. Neurosurg Focus 2007;23:E6.
32. Hoving EW. Pathophysiology and management of tethered cord (including myelomeningocele). In: Jallo GI, Kothbauer KF, Reckons VMR, editors. Handbook of pediatric neurosurgery. New York: Thieme Medical Publishers Inc; 2018. p. 325–31.

33. Di X. Endoscopic spinal tethered cord release: operative technique. Childs Nerv Syst 2009;25:577–81.
34. Jerome EH. Tethered spinal cord. In: Houck PJ, Hache M, Sun LS, editors. Handbook of pediatric anesthesia. New York: McGraw-Hill Education; 2015.
35. Bhimani AD, Selner AN, Patel JB, et al. Pediatric tethered cord release: an epidemiological and postoperative complication analysis. J Spine Surg 2019;5:337–50.
36. Sandrameli SS, Chu JK, Chan TM, et al. Minimally invasive tubular tethered cord release in the pediatric population. World Neurosurg 2019;128:e912–7.
37. Hayashi T, Kimiwada T, Kohama M, et al. Minimally invasive surgical approach to filum lipoma. Neurol Med Chir (Tokyo) 2018;58:132–7.
38. Soundararajan N, Cunliffe M. Anaesthesia for spinal surgery in children. Br J Anaesth 2007;99:86–94.
39. Jiang J, Zhang S, Dai C, et al. Clinical observations on the release of tethered spinal cord in children with intra-operative neurophysiological monitoring: a retrospective study. J Clin Neurosci 2020;71:205–12.
40. Poonia S, Graber S, Wilkinson CC, et al. Outcome of hospital discharge on postoperative day 1 following uncomplicated tethered spinal cord release. J Neurosurg Pediatr 2016;17:651–6.

Pediatric Mass Casualty Preparedness

Alison R. Perate, MD

KEYWORDS

- Pediatric • Disaster medicine • Mass casualty • Disaster preparedness
- Disaster plan • CBRNE • Terrorism

KEY POINTS

- Disaster medicine refers to situations in which the need to care for patients outweighs the available resources.
- It is imperative for anesthesiologists to be involved at a leadership level in mass casualty/disaster preparedness planning.
- Mass casualty disaster plans should be clear, concise, and easy to follow.
- Terror events and natural disasters can differ significantly in anesthesia preparedness.
- Resiliency is an important aspect of the recovery phase that decreases psychological damage in the aftermath of a mass casualty event.

The roots of disaster medicine trace back as the early as the late eighteenth century, when the surgeon in chief to Napoleon created the concept of triage for military injuries.[1] Basic concepts of disaster medicine continued to evolve in the military over time as wars continued to be waged. In the early twentieth century, Heinrich Zangger, one of the founding fathers of disaster preparedness, is credited with building the subspecialty from the study of civilian mine explosions.[2] Much of the early phase of disaster medicine focused solely on the prehospital response due to the military history of assessing viability of soldiers on the battlefield. As modern medicine has continued to become specialized, disaster medicine has become an important subspecialty.

In the United States, it was not until 1984 that the National Medical Disaster Systems (NMDS) developed disaster response protocols at the federal level.[3] As part of the NMDS, Disaster Medicine Assistant Teams (DMATs) were created under the Department of Health and Human Services and the Federal Emergency Management Agency.[3,4] The main purpose of DMATs was to receive and treat war casualties in an efficient and effective manner. Focus was placed on training and standardizing

Department of Anesthesiology and Critical Care Medicine, The Children's Hospital of Philadelphia, The Perelman School of Medicine at the University of Pennsylvania, 3401 Civic Center Boulevard, Philadelphia, PA 19104, USA
E-mail address: peratea@email.chop.edu

Anesthesiology Clin 38 (2020) 509–516
https://doi.org/10.1016/j.anclin.2020.05.002
1932-2275/20/© 2020 Elsevier Inc. All rights reserved.

anesthesiology.theclinics.com

procedures. Due to the lack of war casualties, the roles of these systems evolved to respond to natural disasters and other issues affecting mass populations. The DMATs are located throughout the country and are available for immediate deployment for a variety of situations.

The purpose of the DMATs is to provide support in the early stages of a crisis to facilitate on-scene stability in the prehospital environment.[4] The approach is standardized, allowing for efficient utilization of personnel and organization of the response. The initial actions include mobilization and distribution of resources. Mobile triage units are established on site or at the closest safe location. The goal of the DMAT is to quickly identify, stabilize, and move the affected individuals to the appropriate destination. Within the past decade, there has been a focus on improving the collaboration and communication with the health care system that ultimately receives the patients.

PHILOSOPHIC APPROACH TO DISASTER MEDICINE

The approach to disaster medicine presents a philosophic dilemma. By definition, a disaster is an event where the needs of the situation are greater than the resources available.[5] In a situation where resources are a limiting factor in providing medical care, difficult decisions must be made. There are 3 main philosophies in disaster medical care: utilitarian, egalitarian, and proceduralism. Each of these philosophies has both benefits and drawbacks. Often, the cultural norms of the society, which can change depending on time and place, play a large role in the approach to utilization of resources.

The utilitarian philosophy embraces the basic tenet in trauma medicine, which is to produce the greatest happiness; in medicine, this translates to mean providing the "greatest good to the greatest number."[6,7] The goal is to maximize the number of survivors with a meaningful quality of life. Mathematical metrics, such as years and number of people saved, are used to determine distribution of care. The benefit of this approach is that if employed correctly, it results in the greatest number of survivors. One of the criticisms of the utilitarian method is that some people who could be saved need to be sacrificed in order to save a greater number of people. In this way, the value is placed on the benefit to society and not the individual.[8] In certain cultures, this is a less acceptable approach due to the importance of the individual within its structure. Utilitarian philosophy favors pediatric patients because they have the most years of life to save.

The egalitarian philosophy distributes all resources equally, with an approach of "take anyone, with anything, at anytime."[9] Under this philosophy, there is no rationing of goods or services, and, as a result, there is significant resource utilization on patients who do not survive, often at a cost of those who could have survived. Egalitarian philosophy is at the foundation of the Emergency Medical Treatment and Labor Act (EMTALA) of 1986 that guaranteed medical care in emergency rooms across the United States.[10] As opposed to the utilitarian approach, egalitarianism places the value on the life of the individual. This philosophy often is viewed as the most fair or equitable.

The proceduralism philosophy utilizes predetermined criteria to distribute resources.[11] Usually the decisions are made by inclusion or exclusion criteria. Some systems even use a lottery system to assign priority for resource access. The benefit of such a system is that it takes the human component out of the decision process. This type of system often is seen as the most easily executed because it requires minimal individual thought. Because these systems are not flexible, however, there is a potential for excess resource utilization on patients who meet criteria but are not salvageable.

Disaster medicine involves the intersection of medicine, ethics, and resources.[12,13] Cultural and societal attitudes play a critical role in determining which philosophic approach guides distribution of resources.[14] Determining procedures prior to an event as well as the goal, lives saved versus life years saved, is important to ensure that streamlined procedures are executed in the immediate chaos of a disaster event.

TYPES OF DISASTER EVENTS

A disaster is an event when the needs of the situation outweigh the resources available. There are 3 main categories of disaster events: natural, traumatic terror, and exposure.[15] Each category has considerations for the anesthesiologist as well as unique pediatric considerations. Although a single disaster plan is not sufficient for the response to all events, there is considerable overlap, and the need for a systematic protocol allows for the most effective and efficient action. Understanding the needs of the different types of disasters as well as the available resources is critical to designing the correct plan.

Natural disasters include those that occur due to climate or geologic events. Examples of natural disasters include hurricanes, tornadoes, earthquakes, and similar events. These events have the potential for significant volumes of victims. The anesthesiologist has a role in the entire response, from the site of the event, to the prehospital staging area, to the hospital reception, and through to the postoperative recovery.

In both natural and terror events, geographic location dictates the expected/needed role of the anesthesiologist. For example, in rural settings, the anesthesiologist often plays a significant role in the field, often providing on-site support becuase the responding emergency medical services (EMS) may be limited. In urban areas, there is a robust EMS system and the anesthesiologist is most effective in the perioperative arena. This role can change depending on the event, as witnessed with the attack on the north and south towers of the World Trade Center in New York on September 11, 2001. Because there was a concern for significant volumes of injured patients which would overwhelm the EMS system, anesthesiologists, as part of a multidisciplinary team, were deployed to the site for immediate triage and treatment.[16] Similarly, at the Boston Marathon bombing on April 15, 2013, there were robust medical tents that provided approximately 200 beds available for injured runners.[17] After the bombing, medical staff, including anesthesiologists, were involved in the prehospital triage and stabilization of the victims.

Another factor for consideration in natural disasters is that often the anesthesiologist is located within the disaster red zone. For example, if a tornado hits a town, the physicians and the hospital system are at risk for personal involvement and devastation. In such situations, the ability of anesthesiologists to respond is compromised as they care for their family and possessions. If the hospital structure itself is affected, such as the 1994 Northridge earthquake in California, the safety of the environment in which the anesthesiologist provides care may be compromised. At the epicenter, Northridge Hospital Medical Center (NHMC) suffered severe structural damage, requiring treatment of patients to be moved from the emergency room to tents in the parking lots.[18] Due its proximity to the earthquake, NHMC received many injured patients, treating approximately 200 patients in the first 2 hours and more than 1700 patients during the duration of the event.[18] NHMC sustained significant structural damage that included interruption of electricity. This provided a significant obstacle to the anesthesiologists' ability to provide care in the surgical suite. All disaster plans should include alternative plans for providing anesthesia for critical patients in the situation in which water and electricity are compromised.

Natural disasters also disrupt the normal channels that replenish supplies and personnel to the hospital system. The Joint Commission on Accreditation of Health-care Organizations requires hospitals to have on-hand enough resources and the capability of providing care for 72 hours.[19] Probably the greatest example of the impact on resources and personnel was Hurricane Katrina, which struck New Orleans in 2005. Tulane University Hospital and Memorial Medical Center were 2 hospitals that were significantly affected. The difference between these 2 hospitals highlights the benefits of a well-designed disaster preparedness plan. Tulane Hospital recognized alternative plans for patient transfer and contracted with private helicopter, bus, and ambulance companies. Memorial Medical Center relied solely on governmental re-sources to mobilize patients.[20,21] When Hurricane Katrina hit downtown New Orleans, Tulane was able to evacuate all necessary patients, with no loss of life from the storm. In contrast, Memorial Medical Center was dependent on the arrival of transportation and resources from federal and state government agencies. By day 4 of the storm, all generators had failed. There was complete loss of electricity, sanitation, running water, and heating, ventilation, and air conditioning systems. The staff waited for days for more resources and personnel to arrive from the state and federal aid sour-ces, but none came. Overall, there were 45 patient deaths that were directly attributed to the lack of resources.[20,21] Anesthesia requires a steady supply chain of both medi-cation and equipment. The basic core of medications that are utilized most frequently in anesthesia are quickly exhausted in cases where new supplies cannot be obtained. Pediatric anesthesiology requires the maintenance of a range of equipment due to the age and size ranges of children so that interruption of the supply chain can have a more dramatic effect on the ability to provide care.

Terror events pose a different challenge for the anesthesiologist. These types of events can be broken down into 2 main categories: traumatic and exposure. Although the potential for significant numbers of victims and the resultant drain on resources are similar for both types, there are differences in the considerations for the anesthesiol-ogist. Each disaster plan should account not only for the difference in event type based on the treatment of the patient but also on the self-care of the anesthesiologist.

Traumatic events can quickly overwhelm an operating room due to the increased likelihood for surgical procedures. In the Route 91 Harvest music festival shooting in Las Vegas in October 2017, a total of 515 people were shot at an open air country mu-sic concert. Sunrise Hospital received 200 patients in rapid succession, most arriving in groups of 4 to 5 people transported in the back of pickup trucks.[22] This was an extreme test of the hospital's surge capacity. Staff was quickly overwhelmed while equipment and supplies became a limiting factor in patient care. The anesthesia staff was forced to mobilize both staff and resources to staff multiple operating rooms at the same time. Further compounding the chaos was that this occurred at 10:00 PM, well after normal scheduled hours. Due to the mechanism of injury caused by high-velocity guns, the injury pattern almost exclusively was hemorrhage control. Obtaining significant volumes of compatible blood in a timely fashion for multiple patients was a top priority in the anesthetic set-up. With after-hours staffing numbers, this would be a challenge at most hospitals. Contingency plans for increasing staff numbers for events that happen during times when staff is at a minimum is an important step in any disaster plan. Because a majority of operating suites around the country are coordi-nated by an anesthesia board runner, a system for rapid identification and assignment of available surgeons is necessary for fluid movement of patients.

In the age of the powerful electronic medical record, staff have become overwhelm-ingly dependent on it functioning correctly. A rapid influx of patients needing to be registered is an overwhelming task for even the most robust electronic system.

Many hospitals are paralyzed by the need for complete registration to not only record an intraoperative anesthetic record but also to place orders, obtain blood products or studies, and facilitate patient movement through the system. A reliable alternative to attempting to register large volumes of patients simultaneously is a system that reverts to paper registration. The advantage of a paper system is that packets can be made with preregistered patients with coded generic names. Because the patients are already registered within the hospital system, all that needs to be completed is placing a name band that already has been printed onto the patient. This saves considerable time, effort, and manpower. Within each premade packet is a paper anesthetic record, so that if there is the need for an anesthetic procedure, all documents are located in a solitary place. The disadvantage of this system is that it requires significant effort post-discharge to merge the paper records with their real electronic medical records, and most staff, in particular anesthesia providers, are not as facile with paper records.

The ability of the physicians in the emergency room to efficiently triage and transport the most critical patients to the operating room can have a significant impact on the status of arrival to the operating room. The anesthesia disaster plan for traumatic terror events must start with an effective communication plan with the emergency room so that the reception of patients is well choreographed. The largest obstacle in most disaster events is effective communication. The failure in communication most often is due to staff attempting to utilize standard operating procedure systems. In large-scale events, lines of communication quickly become chaotic and overwhelmed. Large amounts of information are lost or incorrectly conveyed. The most critical line of communication is from the emergency room to the operating room office with the anesthesia board runner. Designing an emergency operating procedure that streamlines this communication allows for operating rooms to be appropriately prepared to receive patients in rapid succession. In pediatric anesthesia, this is even more important because there is considerable difference in the equipment set-up and medication preparation for a 2-year-old child versus a 16-year-old child, thereby requiring correct prior information.

Exposure events produce challenges that are different from traumatic terror events. Such events are abbreviated by the mnemonic, CRBNE, which stands for: chemical, radiological, biological, nuclear, and explosive.[23] In contrast to a traumatic event, where staff often is eager to respond and report to the hospital, exposure events can be a real or perceived threat to the well-being of staff and their families, therefore reducing the amount of voluntary staff available. Exposure events are less likely to need surgical intervention and more likely to require tracheal intubation. Patients who are victims of an exposure event need decontamination prior to any medical treatment. It is imperative that decontamination is performed to prevent compromise of the staff. The benefit of decontamination is that it creates a bottleneck prior to entering the emergency room, thereby causing a pacing system that prevents rapid influx into the hospital. This patient staggering allows more time for the anesthesia team to communicate and prepare for the reception of possible patients as opposed to the uncontrolled patient volume of a traumatic event.

HOW TO DESIGN A DISASTER PLAN FOR THE ANESTHESIOLOGIST

The first step in creating a disaster plan is for the anesthesia department to be involved at a leadership level. Most disaster planning for hospital systems focuses primarily on the emergency room response. As such, emergency room physicians and trauma surgeons dominate the planning committees as well as the leadership positions. By being present at the table, perioperative planning and needs are included in the overall disaster plan, allowing for smooth transitions from the hospital entrance through the operating room complex.

The goal is to create a disaster plan that is simple and easy to follow. In any disaster event, there undoubtedly is chaos and confusion. Simplicity with clear actionable items increases the likelihood of seamless execution. The disaster plan should be easily accessible with both electronic and paper copies in multiple locations. Along with the disaster plan, there should be an extensive list of phone numbers, including numbers for all anesthesia staff, surgical staff, nursing administration, blood banks, hospital administration, command center, and security. Although most hospitals have an electronic staff directory, having a centralized location of needed numbers is invaluable if the electronic systems are slowed or fail.

The same response should be enacted for all disasters with only minor modifications depending on the needs of the situation. The 3 Cs—command, control, and communications—should be the structure used to guide the first step of the disaster plan. *Command* is the establishment of a command structure that clearly delineates the hierarchal plan of leadership. *Control* refers to the identification of the anesthesiologist in charge of the operating room schedule and flow. Anesthesiologists familiar with board running duties often are best suited for this position because they have experience with patient flow and interfacing with different aspects of the perioperative care model. *Communications* identifies the mode of communication that will be utilized and the personnel in charge of said communications.

The second step is to create and communicate situational awareness among the staff. This step is defined by the 4 Ws: who, what, where, and when. This step allows the staff to prepare for surgical cases based on prehospital information from the scene. *Who* is the patients who are expected based on the type of event. In most disaster events, patients sometimes are transported to incorrect hospitals. Adults can end up at pediatric hospitals and vice versa. *What* are the types of injuries most likely to be encountered: blast, penetrating, chemical, and so forth. *Where* describes the location of the scene of the event. This gives an indication of the magnitude of the event as well as provides a broad view of the disaster event. *When* refers to the time of day of the disaster, which has an impact on staffing as well as the timing of the arrival of patients.

The third step is to create an incident action plan, more commonly known as the protocol. The action plan should describe in a clear, concise, step-by-step fashion the duties that should be performed by different roles. These duties should be enumerated and divided by time periods: 1 minute to 15 minutes, 15 minutes to 30 minutes, and 30+ minutes. It is the duty of the anesthesia board runner to ensure that the plan is executed properly. The action plan includes all phases of the response. It is important to include the possibility of a prolonged event, such as a natural disaster, that could last days to weeks. All-important actionable items should be listed as well as plans for disruption of the supply chain and replenishment of resources and personnel.

The final step is called the battle rhythm. This stage refers to the execution of the incident action plan. Having a well-planned and thorough disaster plan and conducting regular drills of the disaster plan enable this step to become routine. Many institutions avoid practice of the disaster plan because disaster drills are time-consuming and resource-intensive endeavors. Exercises are the most effective way to identify areas of deficiency within a plan. If disaster drills are not practiced at regular intervals, much of the information is forgotten because disasters are low-frequency events at most hospitals.

Resiliency is the ability of a person or object to return to its original state after a state of stress. Disaster incidents are profoundly stressful for all staff involved. Often, personnel are pushing to or past the limits of their capability to care for patients. Loss of life takes a significant toll on the morale of staff. Although not a part of the response phase, the recovery phase needs to include plans to maintain the well-being of staff. This portion of the plan involves mobilizing therapists, counselors, and chaplains early on in an event to minimize psychological damage and prevent the loss of personnel postincident.

SUMMARY

In conclusion, disaster incidents occur across the country at a frequency much greater than that appreciated by most people. Historically, anesthesiologists have not been involved at a leadership level of hospital disaster planning. As gatekeepers to the operating rooms, it is imperative that anesthesiologists take an active role in disaster planning and management to provide the most efficient and effective care of patients. It is important that every anesthesia department establish and practice the execution of a well-designed disaster plan. Such planning and preparation allow resources to be maximized and standards of care to be provided for the greater number of patients while minimizing waste.

Clinics care points

- Mass casualty events are a low frequency, yet high impact occurrence.
- The system for allocation of resources and assignment of roles must be established well ahead of an event.
- Standard operating procedures are not sufficient for mass casualty events.
- The Anesthesiologist plays a critical role in facilitating flow of surgical patients drom the emergency room through the perioperative setting.
- Effective execution of disaster plans is highly dependent upon education and practice.

REFERENCES

1. Ian-Robertsobn-Steel. Evolution of triage systems. Emerg Med J 2006;23:154–5.
2. Stehrenberger CS, Goltermann S. Disaster medicine: genealogy of a concept. Soc Sci Med 2014;120:317–24.
3. Franco C, Toner E, Waldhorn R, ct al. The national disaster medical system: past, present, and suggestions for the future. Biosecur Bioterror 2007;5:319–25.
4. The Key Role of NDMS in Disaster Response Kevin Yeskey M.D. Deputy Assistant Secretary, Director, Office of Preparedness and Emergency Operations U.S. Department of Health and Human Services Committee on Homeland Security and Governmental Affairs Subcommittee on State, Local, and Private Sector Preparedness and integration United States Senate. Washington, DC, July 22, 2010.
5. Stehrenberger CS, Goltermann S. Disaster medicine: Genealogy of a concept. Soc Sci Med 2014;120:317–24.
6. Lanken PN, Terry PB, Osborne ML. Ethics of allocating intensive care unit resources. New Horiz 1997;5:38–50.
7. Mill JS. Utilitarianism. 2nd edition. Indianapolis (IN): Hackett Publishing Company; 2001.
8. Sztajnkrycer MD, Madsen BE, Báez AA. Unstable ethical plateaus and disaster triage. Emerg Med Clin North Am 2006;24:749–68.
9. Olsen JA. Theories of justice and their implications for priority setting in health care. Health Econ 1997;16:625–39.

10. Zink B. Anyone, anything, anytime—a history of emergency medicine. Philadelphia: Mosby Elsevier; 2006.
11. Capp S, Savage S, Clarke V. Exploring distributive justice in health care. Aust Health Rev 2001;24:40–4.
12. Rawls J. A theory of justice (revised). New York: Oxford University Press; 1999.
13. Roberts MJ, Reich MR. Ethical analysis in public health. Lancet 2002;359: 1055–9.
14. Society of Critical Care Medicine Ethics Committee. Consensus statement on the triage of critically ill patients. JAMA 1994;271:1200–3.
15. Mohamed Shaluf I. Disaster types. Disaster Prev Manag 2007;16(5):704–17.
16. Simon R, Teperman S. The World Trade Center attack. Lessons for disaster management. Crit Care 2001;5(6):318–20.
17. Walls RM, Zinner MJ. The Boston Marathon response: Why did it work so well? JAMA 2013;309(23):2441–2.
18. Cheevers J, Abrahamson A. Earthquake: The Long Road Back: Hospitals Strained to the Limit by Injured: Medical care: Doctors treat quake victims in parking lots. Details of some disaster-related deaths are released. Los Angeles Times 1994.
19. Aberle V, Anthony R, Bass R, et al. Standing Together: An Emergency Planning Guide for America's Communities. The Joint Commission 2006.
20. Dara SI, Farmer JC. Preparedness Lessons from Modern Disasters and Wars. Crit Care Clin 2009;25(1):47–65.
21. Curiel TJ. Murder or Mercy? Hurricane Katrina and the Need for Disaster Training. N Engl J Med 2006;355:2067–9.
22. American College of Surgeons. Trauma surgeons share lessons learned from the Las Vegas mass shooting tragedy at American College of Surgeons conference. 2017. Available at: https://www.prnewswire.com/news-rel eases/trauma-surgeons-share-lessons-learned-from-the las-vegas-mass-shooting-tragedy-at-american-college-.
23. Baker DJ. Role of the anesthesiologist in the clinical management of hazards and threats from chemical and biological warfare agents. In: Miller RD, Eriksson L, Fleisher L, et al, editors. Miller's anesthesia. 7th edition. Philadelphia: Churchill livingstone/elsevier; 2010. Chap 74.

The Pediatric Burn
Current Trends and Future Directions

David Preston, DO, MPH, Aditee Ambardekar, MD, MSEd*

KEYWORDS

- Pediatric burn • Anesthesia • Analgesia • Anxiolysis • Resuscitation

KEY POINTS

- Pediatric burns represent a significant public health burden with unique challenges in all phases of perioperative care.
- The physiologic changes of injury mandate timely and goal-directed fluid resuscitation, careful airway evaluation, and optimized nutritional support throughout the perioperative period.
- A multimodal approach to anxiety and pain is essential, necessitating an increased emphasis on the use of regional anesthesia and nonpharmacologic adjuncts.
- Overall variability of management and relative paucity of clinical trials reveal the need for further study to establish more concrete standards of care within this population.

INTRODUCTION

Burn injury is one of the most common causes of preventable morbidity and mortality.[1,2] Epidemiologic studies of pediatric burns consistently find that scald injury is the most frequent mechanism (42%) followed by flame (29%) and contact injury (10%).[3–5] Although any burn injury in childhood increases long-term mortality with positive association for size, nonaccidental burns and inhalation injury are associated with greater risk of short-term mortality.[3,6,7] Care of these children in centers experienced in the treatment of burns reduces mortality, yet variability still exists in management protocols.[6,7]

For the anesthesiologist, treating pediatric burn patients presents challenges in all phases of care, from airway management and fluid resuscitation to comprehensive pain control. These challenges necessitate a detailed understanding of the pathophysiology of burns as well as current data regarding clinical management. This article reviews the pathophysiology and initial stabilization of burn injuries, unique airway considerations, fluid resuscitation and transfusion strategies, and finally, pain management of the pediatric burn patient.

Department of Anesthesiology and Pain Management, University of Texas Southwestern Medical Center, 5323 Harry Hines Boulevard, Dallas, TX 75390-9068, USA
* Corresponding author.
E-mail address: aditee.ambardekar@utsouthwestern.edu

Anesthesiology Clin 38 (2020) 517–530
https://doi.org/10.1016/j.anclin.2020.05.003
anesthesiology.theclinics.com
1932-2275/20/© 2020 Elsevier Inc. All rights reserved.

INITIAL STABILIZATION
Physiologic Considerations

Burn injuries present a complex pathophysiologic process with local and systemic effects. Systemic manifestations are typically seen in patients with burn injury at or greater than 30% total body surface area (TBSA) and are mediated by cytokine and catecholamine release.[8] The initial phase, historically called "burn shock," is due to third-spacing of fluid causing hypovolemia.[9] Jeschke and colleagues[8] demonstrated significantly elevated cardiac output at the time of injury that is sustained throughout the acute phase, but systolic dysfunction has also been documented in a small cohort of children in the perioperative period by transesophageal echocardiogram. Basic science models also demonstrate myocardial depression in the setting of burn injury.[10,11]

The hypermetabolic phase, initiated 24 hours after injury and mediated by cortisol, catecholamines, and cytokines, is characterized by hyperdynamic circulation, elevated oxygen consumption, and a catabolic state that can persist for years after burn injury.[11] Changes in circulating volumes owing to large intravascular fluid shifts and variations in organ perfusion decrease circulating concentrations and cause resistance to drugs, namely opioids.[12] Upregulation of extrajunctional acetylcholine receptors is hypothesized as the mechanism for well-documented resistance to nondepolarizing neuromuscular blockers and the contraindication to the use of succinylcholine for paralysis.[13,14] Furthermore, Jeschke[8] has demonstrated infiltrative processes and resultant hepatomegaly in the acute burn phase that may impact drug metabolism.[8]

The short- and long-term sequelae of burn injury portend significant morbidity and mortality, requiring careful attention during all phases of a child's care. In subsequent sections, the authors discuss the implications of these physiologic changes on the perioperative care of these patients.

Evaluation and Extent of Injury

The initial evaluation and stabilization of a burn-injured child are critical given the propensity for rapid airway compromise, increased oxygen demands, and limited hemodynamic reserve. A full trauma evaluation is warranted because coexisting injury is common. Accurate evaluation of percent TBSA involvement of the partial- and full-thickness burn is the next essential step in planning for resuscitation, stabilization, and even prompt referral to a pediatric burn center. The traditional rule of nines estimation of burn injury is less accurate in children, who have relatively large heads and small limbs compared with adults. Lund and Browder reported an age-based algorithm that considers this difference (**Fig. 1**). Despite the importance of TBSA estimation, there is still frequent miscalculation of burn injury in very young or obese children, particularly in centers less familiar with pediatric burn care.[15–17]

Airway and Breathing

The pediatric anesthesiologist may be called on at any stage of the burn injury for assistance with airway management, whether it is during initial stabilization, during rescue of a failed or lost airway, during surgical procedures, or even during extubation planning. The presence of appropriately sized videolaryngoscopic or fiber-optic equipment should be confirmed before any airway manipulation because burn injuries may introduce profound anatomic changes, which can complicate airway management. High oxygen and metabolic requirements in these vulnerable patients further challenge these clinical situations.

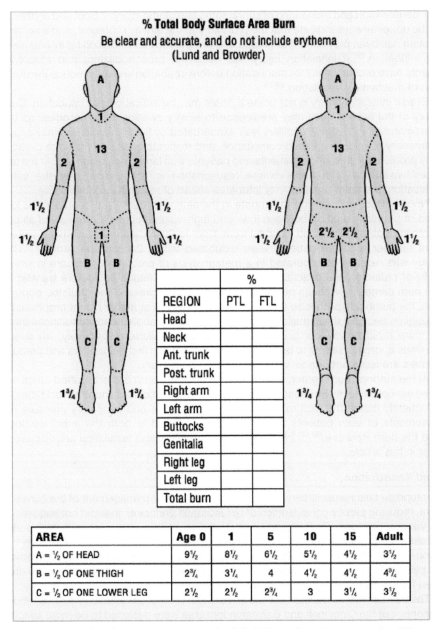

% Total Body Surface Area Burn
Be clear and accurate, and do not include erythema
(Lund and Browder)

	%	
REGION	PTL	FTL
Head		
Neck		
Ant. trunk		
Post. trunk		
Right arm		
Left arm		
Buttocks		
Genitalia		
Right leg		
Left leg		
Total burn		

AREA	Age 0	1	5	10	15	Adult
A = ½ OF HEAD	9½	8½	6½	5½	4½	3½
B = ½ OF ONE THIGH	2¾	3¼	4	4½	4½	4¾
C = ½ OF ONE LOWER LEG	2½	2½	2¾	3	3¼	3½

Fig. 1. Lund-Browder chart. Ant., anterior; FTL, full-thickness loss; Post., posterior; PTL, partial-thickness loss. (*From* Lund CC, Browder NC (1944). "The estimation of areas of burns". Surg Gynecol Obstet. 79: 352–8. *Reprinted with permission from* the Journal of the American College of Surgeons, formerly Surgery Gynecology & Obstetrics.)

The presence of inhalation injury significantly increases morbidity and mortality and should be an early part of the initial assessment.[18,19] Facial burns, carbonaceous sputum, singed nasal hairs, and hoarseness are indicators of possible inhalational injury and need for intubation.[20] Serial fiber-optic bronchoscopy may be useful in the identification and monitoring of supraglottic and glottic injury.[21] Soot and erythema in the upper airways indicate that thermal injury to the airway is present, and a scoring system has been proposed that grades and prognosticates inhalation injury and need for intubation.[22] If inhalation injury has occurred, bronchodilators and mucolytic agents have proven useful for stabilization before intubation and may reduce the duration of mechanical ventilation.[23,24]

Even if inhalation injury is not present, there may be indications for intubation. Burn injury of the face or neck may predispose to airway swelling or compromise as the burn matures.[25] Similarly, capillary leak exacerbated by fluid resuscitation may cause pulmonary edema, decreased compliance, and respiratory failure, which are particularly problematic in younger patients and patients with larger, scald burns.[26] At the authors' institution, if a large-volume resuscitation is anticipated after the initial evaluation, the team preemptively intubates ahead of respiratory compromise.

Nonetheless, the decision to intubate in the setting of burn injury represents a key area of practice variation between low- and high-volume centers. A review of all patients intubated at Parkland Hospital from 1982 to 2005 demonstrated that a significant number of these patients were extubated within 24 hours of arrival.[27] This study was recently corroborated in a metaanalysis of preburn center care in which 31% of patients were described to be "unnecessarily intubated" before transfer to the burn center.[15] Although neither of these studies addressed the pediatric population, the authors hypothesize that pediatric patients are at higher risk of prophylactic intubation because their smaller airways and higher metabolic needs predispose them to more rapid airway compromise and respiratory failure, respectively. An overly cautious approach seems to be chosen particularly when first responders and preburn centers are less comfortable with the pediatric burn injury.

At the authors' burn center, like most large pediatric burn centers, cuffed tubes are used almost exclusively, because the safety and utility of cuffed endotracheal tubes to adequately match the high minute volume and positive-end expiratory pressure requirements of burn patients have been demonstrated in both the anesthesiology and the burn literature.[28–30] Implications of burn injury and ventilation are discussed later in this article.

Fluid Resuscitation

Appropriate fluid resuscitation is the cornerstone of initial management of the burn patient, requiring careful consideration of resuscitation endpoints to avoid consequences of volume overload. Furthermore, early initiation of large-volume resuscitation decreases the incidence of sepsis, renal failure, and overall mortality.[31,32] Although the Lund-Bowder diagram provides a more accurate assessment of overall injury in pediatric patients, this algorithm is not perfect, and erroneous estimates of burn injury in children frequently result in overresuscitation or underresuscitation.[17,33]

The Parkland formula is the best known estimate of fluid resuscitation volumes in burn patients, but the Cincinnati and Galveston formulae were designed to be more specific to the fluid needs of pediatric patients, especially those less than 30 kg. These "two figure formulae" account for the insensible loss caused by the burn injury and also consider the hourly maintenance requirements. No studies to date compare the use of the Cincinnati formula to the Galveston formula with respect to overall outcome.[33] No matter the formula used, it is important to remember that younger and smaller patients are less able to mobilize glycogen stores and maintain euglycemia, necessitating the use of dextrose-containing fluids for maintenance. Isotonic fluids, however, are the mainstay for resuscitation of insensible losses. Finally, colloid use and its role in burn resuscitation have been points of significant debate. Two studies have emerged that point to the potential benefit of early albumin administration in children.[31,34] In fact, adding albumin as early as within 8 hours of burn injury decreased overall volume administered, decreased length of stay, and reduced volume overload.[34]

Despite the risk of respiratory failure, longer ventilatory requirements, compartment syndrome, and overall increased length of hospital stay, overresuscitation is a common occurrence.[35] A metaanalysis revealed that burn centers routinely administer fluids greater than predicted by the Parkland formula, which was also confirmed by Nagpal and colleagues[36] in the pediatric population. Urine output has been the traditional measure of end-organ perfusion with targets between 0.5 and 1.0 mL/kg per hour. Other physical examination findings, such as sensorium, warmth of extremities, pulse rate, and systolic blood pressure, have been cited but may be challenging to assess in the critically ill and hypermetabolic state of a burn-injured child. Lactate and base excess may be physiologic markers of perfusion and could be trended, but no prospective studies support any of these practices in an evidence-based way. One of the more compelling technologies that has recently been studied uses an invasive monitor to measure and trend transcardiopulmonary thermodilution as a surrogate for cardiac output.[33] Kraft and colleagues[37] demonstrated that its use decreased total fluid administration while maintaining cardiovascular parameters and reducing renal and heart failure in the postburn period.

The pediatric anesthesiologist may be asked to care for these critically ill and physiologically vulnerable patients at any stage of their burn injury. Whether for early assistance with a challenging airway or vascular access, monitor insertion for resuscitative efforts, or anesthesia services along the entire spectrum of hospitalization, the pediatric anesthesiologist should know the pathophysiological changes and their implications of care in order to adequately care for these patients.

PERIOPERATIVE MANAGEMENT
Surgical Considerations

After initial stabilization, a pediatric burn patient may require a variety of procedures for which an anesthetic is necessary. Knowledge and understanding of relevant surgical techniques facilitate a team-based approach to care and empower the anesthesiologist in the perioperative management.

Often the first encounter with a burn-injured child, if not for airway management or general stabilization, is for emergent escharotomy or fasciotomy. Circumferential burns or electrical injury to a limb may require fascial release if signs of compartment syndrome are present. Full-thickness burns to the thorax and abdomen can compromise respiratory mechanics, can impair intraabdominal perfusion, and may mandate early escharotomy to provide life-saving improvement in oxygenation, ventilation, and perfusion.[38] Similarly, secondary abdominal compartment syndrome, a result of large volume resuscitation and increased intraabdominal pressures, is relieved by decompressive laparotomy.[39]

Early wound closure through tangential excision and split-thickness skin grafting lowers overall morbidity and mortality in children even though transfusion requirements may be greater.[40] Xiao-Wu and colleagues[41] identified the optimal time for early excision as 48 hours. Wound excision involves removal of nonviable, burned skin to facilitate an optimal environment for reepithelialization via split-thickness skin graft from a healthy donor site. These excisions exacerbate insensible fluid loss and bleeding from injured tissues and result in severe pain from the graft harvest site. The management of bleeding, volume resuscitation, and pain is an important anesthetic consideration of burn surgery, which will be discussed here in further detail.

The severe pain and risk for wound complications associated with split-thickness skin grafting prompted investigation into alternative approaches for reepithelialization. Cultured epithelial cells were first used in the 1990s to decrease the need for large donor sites and achieve improved cosmesis. Coleman and Siwy[42] demonstrated benefit in a small number of children, despite increased time for preparation and significant cost. Recently, the use of an autologous skin cell suspension was reported as a viable alternative with improvement in pain control and wound-healing indices.[43] This skin cell suspension is prepared in real time from less donor skin and does not require the time for cells to culture and grow in vitro.

Surgical strategies are used to minimize blood loss during burn surgery. Tourniquets can be used on limbs for excision or reconstruction surgery, yet can be a source of pain and metabolic consequences. In areas where tourniquets cannot be used, subcutaneous and subdermal tumescent solutions can decrease intraoperative bleeding and postoperative pain.[44] Lidocaine is a safe additive to tumescent solutions with benefit for pain control, but studies investigating the safety and efficacy of other local anesthetics are currently lacking.[44–46] Studies describe the use of both phenylephrine and epinephrine to decrease blood loss.[47,48] Although epinephrine-containing tumescent solutions have minimal hemodynamic consequences, the authors recently reported a high incidence of hypertension and reflex bradycardia in children receiving phenylephrine-containing tumescence.[49,50] In addition, the volume of tumescence used should be monitored because it can exacerbate volume overload when subcutaneous fluid redistributes to the central circulation compartment.

Long-term surgical management of burn injuries involves both contracture release and hypertrophic burn scar rehabilitation. Surgical or fractionated laser treatments result in improved function and cosmesis of the scar site. These treatments can be painful procedures and usually require general anesthesia, especially in children. A recent review identified as many as 26 unique approaches to anesthetics for these patients, underlining the need for further study consensus around anesthetic implication and appropriate anesthetic management.[51]

Operating Room and Patient Preparation

The preparation of the environment and patient for a safe anesthetic in the setting of pediatric burns deserves discussion. Increased ambient temperature prevents the untoward effects of hypothermia, such as altered effects of intravenous and inhalation anesthetics, prolonged neuromuscular blockade, increased bleeding and need for transfusion, and impaired wound healing.[52] Compromised thermoregulatory and hemostasis mechanisms leave burned children at high risk for hypothermia.

Monitor application and intravenous access may be challenging if the entire patient is sterilely prepared for burn surgery because this precludes application of adhesives for electrocardiogram leads and pulse oximetry probes. Similarly, intravenous access and invasive monitors may be prepared into the surgical field. Innovative and creative methods have been reported for securing electrocardiogram leads.[53,54]

Nutritional Support

Adequate nutritional support is vital. The hypermetabolic state precipitated by the systemic catecholamine and cytokine release, especially in burn injuries greater than 30% TBSA, increases energy expenditure up to 130% to 140% above predicted values and can result in protein catabolism and weight loss for up to 2 years after injury.[8] Early initiation of nutritional support in the form of enteral feeds reduces hospitalization and mortality.[55] The frequent interruption of feeds with the nil per os state for procedures may introduce nutritional deficits, which are correlated with mortality.[56] Two recent retrospective analyses have advocated for continuing feeds perioperatively to mitigate these nutritional deficits and report no aspiration events in children with post-pyloric feeds and established airways.[57,58] The authors' burn center maintains full nothing by mouth precautions for surgery in the prone position.

Airway and Ventilation

Although the considerations and challenges of airway management in the setting of acute injury were previously discussed, repetitive anesthetics and airway maneuvers during the care of a burn patient often require modification and contingency planning as burn scars mature. Limited mouth opening, oropharyngeal swelling, neck contrac-tures, and distortions of tracheal anatomy may evolve over the course of burn injury and are predictors of difficult intubation.[59] Laryngeal mask airway placement may be limited by airway distortions and often requires unique approaches.[60] If tolerated, fiber-optic oral intubation is optimal in order to maintain spontaneous ventilation. Sur-geon involvement in airway planning is imperative in case of the need for a definitive surgical airway, but it is important to consider that anatomic distortions also create distinct operative challenges.[61]

Respiratory status and ventilatory challenges should also be considered. Acute res-piratory distress syndrome (ARDS) can occur in up to 50% of pediatric burn patients and may require special ventilatory modes to improve oxygenation. Low-tidal volume strategies, a mainstay in ARDS, have recently been challenged by the use of high-tidal volume in pediatric burn patients.[62] Some centers report successful use of high-frequency oscillatory ventilation in both the intensive care unit and the operating room as a mainstay of ventilation for patients who develop ARDS.[63] Provider unfamil-iarity with this mode of ventilation is cited as an inhibitor to its widespread use in the perioperative setting.[64] In the authors' institution, these children are transported to the operating room with individuals who are expert in the management of these special-ized ventilatory settings.

Extubation of a burn patient requires careful assessment of airway patency. Lack of an air leak and the mechanism of burn injury are key prognostic indicators of extuba-tion failure.[65] Steroids facilitate the reduction of airway edema before extubation, and high-flow nasal cannula may prevent reintubation.[65,66] Tracheostomy may be required to facilitate long-term ventilation with reduction in peak inspiratory pressures and improved chest wall compliance. The proper timing of tracheostomy is debatable. However, recent studies support early tracheostomy to help decrease the risk of sub-glottic stenosis.[66,67]

Hemorrhage and Transfusion

Blood loss is routine in burn surgery, and the nature and frequency of operative pro-cedures warrant frequent and large-volume blood transfusion. Transfusion triggers are debatable in critically ill patients, and pediatric burns are no exception. A retrospective study by Voigt and colleagues[68] reported differences in morbidity and mortality out-comes between a hemoglobin transfusion trigger of 10 and 7 g/dL. Data support a transfusion trigger of 7 g/dL in stable, critically ill children.[69] Although promising, neither study can be generalized to the dynamic and hypermetabolic pathophysiology pediatric anesthesiologists face during the anesthetic care of burn injury.

Transfusion of blood products in a matched ratio of packed red blood cells to plasma during excision and grafting surgery may have benefit. An interim analysis of a prospective study comparing outcomes of 1:1 versus 4:1 ratio has demonstrated safety but is still currently not powered to show differences in coagulation status, blood loss, product use, infection and sepsis, and ventilator days.[70] The results of this study will be important because transfusion of any product puts burn patients at risk for sepsis, metabolic derangements, and increased length of stay.[71,72]

Studies in perioperative, adult burn patients demonstrate the utility of point-of-care testing, such as ROTEM or TEG, to guide intraoperative blood product resuscitation, but such studies in the pediatric burn literature are lacking.[73,74] Pharmacologic mitigation of blood loss may be an optimal strategy in these vulnerable patients. Antifibrinolytics have been used successfully in craniofacial surgery, in which intraoperative blood loss can be similarly rapid and extensive.[75,76] However, prospective studies are needed to demonstrate the safety and efficacy of this strategy in burn patients.

Anxiolysis and Pain Management

The pain experience after a burn injury is a complex pathophysiologic process characterized by 3 distinct types of pain: nociceptive, inflammatory, and neuropathic pain. The inflammatory response produced by burn injury sensitizes peripheral nociceptors resulting in both hyperalgesia and allodynia lasting long after resolution of the initial insult.[76] Procedures only exacerbate the background pain caused by this inflammatory response. It is well accepted that effective pain control throughout the perioperative period diminishes the risk of long-term alterations in sensory and pain processing as well as acute stress and posttraumatic stress disorder (PTSD) development after recovery; however, great variability exists across burn centers on how best to manage the spectrum of pain.[77,78]

A multimodal approach to background pain is essential. Acetaminophen is used quite broadly in this population, yet an overreliance on opioids remains prevalent despite the paucity of prospective studies in this population.[79,80] Although additional pharmacologic agents, such as nonsteroidal anti-inflammatory drugs, gabapentin, and methadone, have been incorporated into pain management strategies, limited evidence exists for their efficacy.[78,81] Dexmedetomidine, because of its alpha-2 agonist activity, has also been shown to decrease opioid requirement when used to sedate an intubated child.[82]

Perioperative and procedural pain management in these children is similarly challenging with little guidance for best practice in the literature.[80] Dexmedetomidine, clonidine, gabapentin, and ketamine have all been described as analgesic adjuvants yet not studied in the pediatric burn population. Extrapolation from other surgical populations suggests equivocal results in decreasing opioid requirements during intraoperative and postoperative care.[80] Perioperative pain management strategies are deserving of more rigorous study to ensure utilization of and efficacy of the practices.

Regional anesthesia techniques offer an area of opportunity for improved analgesia in this population. A recent review identified only 2 randomized controlled trials related to regional anesthesia in burn populations, with only one related to pediatric populations.[83] Ultrasound-guided, catheter-delivered, or single-shot local anesthetic techniques provide superior pain control than local infiltration of donor sites in burn-injured children.[84] A multicenter database of regional anesthesia in children demonstrates good safety profiles in pediatric patients.[85]

Investigation of burn centers' sedation practices for dressing changes identified a ubiquitous use of benzodiazepines for periprocedural anxiety and opiates for pain relief but more variability in the use of ketamine, alpha-2-agonists, and propofol.[86] Reported combinations of sedatives and analgesics include ketamine plus propofol, ketamine plus dexmedetomidine, and remifentanil plus propofol, all with expected relative changes in recovery times or respiratory drive.[87,88] These results reveal a freedom to tailor sedation agent use to patient characteristics and comorbidities while also highlighting the need for further study regarding optimal procedural sedation regimens.

Finally, nonpharmacologic approaches to pain management in pediatric burn patients is a rapidly developing and promising field. Child life therapy significantly reduces pain and anxiety scores with the use of clear and honest communication, engagement, and medical play.[89] Distraction techniques with the use of a tablet decreases anxiety during and after hydrotherapy sessions.[90] Virtual reality has emerged as a useful distraction tool to decrease pain and overall anxiety. A recent metaanalysis of virtual reality use in burn care evaluated 6 randomized trials, four of which showed statistically significant improvement in pain scores when used during burn procedures.[91]

The management of pain and anxiety critically impacts short- and long-term outcome of these vulnerable children, especially because burn care and survival have improved over time.[92] Up to 38% of all pediatric burn victims develop anxiety disorders after hospitalization, with a known contribution of pain to subsequent acute stress and PTSD symptoms.[93,94] Given the promising results of relatively underutilized pharmacologic agents and alternative modalities, pain management research and protocolization within the pediatric burn population should be pursued aggressively, creatively, and in a team-based manner to both optimize the inpatient recovery process and also mitigate the long-term psychological consequences for these patients.

SUMMARY

As experts in airway management, fluid resuscitation, transfusion practices, and pain management, anesthesiologists are in a unique position to cohesively treat key areas of complexity in the burned patient. Open and clear communication with members from the surgical, nursing, and critical care teams promotes the highest standard of care. Despite the burden and the challenge these patients present, there is a paucity of rigorous, prospective studies that guide best practice. Future directions of the field should focus on continued expansion of the standardization of care for pediatric burn patients, formulation of more elegant endpoints of resuscitation, and development of pain management protocols that use modalities of emerging benefit to the burned patient.

Clinics Care Points

- A significant number of burn patients are preemptively intubated without clinical necessity. A greater familiarity with the characterization of burn injuries and serial airway evaluation may prevent unnecessary intubation.

- Fluid resuscitation of pediatric burn patients requires vigilance with respect to accurate TBSA calculation, careful recording of volumes administered, and utility of dextrose-containing maintenance fluids.

- Although in need of confirmation via prospective study, there is likely benefit to continuing postpyloric feeds perioperatively in children with established airways.

- Upcoming data should soon reveal if there is benefit in a 1:1 versus 4:1 transfusion ratio for pediatric burn patients.

- Regional anesthesia is an underutilized technique with proven analgesic benefit in the pediatric burn population.

- Virtual reality is a promising component of anxiolysis and pain control during pediatric burn procedures.

DISCLOSURE

The authors have no financial interests to disclose.

REFERENCES

1. Injury Prevent & Control, Fatal Injury Data. 2019. 2020. Available at: https://www.cdc.gov/injury/wisqars/fatal.html. Accessed Jauary 5, 2020.
2. Burns. 2018. 2020. Available at: https://www.who.int/news-room/fact-sheets/detail/burns. Accessed January 5, 2020.
3. Saeman MR, Hodgman EI, Burris A, et al. Epidemiology and outcomes of pediatric burns over 35 years at Parkland Hospital. Burns 2016;42:202–8.
4. Lee CJ, Mahendraraj K, Houng A, et al. Pediatric burns: a single institution retrospective review of incidence, etiology, and outcomes in 2273 burn patients (1995-2013). J Burn Care Res 2016;37:e579–85.
5. Avci V, Kocak OF. Treatment algorithm in 960 pediatric burn cases: a review of etiology and epidemiology. Pak J Med Sci 2018;34:1185–90.
6. Palmieri TL, Taylor S, Lawless M, et al. Burn center volume makes a difference for burned children. Pediatr Crit Care Med 2015;16:319–24.
7. Kazis LE, Sheridan RL, Shapiro GD, et al. Development of clinical process measures for pediatric burn care: understanding variation in practice patterns. J Trauma Acute Care Surg 2018;84:620–7.
8. Jeschke MG, Chinkes DL, Finnerty CC, et al. Pathophysiologic response to severe burn injury. Ann Surg 2008;248:387–401.
9. Monafo WW. Initial management of burns. N Engl J Med 1996;335:1581–6.
10. Howard TS, Hermann DG, McQuitty AL, et al. Burn-induced cardiac dysfunction increases length of stay in pediatric burn patients. J Burn Care Res 2013;34:413–9.
11. Jeschke MG, Gauglitz GG, Kulp GA, et al. Long-term persistance of the pathophysiologic response to severe burn injury. PLoS One 2011;6:e21245.
12. Kaneda K, Han TH. Comparative population pharmacokinetics of fentanyl using non-linear mixed effect modeling: burns vs. non-burns. Burns 2009;35:790–7.
13. Martyn JA, White DA, Gronert GA, et al. Up-and-down regulation of skeletal muscle acetylcholine receptors. Effects on neuromuscular blockers. Anesthesiology 1992;76:822–43.
14. Uyar M, Hepaguşlar H, Uğur G, et al. Resistance to vecuronium in burned children. Paediatr Anaesth 1999;9:115–8.
15. Harshman J, Roy M, Cartotto R. Emergency care of the burn patient before the burn center: a systematic review and meta-analysis. J Burn Care Res 2019;40:166–88.
16. McCulloh C, Nordin A, Talbot LJ, et al. Accuracy of prehospital care providers in determining total body surface area burned in severe pediatric thermal injury. J Burn Care Res 2018;39:491–6.
17. Goverman J, Bittner EA, Friedstat JS, et al. Discrepancy in initial pediatric burn estimates and its impact on fluid resuscitation. J Burn Care Res 2015;36:574–9.
18. Sutton T, Lenk I, Conrad P, et al. Severity of inhalation injury is predictive of alterations in gas exchange and worsened clinical outcomes. J Burn Care Res 2017;38:390–5.
19. Tan A, Smailes S, Friebel T, et al. Smoke inhalation increases intensive care requirements and morbidity in paediatric burns. Burns 2016;42:1111–5.
20. Madnani DD, Steele NP, de Vries E. Factors that predict the need for intubation in patients with smoke inhalation injury. Ear Nose Throat J 2006;85:278–80.

21. Muehlberger T, Kunar D, Munster A, et al. Efficacy of fiberoptic laryngoscopy in the diagnosis of inhalation injuries. Arch Otolaryngol Head Neck Surg 1998;124: 1003–7.

22. Spano S, Hanna S, Li Z, et al. Does bronchoscopic evaluation of inhalation injury severity predict outcome? J Burn Care Res 2016;37:1–11.

23. Desai MH, Mlcak R, Richardson J, et al. Reduction in mortality in pediatric patients with inhalation injury with aerosolized heparin/N-acetylcystine [correction of acetylcystine] therapy. J Burn Care Rehabil 1998;19:210–2.

24. McGinn KA, Weigartz K, Lintner A, et al. Nebulized heparin with N-acetylcysteine and albuterol reduces duration of mechanical ventilation in patients with inhalation injury. J Pharm Pract 2019;32:163–6.

25. Hyland EJ, Harvey JG, Martin AJ, et al. Airway compromise in children with anterior neck burns: beware the scalded child. J Paediatr Child Health 2015;51: 976–81.

26. Zak AL, Harrington DT, Barillo DJ, et al. Acute respiratory failure that complicates the resuscitation of pediatric patients with scald injuries. J Burn Care Rehabil 1999;20:391–9.

27. Eastman AL, Arnoldo BA, Hunt JL, et al. Pre-burn center management of the burned airway: do we know enough? J Burn Care Res 2010;31:701–5.

28. Khine HH, Corddry DH, Kettrick RG, et al. Comparison of cuffed and uncuffed endotracheal tubes in young children during general anesthesia. Anesthesiology 1997;86:627–31 [discussion: 27A].

29. Sheridan RL. Uncuffed endotracheal tubes should not be used in seriously burned children. Pediatr Crit Care Med 2006;7:258–9.

30. Dorsey DP, Bowman SM, Klein MB, et al. Perioperative use of cuffed endotracheal tubes is advantageous in young pediatric burn patients. Burns 2010;36: 856–60.

31. Huang M, Chen JF, Chen LY, et al. A comparison of two different fluid resuscitation management protocols for pediatric burn patients: a retrospective study. Burns 2018;44:82–9.

32. Barrow RE, Jeschke MG, Herndon DN. Early fluid resuscitation improves outcomes in severely burned children. Resuscitation 2000;45:91–6.

33. Romanowski KS, Palmieri TL. Pediatric burn resuscitation: past, present, and future. Burns Trauma 2017;5:26.

34. Muller Dittrich MH, Brunow de Carvalho W, Lopes Lavado E. Evaluation of the "early" use of albumin in children with extensive burns: a randomized controlled trial. Pediatr Crit Care Med 2016;17:e280–6.

35. Shah A, Pedraza I, Mitchell C, et al. Fluid volumes infused during burn resuscitation 1980-2015: a quantitative review. Burns 2019;46(1):52–7.

36. Nagpal A, Clingenpeel M-M, Thakkar RK, et al. Positive cumulative fluid balance at 72h is associated with adverse outcomes following acute pediatric thermal injury. Burns 2018;44:1308–16.

37. Kraft R, Herndon DN, Branski LK, et al. Optimized fluid management improves outcomes of pediatric burn patients. J Surg Res 2013;181:121–8.

38. Tsoutsos D, Rodopoulou S, Keramidas E, et al. Early escharotomy as a measure to reduce intraabdominal hypertension in full-thickness burns of the thoracic and abdominal area. World J Surg 2003;27:1323–8.

39. Jensen AR, Hughes WB, Grewal H. Secondary abdominal compartment syndrome in children with burns and trauma: a potentially lethal complication. J Burn Care Res 2006;27:242–6.

40. Pietsch JB, Netscher DT, Nagaraj HS, et al. Early excision of major burns in children: effect on morbidity and mortality. J Pediatr Surg 1985;20:754–7.

41. Xiao-Wu W, Herndon DN, Spies M, et al. Effects of delayed wound excision and grafting in severely burned children. Arch Surg 2002;137:1049–54.

42. Coleman JJ 3rd, Siwy BK. Cultured epidermal autografts: a life-saving and skin-saving technique in children. J Pediatr Surg 1992;27:1029–32.

43. Holmes Iv JH, Molnar JA, Carter JE, et al. A comparative study of the ReCell(R) device and autologous spit-thickness meshed skin graft in the treatment of acute burn injuries. J Burn Care Res 2018;39:694–702.

44. Bashir MM, Sohail M, Wahab A, et al. Outcomes of post burn flexion contracture release under tourniquet versus tumescent technique in children. Burns 2018;44: 678–82.

45. Bussolin L, Busoni P, Giorgi L, et al. Tumescent local anesthesia for the surgical treatment of burns and postburn sequelae in pediatric patients. Anesthesiology 2003;99:1371–5.

46. Bussolin L, Serio P, Busoni P, et al. Plasma levels of lignocaine during tumescent local anaesthesia in children with burns. Anaesth Intensive Care 2010;38: 1008–12.

47. Mitchell RTM, Funk D, Spiwak R, et al. Phenylephrine tumescence in split-thickness skin graft donor sites in surgery for burn injury- a concentration finding study. J Burn Care Res 2011;32:129–34.

48. Allorto NL, Bishop DG, Rodseth RN. Vasoconstrictor clysis in burn surgery and its impact on outcomes: systematic review and meta-analysis. Burns 2015;41: 1140–6.

49. Cartotto R, Kadikar N, Musgrave MA, et al. What are the acute cardiovascular effects of subcutaneous and topical epinephrine for hemostasis during burn surgery? J Burn Care Rehabil 2003;24:297–305.

50. Weis HB, Meinhardt KE, Minhajuddin A, et al. Administration of tumescence in pediatric burn patients causes significant hypertension. J Burn Care Res 2019; 40:752–6.

51. Wong BM, Keilman J, Zuccaro J, et al. Anesthetic practices for laser rehabilitation of pediatric hypertrophic burn scars. J Burn Care Res 2017;38:e36–41.

52. Reynolds L, Beckmann J, Kurz A. Perioperative complications of hypothermia. Best Pract Res Clin Anaesthesiol 2008;22:645–57.

53. Ravindran RS. A solution to monitoring the electrocardiograph in patients with extensive burn injury. Anesthesiology 1997;87:711–2.

54. Sofos SS, Tehrani H, Shokrollahi K, et al. Surgical staple as a transcutaneous transducer for ECG electrodes in burnt skin: safe surgical monitoring in major burns. Burns 2013;39:818–9.

55. Khorasani EN, Mansouri F. Effect of early enteral nutrition on morbidity and mortality in children with burns. Burns 2010;36:1067–71.

56. Czapran A, Headdon W, Deane AM, et al. International observational study of nutritional support in mechanically ventilated patients following burn injury. Burns 2015;41:510–8.

57. Sunderman CA, Gottschlich MM, Allgeier C, et al. Safety and tolerance of intra-operative enteral nutrition support in pediatric burn patients. Nutr Clin Pract 2019;34:728–34.

58. Imeokparia F, Johnson M, Thakkar RK, et al. Safety and efficacy of uninterrupted perioperative enteral feeding in pediatric burn patients. Burns 2018;44:344–9.

59. Jeong IM, Seo WG, Woo CH, et al. Prediction of difficult intubation in patients with postburn sternomental contractures: modified Onah class. Korean J Anesthesiol 2009;57:290–5.

60. Khan RM, Kaul N, Aziz H, et al. A pathfinder technique of laryngeal mask airway placement in an infant with severe contracture of face, neck, and chest. Paediatr Anaesth 2014;24:339–40.

61. Schlossmacher P, Martinet O, Testud R, et al. Emergency percutaneous tracheostomy in a severely burned patient with upper airway obstruction and circulatory arrest. Resuscitation 2006;68:301–5.

62. Sousse LE, Herndon DN, Andersen CR, et al. High tidal volume decreases adult respiratory distress syndrome, atelectasis, and ventilator days compared with low tidal volume in pediatric burned patients with inhalation injury. J Am Coll Surg 2015;220:570–8.

63. Greathouse ST, Hadad I, Zieger M, et al. High-frequency oscillatory ventilators in burn patients: experience of Riley Hospital for Children. J Burn Care Res 2012;33:425–35.

64. Walia G, Jada G, Cartotto R. Anesthesia and intraoperative high-frequency oscillatory ventilation during burn surgery. J Burn Care Res 2011;32:118–23.

65. Byerly FL, Haithcock JA, Buchanan IB, et al. Use of high flow nasal cannula on a pediatric burn patient with inhalation injury and post-extubation stridor. Burns 2006;32:121–5.

66. Silver GM, Freiburg C, Halerz M, et al. A survey of airway and ventilator management strategies in North American pediatric burn units. J Burn Care Rehabil 2004;25:435–40.

67. Palmieri TL, Jackson W, Greenhalgh DG. Benefits of early tracheostomy in severely burned children. Crit Care Med 2002;30:922–4.

68. Voigt CD, Hundeshagen G, Malagaris I, et al. Effects of a restrictive blood transfusion protocol on acute pediatric burn care: Transfusion threshold in pediatric burns. J Trauma Acute Care Surg 2018;85:1048–54.

69. Lacroix J, Hebert PC, Hutchison JS, et al. Transfusion strategies for patients in pediatric intensive care units. N Engl J Med 2007;356:1609–19.

70. Tejiram S, Sen S, Romanowski KS, et al. Examining 1:1 versus 4:1 packed red blood cell to fresh frozen plasma ratio transfusion during pediatric burn excision. J Burn Care Res 2020;41(3):443–9.

71. Galganski LA, Greenhalgh DG, Sen S, et al. Randomized comparison of packed red blood cell-to-fresh frozen plasma transfusion ratio of 4: 1 vs 1: 1 during acute massive burn excision. J Burn Care Res 2017;38:194–201.

72. Jeschke MG, Chinkes DL, Finnerty CC, et al. Blood transfusions are associated with increased risk for development of sepsis in severely burned pediatric patients. Crit Care Med 2007;35:579–83.

73. Schaden E, Kimberger O, Kraincuk P, et al. Perioperative treatment algorithm for bleeding burn patients reduces allogeneic blood product requirements. Br J Anaesth 2012;109:376–81.

74. Huzar TF, Martinez E, Love J, et al. Admission rapid thrombelastography (rTEG®) values predict resuscitation volumes and patient outcomes after thermal injury. J burn Care Res 2018;39:345–52.

75. Engel M, Bodem JP, Busch CJ, et al. The value of tranexamic acid during fronto-orbital advancement in isolated metopic craniosynostosis. J Craniomaxillofac Surg 2015;43:1239–43.

76. Hsu G, Taylor JA, Fiadjoe JE, et al. Aminocaproic acid administration is associated with reduced perioperative blood loss and transfusion in pediatric craniofacial surgery. Acta Anaesthesiol Scand 2016;60:158–65.
77. Nelson S, Conroy C, Logan D. The biopsychosocial model of pain in the context of pediatric burn injuries. Eur J Pain 2019;23:421–34.
78. Gamst-Jensen H, Vedel PN, Lindberg-Larsen VO, et al. Acute pain management in burn patients: appraisal and thematic analysis of four clinical guidelines. Burns 2014;40:1463–9.
79. Martin-Herz SP, Patterson DR, Honari S, et al. Pediatric pain control practices of North American burn centers. J Burn Care Rehabil 2003;24:26–36.
80. Pardesi O, Fuzaylov G. Pain management in pediatric burn patients: review of recent literature and future directions. J Burn Care Res 2017;38:335–47.
81. Rimaz S, Alavi CE, Sedighinejad A, et al. Effect of gabapentin on morphine consumption and pain after surgical debridement of burn wounds: a double-blind randomized clinical trial study. Arch Trauma Res 2012;1:38–43.
82. Martin E, Ramsay G, Mantz J, et al. The role of the alpha2-adrenoceptor agonist dexmedetomidine in postsurgical sedation in the intensive care unit. J Intensive Care Med 2003;18:29–41.
83. Town CJ, Johnson J, Van Zundert A, et al. Exploring the role of regional anesthesia in the treatment of the burn-injured patient: a narrative review of current literature. Clin J Pain 2019;35:368–74.
84. Shank ES, Martyn JA, Donelan MB, et al. Ultrasound-guided regional anesthesia for pediatric burn reconstructive surgery: a prospective study. J Burn Care Res 2016;37:e213–7.
85. Walker BJ, Long JB, Sathyamoorthy M, et al. Complications in pediatric regional anesthesia: an analysis of more than 100,000 blocks from the pediatric regional anesthesia network. Anesthesiology 2018;129:721–32.
86. Hansen JK, Voss J, Ganatra H, et al. Sedation and analgesia during pediatric burn dressing change: a survey of american burn association centers. J Burn Care Res 2019;40:287–93.
87. Canpolat DG, Esmaoglu A, Tosun Z, et al. Ketamine-propofol vs ketamine-dexmedetomidine combinations in pediatric patients undergoing burn dressing changes. J Burn Care Res 2012;33:718–22.
88. Seol TK, Lim JK, Yoo EK, et al. Propofol-ketamine or propofol-remifentanil for deep sedation and analgesia in pediatric patients undergoing burn dressing changes: a randomized clinical trial. Paediatr Anaesth 2015;25:560–6.
89. Moore ER, Bennett KL, Dietrich MS, et al. The effect of directed medical play on young children's pain and distress during burn wound care. J Pediatr Health Care 2015;29:265–73.
90. Burns-Nader S, Joe L, Pinion K. Computer tablet distraction reduces pain and anxiety in pediatric burn patients undergoing hydrotherapy: a randomized trial. Burns 2017;43:1203–11.
91. Eijlers R, Utens E, Staals LM, et al. Systematic review and meta-analysis of virtual reality in pediatrics: effects on pain and anxiety. Anesth Analg 2019;129:1344–53.
92. Barrett LW, Fear VS, Waithman JC, et al. Understanding acute burn injury as a chronic disease. Burns Trauma 2019;7:23.
93. Meyer WJ, Blakeney P, Thomas CR, et al. Prevalence of major psychiatric illness in young adults who were burned as children. Psychosom Med 2007;69:377–82.
94. Rimmer RB, Bay RC, Alam NB, et al. Burn-injured youth may be at increased risk for long-term anxiety disorders. J burn Care Res 2014;35:154–61.

Perioperative Considerations for the Fontan Patient Requiring Noncardiac Surgery

Adam C. Adler, MS, MD[a],*, Aruna T. Nathan, MD[b]

KEYWORDS

- Pediatrics • Pediatric anesthesiology • Congenital heart disease • Fontan
- Noncardiac surgery • Risk assessment

KEY POINTS

- Children and adults with congenital heart disease undergoing noncardiac surgery are at higher risk of perioperative adverse events.
- Patients have significant comorbidities and syndromic associations that increase perioperative risk further.
- The complexity of congenital heart disease requires a thorough understanding of lesion-specific pathophysiology in order to provide safe care.
- Comprehensive multidisciplinary planning and the use of skilled and experienced teams achieve the best outcomes.
- The anesthesiologist is a perioperative physician charged with providing safe anesthesia care, instituting appropriate hemodynamic monitoring, and determining appropriate postoperative disposition on an individual basis.

INTRODUCTION

Assessment of children with varying severity of congenital heart disease in phases of surgical and medical management can prove challenging for the anesthesia provider. Certainly, with the variability in anatomic morphology coupled with the individualized response to treatment, it is not possible to define all patients homogenously. Therefore, this review focuses on assessing patients with congenital heart disease having undergone the Fontan procedure, the anatomic endpoint for several congenital heart

[a] Department of Anesthesiology, Perioperative and Pain Medicine, Texas Children's Hospital, Baylor College of Medicine, 6621 Fannin Street, Houston, TX 77030, USA; [b] Department of Anesthesia, Stanford University Medical Center, 300 Pasteur Drive, Room H3580, MC 5640, Stanford, CA 94304, USA
* Corresponding author.
E-mail address: adamcadler@gmail.com

Anesthesiology Clin 38 (2020) 531–543
https://doi.org/10.1016/j.anclin.2020.04.001
1932-2275/20/© 2020 Elsevier Inc. All rights reserved.

anesthesiology.theclinics.com

defects. Specifically, the focus is on patients with Fontan physiology in the context of the perioperative evaluation and conduct of anesthesia for noncardiac surgery.

With increasing survival for patients with Fontan circulation, the number of noncardiac surgical encounters is increasing, necessitating detailed understanding of this physiology and the interplay with anesthesia and surgery.

INCIDENCE AND EPIDEMIOLOGY

The overall incidence of congenital heart disease is approximately 8 per 1000 live births, although with significant interlesion variability.[1] Cardiac lesions may be found in association with several syndromes or occur in isolation. Lesions also may be simple (eg, atrial septal defect) or complex (eg, tricuspid atresia). With advances in surgical and medical management, the number of children and adults living with all forms of congenital heart disease, in particular, Fontan circulation, has increased. Although transplant-free survival for patients with Fontan circulation continues to increase, there are several morbidities specific to this population that require consideration during the conduct of the perioperative evaluation.

FONTAN ANATOMY AND PHYSIOLOGIC CONSIDERATIONS

The Fontan operation is performed for patients with congenital heart lesions for which a 2-ventricle repair is not achievable (**Box 1**). This operation consists of a total cavopulmonary anastomosis establishing series circulation whereby venous return to the lungs is passive via the cavopulmonary anastomoses instead of utilizing the normal right ventricular pump, and the single ventricle provides the oxygenated blood systemically. There is significant presurgical anatomic variation, however, in patients with Fontan circulation based on the underlying pathology. Both right ventricular hypoplasia and left ventricular hypoplasia are indications for a Fontan procedure. For example, a patient with tricuspid atresia (hypoplastic right ventricle) and a patient with hypoplastic left heart syndrome (HLHS) (hypoplastic left ventricle) both are candidates for Fontan surgical palliation. The 2 most common types of Fontan procedures are the fenestrated intra-atrial Fontan and the unfenestrated extracardiac Fontan (**Fig. 1**). A fenestration is a connection between the Fontan circuit and the common atrium that serves as a pop-off for maintenance of cardiac output during times of increased pulmonary pressure. The atriopulmonary Fontan is an older technique that involved anastomosis of the right atrium directly to the pulmonary artery. This procedure no longer is performed; however, this anatomic type of Fontan may be observed in older patients.

The physiology with regard to pulmonary blood flow in a Fontan circuit is unique. As the single ventricle becomes dedicated to providing systemic blood flow, blood return

---

Box 1
Common anatomic pathologies requiring the Fontan operation

- Double-inlet left ventricle
- Double-outlet right ventricle
- HLHS
- Pulmonary atresia with intact ventricular septum
- Tricuspid atresia
- Unbalanced AV canal defect

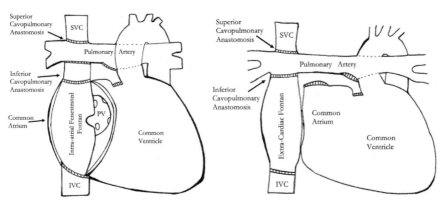

Fig. 1. Illustration of intra-atrial (lateral tunnel) fenestrated Fontan (*left*) and extracardiac Fontan (*right*). IVC, inferior vena cava; PV, pulmonary veins; SVC superior vena cava.

to the lungs becomes passive from the upper body and lower body from the superior vena cava and inferior vena cava, respectively. As the child grows, the percentage of total venous return from the lower body via the inferior vena cava increases.[2,3] Factors that increase pulmonary vascular pressures, either transient or persistent, over time lead to reduced pulmonary blood flow and contribute to Fontan failure. These factors include recurrent exercise, gravitational forces, pregnancy, pulmonary venous obstruction, ventricular failure, valvular regurgitation, constipation, obstructive sleep apnea, and obesity. Failure is characterized by inadequate cardiac output, the sequelae of which include elevated central venous pressure: pleural effusions, ascites, and peripheral edema.

A normal Fontan patient should have a normal oxygen saturation. Patients with Fontan fenestrations may have slightly reduced oxygen saturations due to a small degree of right to left shunting across the fenestration. Persistent oxygen desaturation should raise concern for a failing Fontan circulation.

PREOPERATIVE ASSESSMENT OF THE FONTAN PATIENT

When conducting a preanesthetic evaluation, there are several considerations specific to patients with Fontan circulation (**Table 1**). The aim of the preoperative assessment is to identify factors suggestive of a failing Fontan. The main issues during the basic perioperative examination should include assessment of the underlying cardiac lesion and timing of the previous surgical interventions. The recent echocardiogram and electrocardiograms should be reviewed in addition to home medications, recent illness, exercise capacity, and the need for infective endocarditis prophylaxis.

Cardiac History

A complete medical history with details of the underlying pathology, timing of each stage of palliation of the single-ventricle disease, additional surgeries to address arrhythmias (eg, pacemaker insertion), diaphragmatic plication, airway surgeries, cardiac catheterizations, and interventions must be reviewed. Residual lesions and physiologic burden of those procedures should be assessed. The most important information is gleaned from a patient's cardiologist and the most recent cardiac catheterization report. Any recent changes in a patient's exercise tolerance, functional ability, restriction of physical exercise, or escalation of therapy might indicate a

Table 1
Basic perioperative considerations for patients with Fontan circulation requiring non-cardiac surgery

Preoperative	Intraoperative	Postoperative
Identification of	Premedication	Disposition
Underlying cardiac pathology	Fluid management	Resumption of
Associated syndromes	Pacemaker location for	anticoagulation
Exercise tolerance	electrocautery interference and	Pain management
Physical status	ground pad placement	Pulmonary toilet
Difficult airway history	Central venous access	
Echocardiography	Ventilation Strategies	
Ventricular and valvular	Tidal volume	
function	Respiratory rate	
Residual lesions	Inspiratory time	
Areas of obstruction	Positive End-expiratory Pressure	
Electrocardiography	Abdominal insufflation	
Underlying conduction	Regional Anesthesia	
anomalies	Neuraxial anesthesia	
Previous arrythmias	Infective endocarditis-	
Pacemaker/Defibrillator	requirement	
Location	Blood product availability	
Setting		
Battery life		
Home medications		
Anticoagulation		
Laboratory examinations		
Complete blood cell count/		
chemistry		
Type and screen/cross		
Liver and kidney function		
Albumin		
Coagulation studies		

worsening of cardiac dysfunction. Prior cardiac catheterization data, access sites, patency of veins and arteries, cardiac index, the integrity of the Fontan pathway, presence of a fenestration if any, pressures along the Fontan pathway, transpulmonary gradient, ventricular end-diastolic pressure, pulmonary vascular resistance, and status of the atrioventricular (AV) valve all are useful information.

Morphologically, the right and left ventricles are vastly different, with the right being thin walled and highly trabeculated and the left more muscular and conical shaped. The result is a right ventricle being apt to deal with volume loads and the left suited for ejecting against high pressures. Additionally, both the timing of the initial Fontan completion and the time since Fontan completion are important when considering risk. A study of long-term outcomes for patients with Fontan operations has shown that Fontan completion after age 7 (rather than ages 2–4 years) is associated with worse long-term complications.[4] Delayed Fontan completion often is accompanied by formation of aortopulmonary collaterals, which serve as a source of persistent desaturation (right to left shunt). Additionally, patients with systemic left ventricles have improved outcomes (failure-free survival) compared with non-HLHS patients with systemic right ventricles.[4] Patients with HLHS and, therefore, systemic right ventricles have significantly worse long-term outcomes compared with patients with non-HLHS systemic right ventricles. By comparison, the hazard ratio for Fontan failure is

3.8 (95% CI, 2.0–7.1) for patients with HLHS compared with single-LV Fontan patients.[4]

For all Fontan patients, in particular those with HLHS, time since Fontan completion correlates with the rate of long-term complications and should be considered when conducting the preoperative evaluation. The 10-year freedom from failure rate was 79% for patients with HLHS compared with non-HLHS Fontan patients.[4] There are several factors that contribute to long-term Fontan failure, discussed later.

Echocardiographic Assessment

The most recent echocardiogram should be reviewed with a specific focus on ventricular function as well as function of the AV and semilunar valves. Patients with cardiac failure as evidenced by poor or declining ventricular function are at greater risk of anesthesia-related complications.

Echocardiography should assess for systolic and diastolic ventricular dysfunction, AV valve and semilunar valve function, flow through the atrial septum and patency of pulmonary veins, cavopulmonary connections, and pulmonary arteries. Flow limitations at any level of the Fontan pathway have the potential to impede pulmonary blood flow as well as reduce effective cardiac output.

It must be considered that the single ventricle in the Fontan patient is not equivocal to the corresponding ventricle in a 2-ventricle patient in structure and function.[5] In patients' pre-Fontan years, the single ventricle is subjected to chronic myocardial hypoxia as well as volume overload, which leads to altered myocardial architecture and function.[5,6] Additionally, the geometric architecture of the single ventricle is vastly different when compared with the 2-ventricle inter-relationship. These factors contribute to increased systolic and diastolic dysfunction in the Fontan population, which can be exacerbated during periods of volume expansion and stress, such as the perioperative period.[7] Ventricular assessment is important especially in patients with distant Fontan completion because function is known to decline over time.[8] Similarly, valvulopathy places additional stress on the single ventricle and can be exacerbated during anesthesia. Moderate to severe AV valve or semilunar valve regurgitation and/or presence of pulmonary artery, pulmonary vein, or cavopulmonary anastomosis stenosis may require intervention prior to elective noncardiac surgery.[5]

Arrythmia in Patients with Fontan Physiology

Patients with Fontan circuits are at high risk for several arrythmias, with the incidence correlating with the type of Fontan operation performed.[5,9] Generally, arrythmias in Fontan patients are atrial in origin with sinus node dysfunction. Supraventricular tachycardia is the most common although ventricular arrythmias may occur. Arrythmias may be due to conduction disturbance during surgical intervention or as a sequela of Fontan physiology.[10] Patients with extracardiac conduits have less incidence of arrythmia compared with those with lateral tunnel connection and significantly fewer episodes than those with an atriopulmonary connection.

The etiology and prior treatment of arrythmias should be assessed in the perioperative evaluation. A detailed assessment of the therapies used, such as antiarrhythmics, electrophysiology studies and ablation of pathways, cardioversions, and pacemaker insertion, should be performed. If a patient has an implantable pacemaker or automated implantable cardioverter-defibrillators, the device location, mode of function, and response to tachycardia should be determined. Smaller pediatric patients often have epicardial pacemakers with generators located in the subcostal/abdominal region. Generator location, baseline setting, and response to overlying magnet should be considered. The anesthesia provider should notify the surgeon as to the presence of an intra-abdominal pacemaker so that damage to the unit or leads does not inadvertently occur during a procedure. A conversation with the patient's electrophysiologist should incorporate discussion regarding the status and perioperative reprogramming of the pacemaker to mitigate the effects of interference by electrocautery.

Functional Assessment of the Fontan Patient

Preoperative assessment should elicit signs and symptoms suggestive of cardiac dysfunction and include assessment of underlying exercise capacity and baselines of blood pressure and oxygen saturation. Poor or worsening exercise tolerance and/or dyspnea with exertion may suggest ventricular dysfunction. Poor growth (height) and increasing weight are suggestive of chronically reduced cardiac output and ascites formation, respectively. New-onset or increased frequency of arrythmia may be suggestive of chronic ventricular failure and atrial dilatation.

Oxygen saturation should be assessed in the context of the type of Fontan operation that was performed. Although persistent desaturation may be due to presence of a fenestration, desaturation also may be suggestive of elevated pulmonary venous pressures, collateral formation, and/or ventricular dysfunction.[5]

Although most Fontan patients do not require routine anticoagulation, the risk of stopping these medications must be considered on a case-by-case basis, specifically for patients with persistent arrythmia at risk for thrombogenesis.

Fontan patients with AV valve regurgitation and arrythmia often are managed using diuretic and afterload reduction agents as well as antiarrhythmics, respectively. These medications should be continued perioperatively. Fontan patients lack a ventricle to provide pulmonary blood flow and are reliant on passive flow to the lungs, therefore, adequate preload is critical in maintaining cardiac output. With prolonged nil per os (NPO) times, however, patients may become excessively volume depleted. Long NPO times should be avoided when possible and/or the patients should be started on intravenous fluid to maintain intravascular volume homeostasis.

Preoperative Laboratory Assessment of the Fontan Patient

Laboratory studies should be used to help determine a patient's physiologic status and ability to tolerate the proposed surgical procedure. Typically, a complete blood cell count, chemistry panel, and type and screen suffice for most procedures that are minor. Evaluation of renal and hepatic function should be considered, particularly for those with distant Fontan corrections.

Patients with Fontan physiology are prone to chronic hypoxemia and, therefore, tend to have higher hematocrit levels than normal values. Baseline hemoglobin and hematocrit should be assessed and maintained perioperatively. Fontan patients are prone to excessive surgical bleeding from persistently high venous pressures, anticoagulant therapy, liver involvement, and intrinsic coagulation factor abnormalities.[11] These patients should have cross-matched blood available for surgeries with anticipated blood loss, especially because they might have antibodies that make cross-matching difficult in an urgent situation.

Fontan patients, in particular those with chronically elevated venous pressures, are at risk for Fontan-associated liver disease (FALD).[12] FALD may range from mild hepatic fibrosis to end-stage liver disease and potentially the development of hepatocellular carcinoma. Basic tests of liver function tests, such alanine aminotransferase (ALT) and aspartate aminotransferase (AST) as well as γ-glutamyl transferase, often are elevated.[13] With prolonged hepatic congestion, worsening liver fibrosis can lead to hepatic failure and the sequalae of end-stage liver disease. Testing for coagulopathy should be considered in patients with features suggestive of advanced liver disease.

Patients with Fontan circulation also are at risk for multifactorial chronic kidney disease; the incidence increases with age. Reduced cardiac output, use of nephrotoxic medications, and repeated episodes of cardiopulmonary bypass result in increased incidence of renal dysfunction after the Fontan operation.[14,15] Baseline renal function should be assessed in Fontan patients prior to elective surgery. Adequate hydration, avoidance of prolonged NPO times, and avoidance of hypotension are crucial in perioperative management.

Protein-losing enteropathy (PLE) has been reported in up to 12% of patients with Fontan palliation and is a major source of morbidity.[16,17] Although the exact etiology is unknown, it is suspected that lymphatic congestion results from both reduced cardiac output and chronic venous congestion.[18] The loss of protein in PLE can lead to ascites, hypotension (from oncotic pressure reduction), malabsorption, and intestinal failure. Diffuse ascites and hypoalbuminemia may suggest PLE. The management of PLE is incredibly challenging and should be deferred to centers that routinely provide care to complex congenital heart patients.

Plastic bronchitis (PB) is reported in up to 5% of Fontan patients and characterized by production of thick casts within the airway.[19,20] These protein and lymphatic-rich casts, when expectorated from the airway, are thought to result from elevated venous and lymphatic pressure similar to that occurring in PLE. The presence of PB is suggestive of Fontan failure with management similarly deferred to congenital heart disease centers. PB leads to airway inflammation, chronic cough, and hypoxemia and is a major source of morbidity and mortality for these patients.

Home Medications

These patients often receive multiple medications, cardiac and others, as part of their multidisciplinary medical care. In addition, some patients take herbal medications. It is important to review all medications in detail and determine drug interactions with commonly used anesthetic drugs. Common medications include diuretics, angiotensin-converting enzyme (ACE) inhibitors, inotropes, pulmonary vasodilators, antihypertensives, anticoagulants, antiarrhythmic drugs, antibiotics, and psychotropic medications. Some patients might require oxygen therapy at home. Diuretics probably are best withheld on the morning of surgery to preempt the risk of dehydration. Other medications should be continued based on the cardiologist's recommendations. Generally, ACE inhibitors are withheld on the day of surgery due to concern for refractory hypotension.

Anesthesia and the Fontan Patient

Anesthetic history

Prior anesthetic records should be perused, especially if there are any related to noncardiac surgery after Fontan completion. An indication of the type and amount of premedication that were effective for anxiolysis, which form of induction was better tolerated hemodynamically, and intraoperative course can be ascertained. Difficulties with vascular access, both venous and arterial, and with airway management can be anticipated. Prior airway history should be ascertained, because patients with multiple congenital heart surgeries may have residua, such as subglottic stenosis, vocal cord paralysis or granulomas, and diaphragmatic issues, and might have had tracheostomies in the past. Careful historical and clinical assessment of the airway and planning for additional resources, such as videolaryngoscopy or fiber-optic bronchoscopy, ensure a smooth transition from a natural airway to a secured airway after induction of anesthesia. Also, the postoperative course after prior anesthetics is suggestive of the current postoperative course and assists with disposition planning and the need for additional monitoring or support.

Recent illnesses

Recovery from recent upper respiratory and gastrointestinal illnesses must be optimized prior to elective noncardiac surgery, even if it means surgery is delayed. Because pulmonary blood flow and hence systemic cardiac output are dependent on the transpulmonary gradient, laryngospasm and bronchospasm associated with an intercurrent upper respiratory illness in patients with Fontan physiology can precipitate both respiratory failure and cardiac failure. It is best to wait at least 4 weeks after a patient becomes asymptomatic to schedule elective, noncardiac surgery. Gastrointestinal illnesses with loss of fluid from the gastrointestinal tract leaves a Fontan patient dehydrated, with inadequate preload. Achieving and maintaining adequate intravascular volume aids the anesthetic course in these patients, and it is prudent to ensure full recovery from acute gastrointestinal processes prior to elective surgery.

The anesthetic care of the Fontan patient should be planned with consideration of the surgery required in conjunction with the patient-specific aberrations, as discussed previously. Prolonged NPO times should be avoided because these may lead to dehydration, reduced pulmonary venous return, decreased cardiac output, and exaggerated hypotension with induction of anesthesia. Children demonstrating normal function of the Fontan circuit may be suitable for inhalation induction. When performing intravenous induction of anesthesia, underlying aberrations must be considered (eg, ventricular function, AV valve regurgitation, and pulmonary hypertension). Although all medications have been used, benzodiazepines, ketamine, opioids, and dexmedetomidine often are administered in combination. Additionally, induction of anesthesia can be met with exaggerated hypotension from reduced pulmonary venous return. Although intravenous hydration is appropriate, aggressive fluid administration may be poorly tolerated, particularly in patients with underlying diastolic dysfunction. Due to chronically high venous pressures, Fontan patients generally have ample sites for peripheral venous access. Central venous access should be performed with caution with consideration for femoral access to avoid direct catherization of the cavopulmonary anastomosis.

Ventilation can have exaggerated effects on patients with Fontan physiology. In particular, large tidal volumes, rapid respiratory rates, high positive end-expiratory pressures, and long inspiratory times all contribute to reduced pulmonary venous return. Similarly, factors contributing to elevated pulmonary vascular resistance, especially in patients with underlying pulmonary hypertension, should be avoided (**Table 2**). Although preexisting pulmonary hypertension may preclude the Fontan completion, over time, multifactorial changes to the pulmonary vasculature often result in elevated pulmonary pressures.

Regional anesthesia may be considered in patients with Fontan circulation. Neuraxial anesthesia with resultant sympathectomy, however, has the potential to greatly reduce pulmonary venous return. Similarly, steep reverse Trendelenburg positioning may precipitate venous pooling. Additionally, abdominal and thoracic insufflation greatly reduces pulmonary venous return. When laparoscopic approaches are considered, insufflation should be gradual and with the minimal acceptable pressures to provide adequate surgical conditions.

Postoperative recovery ideally should involve providers adept at caring for Fontan patients. Maintenance of adequate hydration, pain control, and aggressive pulmonary toilet is vital to preserve pulmonary blood flow.

Table 2
Principles of anesthetic management in patients with pulmonary hypertension

Preoperative	• Continue all pulmonary hypertension medications • Monitor for hypoventilation after premedication administration • Consider preinduction intravenous access	• Pulmonary vasodilators (milrinone, nitric oxide, and epoprostenol) • ECMO standby • Discuss with surgeon of specific operative concerns and effects on pulmonary vascular pressures (eg, abdominal insufflation)
Intraoperative	• Avoid excessive PEEP, TV, and inspiratory time • Ensure adequate anesthetic depths in anticipation of intubation and surgical manipulations	
Postoperative	• Consider NPPV as needed to avoid respiratory obstruction[a] • Disposition planning to providers skilled in caring for children with PH (eg, ICU)	
Pulmonary hypertension triggers	• Hypoxemia • Hypercarbia • Acidosis • Hypothermia	• Hypovolemia • Sympathetic stimulation • Pain, shivering, and anxiety

Abbreviations: ECMO, extracorporeal membrane oxygenation; ICU, intensive care unit; NPPV, noninvasive positive pressure ventilation; PEEP, positive end-expiratory pressure; PH, pulmonary hypertension; TV, tidal volume.
[a] Affects both pulmonary reactivity with elevated CO_2 and promotes mechanical obstruction to right ventricular flow.

Syndromic associations

Syndromic associations, if any, should be further explored. There might be other associated anomalies, such as cervical spine instability, a potentially difficult airway, smaller airway size, and other multiorgan issues. These children also can prove very challenging for procurement of vascular access. Factoring the complexities and risk of associated syndromes into the anesthetic care plan helps increase patient safety.[21]

Infective endocarditis prophylaxis

Infective endocarditis prophylaxis is recommended for patients undergoing high-risk procedures, such as dental restoration.
Indications for antibiotic administration for endocarditis prophylaxis include[22]

- A prosthetic heart valve or patients who have had a heart valve repaired with prosthetic material
- A history of bacterial endocarditis
- A heart transplant with abnormal heart valve function
- Certain congenital heart defects, including
  o Cyanotic congenital heart disease that has not been fully repaired, including children who have had a surgical shunts and conduits
  o A congenital heart defect that has been completely repaired with prosthetic material or a device for the first 6 months after the repair procedure
  o Repaired congenital heart disease with residual defects, such as persisting leaks or abnormal flow at or adjacent to a prosthetic patch or prosthetic device

Risk Assessment in Fontan Patients

Multiple studies have assessed the risk of late mortality and significant morbidity after the Fontan procedure. A single-institution review of 773 patients who underwent Fontan procedures in the current era described a freedom from a composite medical morbidity outcome (PLE, plastic bronchitis, serious thromboembolic event, or tachyarrhythmia) of 47% at 20 years.[19] Independent risk factors for morbidity included pre-Fontan AV valve regurgitation, pleural drainage greater than 14 days, and longer cross-clamp times (hazard ratio of 1.2 per 10 minutes).[19] Significantly, the presence of Fontan-associated morbidity was associated with a 36-fold increase in the risk of subsequent Fontan takedown, heart transplantation, or death.[19] Data from the Australia & New Zealand Fontan Registry show that of 683 patients greater than or equal to 16 years old, only 41% were free of serious adverse events at 40 years of age.[23]

A recent systematic review of 28 published studies evaluating long-term mortality and/or heart transplantation in Fontan patients evaluated the risk factors for mortality in this population.[24] There were 1000 deaths out of a total of 6707 patients, with an average follow-up time of 8.23 years ± 5.42 years.[24] The 5 most common causes of death were heart failure, arrhythmia, respiratory failure, renal disease, and thrombosis/bleeding. Obviously, these patients are at high risk of adverse events during general anesthesia. These same patients, however, also need multiple cardiac and noncardiac surgical procedures to monitor the course and effects of the Fontan physiology on end-organ structure and function (eg, liver biopsies, gastrointestinal endoscopies, magnetic resonance imaging scans, cardiac catheterization, and airway examinations). Furthermore, they also are prone to the usual emergencies that other children face, such as orthopedic surgeries, appendectomies, and laparoscopic procedures. Recently, these patients also have undergone more extensive noncardiac procedures, such as spinal fusions. As the Fontan population increasingly reaches adulthood, women with this physiology also face unique physiologic challenges associated with pregnancy and childbirth.

It is essential to understand how to assess anesthetic risk in this population. There is not yet a Fontan risk score, although several studies point toward higher risk of mortality over time. Anesthesia-related risk is highest in patients with single-ventricle physiology and heart failure.[25,26] When assessing the Fontan patient, thorough anesthetic evaluation should include an understanding of their Fontan history (baseline heart defect), presence of Fontan-related morbidities (eg, arrythmia), presence of comorbidities, for example, obstructive sleep apnea, asthma, diabetes, genetic disorders (trisomy 21, 22 q11 deletion syndromes, Turner syndrome, and others), current functional status, and compliance with medications.

Faraoni and colleagues[26,27] have described a risk score for congenital heart disease and noncardiac surgery. The investigators reviewed the National Surgical Quality Improvement Program data for 3 consecutive years (2012–2014) in 4375 children with major or severe congenital heart disease undergoing noncardiac surgery in an attempt to ascertain risk stratification for this group of patients.[26,27] They used preoperative predictors, such as emergency procedure, severe congenital heart disease, single-ventricle physiology, prior surgery within 30 days, inotropic support, preoperative cardiopulmonary resuscitation, acute/chronic kidney injury, and concurrent mechanical ventilation, as risk factors. They derived a risk stratification score of 0 to 10 from the presence of these factors; a score of 4 to 6 was considered medium risk and a score greater than or equal to 7 high risk.[27] Factors that increased risk of in-hospital mortality included preoperative markers of critical illness, complexity of cardiac lesion (eg, single ventricle physiology), and functional severity of congenital heart disease.

Any recent clinical deterioration or new onset of symptoms pertinent to the Fontan physiology should not be ignored. After a preliminary evaluation of a patient's chart, a thorough discussion with the patient's cardiologist is vital to the provision of good clinical care, given the longitudinal view of the patient they possess.

Consideration of high-risk Fontan patients within this schema helps mitigate perioperative complications. These patients need to be assessed in the preoperative clinic well in advance of the planned date of surgery. As the sequelae of Fontan physiology manifest themselves, multidisciplinary planning is necessary. Multiple studies have described multifactorial coagulation abnormalities and prothrombotic tendencies in the Fontan patient. Consulting with a primary cardiologist and surgeon as to when anticoagulation can be safely stopped and reinstituted after surgery is prudent. Bridging to unfractionated or low-molecular-weight heparin before and after surgery may be necessary. Larger centers that care for significant volumes of single-ventricle patients have protocols and procedures that help guide perioperative anticoagulation in these patients. Another significant concern is renal insufficiency. In collaboration with a patient's cardiologist and nephrologist, a perioperative plan for renal preservation can be instituted per institutional criteria. At a minimum, these measures involve intravascular hydration, avoiding nephrotoxic agents, and minimizing contrast exposure.

Pregnant women with Fontan physiology seem at high risk of atrial arrhythmia. Preterm labor is common. They usually are cared for in adult congenital cardiac centers with multidisciplinary teams caring for both mother and baby. Early institution of epidural analgesia is thought to be helpful.

SUMMARY

The Fontan operation presents a unique solution for several complex congenital heart lesions. Absence of a subpulmonary ventricle presents several long-term physiologic issues. As post-Fontan survival continues to increase, presentation for noncardiac surgery will continue to grow. Understanding the physiologic complexities as well as long-term sequalae will allow anesthesia providers to conduct a more informed and comprehensive perioperative evaluation as well as tailor the anesthetic to the challenges of these patients.

Clinics Care Points

- The anatomy underlying a Fontan circulation is highly variable.
- Preoperative desaturation in the unfenestrated Fontan patient should raise concern for elevated pulmonary pressures, significant collateral burden, or failing Fontan.
- Review of a recent echocardiogram should provide critical assessment of the ventricular function, valvular regurgitation, and Fontan circuit patency.
- PLE, plastic bronchitis, and liver dysfunction suggest failing Fontan physiology.

REFERENCES

1. van der Linde D, Konings EE, Slager MA, et al. Birth prevalence of congenital heart disease worldwide: a systematic review and meta-analysis. J Am Coll Cardiol 2011;58(21):2241–7.
2. Jolley M, Colan SD, Rhodes J, et al. Fontan physiology revisited. Anesth Analg 2015;121(1):172–82.
3. Yuki K, Casta A, Uezono S. Anesthetic management of noncardiac surgery for patients with single ventricle physiology. J Anesth 2011;25(2):247–56.
4. d'Udekem Y, Iyengar AJ, Galati JC, et al. Redefining expectations of long-term survival after the Fontan procedure: twenty-five years of follow-up from the entire

population of Australia and New Zealand. Circulation 2014;130(11 Suppl 1): S32–8.

5. Rychik J, Atz AM, Celermajer DS, et al. Evaluation and management of the child and adult with fontan circulation: a scientific statement from the American Heart Association. Circulation 2019;140:e234–84.

6. Ho PK, Lai CT, Wong SJ, et al. Three-dimensional mechanical dyssynchrony and myocardial deformation of the left ventricle in patients with tricuspid atresia after Fontan procedure. J Am Soc Echocardiogr 2012;25(4):393–400.

7. Averin K, Hirsch R, Seckeler MD, et al. Diagnosis of occult diastolic dysfunction late after the Fontan procedure using a rapid volume expansion technique. Heart 2016;102(14):1109–14.

8. Anderson PA, Sleeper LA, Mahony L, et al. Contemporary outcomes after the Fontan procedure: a Pediatric Heart Network multicenter study. J Am Coll Cardiol 2008;52(2):85–98.

9. Diller GP, Giardini A, Dimopoulos K, et al. Predictors of morbidity and mortality in contemporary Fontan patients: results from a multicenter study including cardiopulmonary exercise testing in 321 patients. Eur Heart J 2010;31(24):3073–83.

10. Guichard JB, Nattel S. Atrial cardiomyopathy: a useful notion in cardiac disease management or a passing fad? J Am Coll Cardiol 2017;70(6):756–65.

11. Odegard KC, McGowan FX Jr, Zurakowski D, et al. Procoagulant and anticoagulant factor abnormalities following the Fontan procedure: increased factor VIII may predispose to thrombosis. J Thorac Cardiovasc Surg 2003;125(6):1260–7.

12. Ghaferi AA, Hutchins GM. Progression of liver pathology in patients undergoing the Fontan procedure: chronic passive congestion, cardiac cirrhosis, hepatic adenoma, and hepatocellular carcinoma. J Thorac Cardiovasc Surg 2005;129(6): 1348–52.

13. van Nieuwenhuizen RC, Peters M, Lubbers LJ, et al. Abnormalities in liver function and coagulation profile following the Fontan procedure. Heart 1999; 82(1):40–6.

14. Blinder JJ, Goldstein SL, Lee VV, et al. Congenital heart surgery in infants: effects of acute kidney injury on outcomes. J Thorac Cardiovasc Surg 2012;143(2): 368–74.

15. Esch JJ, Salvin JM, Thiagarajan RR, et al. Acute kidney injury after Fontan completion: Risk factors and outcomes. J Thorac Cardiovasc Surg 2015; 150(1):190–7.

16. Mertens L, Hagler DJ, Sauer U, et al. Protein-losing enteropathy after the Fontan operation: an international multicenter study. PLE study group. J Thorac Cardiovasc Surg 1998;115(5):1063–73.

17. Atz AM, Zak V, Mahony L, et al. Longitudinal outcomes of patients with single ventricle after the Fontan procedure. J Am Coll Cardiol 2017;69(22):2735–44.

18. Itkin M, Piccoli DA, Nadolski G, et al. Protein-losing enteropathy in patients with congenital heart disease. J Am Coll Cardiol 2017;69(24):2929–37.

19. Allen KY, Downing TE, Glatz AC, et al. Effect of Fontan-associated morbidities on survival with intact Fontan circulation. Am J Cardiol 2017;119(11):1866–71.

20. Caruthers RL, Kempa M, Loo A, et al. Demographic characteristics and estimated prevalence of Fontan-associated plastic bronchitis. Pediatr Cardiol 2013;34(2):256–61.

21. Baum VC, Barton DM, Gutgesell HP. Influence of congenital heart disease on mortality after noncardiac surgery in hospitalized children. Pediatrics 2000; 105(2):332–5.

22. Wilson W, Taubert KA, Gewitz M, et al. Prevention of infective endocarditis: guidelines from the American Heart Association: a guideline from the American Heart Association Rheumatic Fever, Endocarditis, and Kawasaki Disease Committee, Council on Cardiovascular Disease in the Young, and the Council on Clinical Cardiology, Council on Cardiovascular Surgery and Anesthesia, and the Quality of Care and Outcomes Research Interdisciplinary Working Group. Circulation 2007;116(15):1736–54.
23. Dennis M, Zannino D, du Plessis K, et al. Clinical outcomes in adolescents and adults after the fontan procedure. J Am Coll Cardiol 2018;71(9):1009–17.
24. Alsaied T, Bokma JP, Engel ME, et al. Factors associated with long-term mortality after Fontan procedures: a systematic review. Heart 2017;103(2):104–10.
25. Ramamoorthy C, Haberkern CM, Bhananker SM, et al. Anesthesia-related cardiac arrest in children with heart disease: data from the Pediatric Perioperative Cardiac Arrest (POCA) registry. Anesth Analg 2010;110(5):1376–82.
26. Faraoni D, Zurakowski D, Vo D, et al. Post-operative outcomes in children with and without congenital heart disease undergoing noncardiac surgery. J Am Coll Cardiol 2016;67(7):793–801.
27. Faraoni D, Vo D, Nasr VG, et al. Development and validation of a risk stratification score for children with congenital heart disease undergoing noncardiac surgery. Anesth Analg 2016;123(4):824–30.

Modernizing Education of the Pediatric Anesthesiologist

Tanna J. Boyer, DO, MS*, Jian Ye, MD, Michael Andrew Ford, DO,
Sally A. Mitchell, EdD, MMSc

KEYWORDS

- Anesthesia • Anesthesiology • Education • Pediatric anesthesiology • Fellowship
- Training • ABA • ACGME

KEY POINTS

- There are clear requirements to become an American Board of Anesthesiology–certified pediatric anesthesiologist in the United States.
- Unfortunately, most of these requirements have not been validated or supported via educational research methodology.
- Second-year fellowships in pediatric anesthesiology are not common, with the exception of the second-year congenital cardiac anesthesia fellowship.
- Future training and accreditation in pediatric anesthesiology should be driven by competencies and entrustable professional activities versus the traditional time in training methodology.
- The pediatric anesthesia community would benefit from collaboration at a national level to study and create reliable and validated curricula for residents, fellows, and practicing pediatric anesthesiologists.

BACKGROUND

Current Requirements to Become a United States Pediatric Anesthesiologist

After graduation from medical school, a physician-in-training must complete an accredited, 4-year residency in anesthesiology that meets the requirements set forth by the Accreditation Council for Graduate Medical Education (ACGME) and its subgroup, the Review Committee for Anesthesiology.[1] The first year is fundamental clinical skills of medicine (post graduate year [PGY]1) followed by 36 months of clinical anesthesia (CA) (CA1–CA3/PGY2–PGY4).[1] During graduate medical education (GME) training, the physician-in-training must complete (a) rotations in pediatric

Department of Anesthesia, Indiana University School of Medicine, 1130 West Michigan Street, Fesler Hall 204, Indianapolis, IN 46202, USA
* Corresponding author.
E-mail address: tjboyer@iu.edu

Anesthesiology Clin 38 (2020) 545–558
https://doi.org/10.1016/j.anclin.2020.06.005   anesthesiology.theclinics.com
1932-2275/20/© 2020 Elsevier Inc. All rights reserved.

anesthesia (minimum 2 months and maximum 6 months; can be discontinuous), and (b) 100 total patients 12 years old or younger, 20 of whom must be 3 years old or younger, and 5 of whom must be less than 3 months old.[1] From December through May of each year, CA2/PGY3 residents apply to pediatric anesthesiology fellowships using the Electronic Residency Application System[2] and enter the National Residency Matching Program (NRMP).[3] Fellowship match results are announced in October.[3] Anesthesiology residents typically graduate June 30 and then begin fellowship training in July or August.

Pediatric anesthesiology fellows complete 12 months of training (PGY5), specializing in the perioperative and intraoperative care of medically complex children, infants, and neonates. Fellows are assessed by a clinical competency committee and a program director[4] for achievements on milestones,[5] minimum case log requirements[6] (**Table 1**), and an institutionally defined list of must-see index cases. Pediatric anesthesiology fellows complete 1 month of pediatric or neonatal intensive care training, the distribution of which varies among programs.

Since the introduction of the subspecialty examination in 2013, eligibility to sit for the American Board of Anesthesiology (ABA) Pediatric Anesthesiology Certification

Table 1
Pediatric anesthesiology fellowship minimum case numbers

Category	Minimum Case Number	Category	Minimum Case Number
Total number of patients	240	*Procedures (cont.)*	
Age of patient		Arterial cannulation	30
Neonates	15	Central venous cannulation	12
1–11 mo	40	Fiberoptic intubation	4
1–2 y	40	*Type of surgery*	
3–11 y	75	Airway[a]	7
12–17 y	30	Cardiac with bypass	15
ASA physical status		Cardiac without bypass	5
1	25	Craniofacial without cleft	3
II	42	Intra-abdominal/intracavitary	12
III	50	Intracranial neurosurgery	9
IV	20	Intrathoracic noncardiac	5
V	0	Major orthopedic	5
VI	0	Total neonate emergency	3
Procedures		Total solid organ transplant	0
Epidural/caudal	10	Other operative	55
General	200	Other nonoperative	10
Intrathecal	0	*Pain management*	
Peripheral nerve block	11	Consultations and patient-controlled analgesia	17

[a] Except tonsillectomy and adenoidectomy.

Data from Accreditation Council for Graduate Medical Education, Review Committee for Anesthesiology. Pediatric anesthesiology fellowship minimum case numbers. In: Program Requirements for Graduate Medical Education in Pediatric Anesthesiology (Subspecialty of Anesthesiology). 2016;1-2. Available at: https://www.acgme.Org/Portals/0/PFAssets/ProgramResources/042_Peds_AN_Minimums.pdf?ver=2016-01-07-124928-940. Accessed November 16, 2019.

Examination requires both completion of an ACGME-accredited pediatric anesthesiology fellowship and achievement of ABA diplomate status through ABMS certification in anesthesiology.[7] Although a grandfather option was offered to non–fellowship-trained anesthesiologists practicing pediatric anesthesiology to register for the examination between 2013 and 2015, some elected to not register or sit the certification examination prior to the deadline of January 1, 2019.[8]

History of Pediatric Anesthesiology Training in the United States

The historical evolution of postgraduate anesthesiology education literature has been curated and well documented by secondary authors.[9,10] This article focuses on how the changes to core residency requirements and subspecialty certification served as influences on the development of the pediatric anesthesiology fellowship. Since 1964, the accreditation of the core anesthesiology residency training included an intern/PGY1 and 2 additional years of CA training[9] **(Fig. 1)**. The first nonaccredited pediatric anesthesiology fellowships emerged in the 1970s.[10] In 1980, the ACGME changed the core residency requirements to include a clinical base year followed by 36 months of CA training.[9] This change also prescribed a minimum of 2 months of pediatric anesthesiology training and permitted a maximum of 6 months during residency, which led to an embedded fellowship opportunity for those residents seeking such a pathway.[10] The fellowship became ACGME accredited in 1997, and, 15 years later, the ABA agreed to establish subspecialty board certification[10] **(Fig. 2)**.

Aside from this traditional training pathway, the American Board of Pediatrics (ABP) and the ABA established combined training in pediatrics and anesthesiology in 2009. The program is 5 years in duration, substitutes many pediatric rotations for adult requirements (ie, pediatric intensive care unit for adult intensive care unit), and qualifies graduates to sit for both ABP and ABA primary certifications.[11] As of 2019, there are 7 training programs.[11] Despite the intense pediatric-focused training however, the graduates are not qualified to sit the ABA pediatric anesthesiology subspecialty

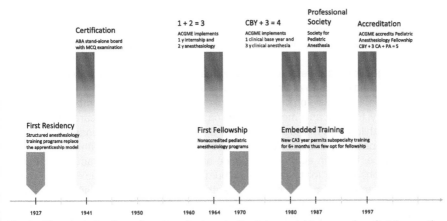

Fig. 1. Historical timeline of postgraduate anesthesiology residency and pediatric anesthesiology fellowship training in the United States. CBY, clinical base year; MCQ, multiple choice questions; PA, pediatric anesthesia fellowship. (*Data from* Ahmad M, Tariq R. History and evolution of anesthesia education in United States. J Anesth Clin Res. 2017;8(6) and Cladis F, Yanofsky S. Education in pediatric anesthesiology: the evolution of a specialty. Int Anesthesiol Clin. 2019 Oct 1;57(4):3-14.)

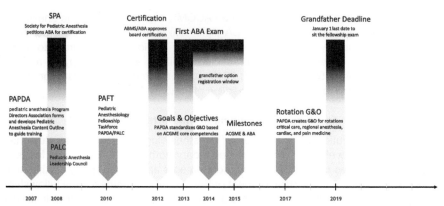

Fig. 2. Historical timeline of pediatric anesthesiology fellowship drivers and evolution in the United States. G&O, Goals and Objectives. (*Data from* Ahmad M, Tariq R. History and evolution of anesthesia education in United States. J Anesth Clin Res. 2017;8(6) and Cladis F, Yanofsky S. Education in pediatric anesthesiology: the evolution of a specialty. Int Anesthesiol Clin. 2019 Oct 1;57(4):3-14.)

examination.[7] Although lack of certification may not pose a practical challenge to producing anesthesiologists highly trained to provide anesthesia for pediatric patients, it does pose a credentialing barrier to obtaining employment at pediatric hospitals that require board-certified/board-eligible status in the subspecialty.

Goals and Objectives of Pediatric Anesthesiology Fellowship Training

As background, current practice models and case mixes of pediatric anesthesiology groups are described. Muffly and colleagues[12] estimated that fellowship-trained pediatric anesthesiologists function in 3 models, where one-third work in academic settings of tertiary-care hospitals, which necessitates fellowship training; one-third work in private practice settings that include some tertiary-care hospitals, which necessitates fellowship training; and the remaining one-third work in private practice caring for healthy children, which generally does not require the depth and breadth of knowledge and skills gained in fellowship. The question then becomes, "Is the training received in residency sufficient to care for this population of healthy pediatric patients?"

Thus, the goal of the core anesthesiology residency with respect to preparing any and all anesthesiologists to provide care to healthy pediatric patients also is considered. Are those anesthesiologists who completed the minimum 2 months of pediatric anesthesiology training and met minimum case logs expected to care for healthy, school-aged children? What about children under 2 years old? Neonates? A recent survey of US pediatric anesthesiologists revealed that compared with physicians in private practice, those in academic practice and those in private practice with academic affiliations cared for both a higher number of fellow-level index cases and a higher percentage of younger patients under the age of 18.[13] Additionally, 64% of academic practice physicians reported spending 50% of their time in free-standing children's hospitals. This is similar to 47% of private practice anesthesiologists with academic affiliations and much higher than 17% of private practice physicians.[13] Perhaps future studies will report morbidity and mortality data for these various practice groups.

Unfortunately, many questions remain unanswered in current literature. In the specialty of pediatric anesthesiology, traditionally the decision of readiness for practice has been left up to individual pediatric anesthesiologists, hospital credentialing committees, and healthcare institutions. Pressing questions to think about deeply and consider are, "What are the qualifications you want in an anesthesiologist to deliver an anesthetic to your child or grandchild? and Is the pediatric anesthesiology community currently meeting the standards for all children everywhere or just those patients who come to children's hospitals for their care?"

Given that approximately two-thirds of those who have completed pediatric anesthesiology fellowships do not work in large, tertiary care academic jobs,[12,13] should the primary goal of fellowship be to train pediatric anesthesiologists to provide superb clinical care for children of all ages and medical complexities? Or is fellowship training intended to cater to the one-third who work in pediatric anesthesia academia, to prepare clinical and educational instructors and scholars who will advance the practice of pediatric anesthesiology as academicians? A Canadian survey of practicing pediatric anesthesiologists[14] found that a large proportion of respondents did not feel competent enough to take care of children with congenital heart disease (CHD) or to perform ultrasound-guided regional anesthesia despite the fact that they routinely take care of CHD children and perform blocks. Even in outpatient pediatric surgeries routinely performed by general anesthesiologists, such as tonsillectomy and adenoidectomy, the available data show improved operating room efficiency with a fellowship-trained anesthesiologist.[15] Further studies need to be conducted to assess if there is a difference in outcome between fellowship-trained and general anesthesiologists.

The Pediatric Anesthesia Program Directors Association (PAPDA) and Pediatric Anesthesia Leadership Council (PALC) have tried to start answering these questions, creating notable strife amongst their group members. It has become clear that a majority of practicing pediatric anesthesiologists and pediatric anesthesiology programs see their goal as teaching fellows how to deliver the best clinical care possible. Where did the secondary goal originate from and why? To answer these questions, the development of the second-year pediatric fellowships must first be examined and discussed.

Optional Second-Year Pediatric Anesthesiology Fellowship

There is a push by some members in the pediatric anesthesiology community to move all fellowships to a 2-year curriculum. The Pediatric Anesthesiology Fellowship Task Force (PAFT) was formed through a collaboration with PALC and PAPDA in 2010.[9,10] After extensive work and careful consideration, the 2014 PAFT recommendation was to create optional second-year fellowships in cardiac, pain, regional, research, quality, and education.[16] Fellowship Year 1 and clinical case numbers would stay the same, and second-year tracks would be established to facilitate training of academic pediatric anesthesiologists with emphasis in leadership and scholarship.[16] The PALC also raised concerns from fellowship program directors and subspecialty leaders that pediatric anesthesiology fellows were not properly educated on how to conduct research, and furthermore, that the pediatric anesthesiology fellowship did not have a scholarship timeline requirement, as other pediatric subspecialties prescribe.[16] Their stated goals were to "improve the education, training, and preparation of the pediatric anesthesia workforce for the future of the specialty in healthcare, especially academic leaders...and to advance the knowledge of the specialty to improve outcomes of pediatric patients."[16]

Since the PAFT recommendation in 2014, pediatric cardiac anesthesiology second-year fellowships have flourished. The Congenital Cardiac Anesthesia Society (CCAS) has developed an organized, national curriculum with specialty-specific milestones and competencies.[17,18] There is discussion of seeking ACGME accreditation for the pediatric cardiac anesthesiology second-year fellowship. The success of second-year congenital cardiac fellowships is attributed to the high level of collaboration by the CCAS membership, as evidenced by the published template and milestones.[17,18] Despite the development of a community of practice with The Second Year Advanced Pediatric Anesthesiology Fellowship Network, no similar coordination in training exist for the other advanced fellowships. This possibly is due to lack of specialized professional societies and low participation by fellowship program directors.[19]

Recruitment Challenges

In the debate over whether second-year pediatric anesthesiology fellowships are necessary, a frequently overlooked aspect is the opinion of the trainees themselves. In order to attract residents and pediatric anesthesiologists to the advanced clinical fellowships, there has to be a demonstrated benefit beyond simply more clinical experience.[20] Fellowships need to be structured to further advance the career of these trainees who will likely become leaders in academic medicine. One of the goals of the advanced fellowship, regardless of its primary focus, should be on building leadership skills and networks.[20] Yet another challenge to recruitment necessitates addressing the newly created pay gap, because accreditation removes the option of supplemental pay and requires adherence to the standard PGY5 and PGY6 salary rates. It must be accepted that participation in pediatric anesthesiology and advanced fellowships is stagnant at best and possibly decreasing at a national level.

Over the past 20 years, there has been a steady increase in the number of pediatric anesthesiology fellowship programs and the number of positions offered. Cladis and colleagues[21] described a 150% increase in positions since the late 1990s, up from 100 to 259. The fill rate in the 2020 pediatric anesthesiology match was 166/220 positions, or 75%.[22] The NRMP listed 57 pediatric anesthesiology fellowship programs for the 2020 match.[22] In the 2019 match, 15 fellowship programs did not fill any positions, and an additional 9 programs had between 1 and 3 empty positions.[21] This represents 52% of pediatric anesthesiology fellowship programs with unfilled spots in 2020.[22]

Is it an achievement if all applicants who want a pediatric anesthesiology fellowship are able to match? If 97.8% of all applicants match,[21] are the best and brightest candidates chosen or are bodies chosen to fill the operating rooms and call schedules of academic pediatric hospitals across the country? Given that ABA board certification in pediatric anesthesiology is a written/computer-based examination and does not contain an oral or objective structured clinical examination (OSCE) section,[23] each individual program is trusted to verify that graduating fellows meet all clinical expectations and milestones.

The massive education debt of current trainees also must be taken into account. The Association of American Medical Colleges reported the average medical education debt at graduation was $200,000 in June 2019.[24] Is it appropriate to ask fellows to carry more debt and push off a substantial salary increase to gain knowledge of research and develop academic leadership qualities when only one-third of them enter academic pediatric anesthesiology? Would these important topics not be better taught in the first few years of faculty appointment? For example, consider if pediatric anesthesiology departments across the country offered graduating fellows 80% full-time equivalent (FTE) clinical appointments and 20% FTE academic time to grow and develop with structured, effective mentorship?

The Society for Pediatric Anesthesia (SPA) has convened its own GME Task Force to help address the second-year fellowship issue as well as pressing concerns related to the specialty. It is vitally important and necessary work. Brock-Utne and Jaffe ask this question in their recent *Anesthesiology News* article, "Is the Golden Age of

Academic Anesthesia Over?"[25] They state that "anesthesiology is losing its position as a respected academic discipline" and that many medical schools and hospital leadership view departments of anesthesiology as necessary for hospital surgery services, their greatest revenue source.[25] According to Brock-Utne and Jaffe,[25] some academic anesthesiology department services are offered to insurers below cost in contract negotiations because the hospital fee is by far the largest and most valuable to obtain. This is a dagger to academic anesthesiology practices, making departments indebted to deans and chief executive officers for any academic time.[25] Many academic anesthesiologists must use their free time (ie, vacation) if they wish to develop professionally, obtain promotion, publish, and advance the specialty.[25] These brilliant academic anesthesiologists go on to suggest a plan for the Association of University Anesthesiologists (AUA) to champion academic anesthesiology practices.[25] Perhaps the SPA should consider joining forces with Brock-Utne, Jaffe, and the AUA. The authors agree with their contention that "many academic anesthesia departments in the United States function simply as hospital revenue-generating training camps for Medicare-funded anesthesia residents."[25]

EXTERNAL DRIVERS AFFECTING PEDIATRIC ANESTHESIA EDUCATION
American College of Surgeons

More than 1 million anesthetics are delivered each year to children 18 years old and younger in children's hospitals in the United States.[26] The American College of Surgeons (ACS) launched a Task Force for Children's Surgical Care in 2012 to review the available evidence and establish standards for surgical care of children.[27] In 2017, ACS launched verifications for Levels I, II, and III children's surgical centers with the stated goal of "ensuring that pediatric surgical patients have access to high-quality care,"[28] similar to the ACS Trauma Verification program that was established 40 years ago. If all of the estimated 70 children's hospitals participate in this verification process, then every anesthetic for children less than 6 months old or American Society of Anesthesiologists (ASA) physical status classification III or higher will require a pediatric anesthesiologist to perform or supervise care.[28] As of January 2020, 21 out of 70 children's hospitals already were participating in this program.[28] Given this information, there may be an increased clinical need for pediatric anesthesiologists, especially if smaller and more rural hospitals begin participating in the ACS verification program.

Workforce

A 2016 publication[13] reported the demographics of US pediatric anesthesiologists. Muffly and colleagues[13] estimated 4048 anesthesiologists practicing pediatric anesthesiology in some capacity. This number comprises 8.8% of the anesthesiologist workforce and 0.5% of the physician workforce.[13] Of these, two-thirds (2672) are board certified in pediatric anesthesiology.[13] Looking at these numbers, it would appear that more pediatric anesthesiologists will be needed. According to a 2018 article by Muffly and colleagues,[26] however, the pediatric anesthesiology workforce supply may outpace the need from 2015 to 2035. One aspect not accounted for in the Muffly and colleagues[26] algorithm is outpatient surgeries. They were only able to estimate needs based on current cases in freestanding children's hospitals, not including ambulatory surgery centers.[26] This information is vital to pediatric anesthesiology fellowship planning, and there is a gap in the literature. It is problematic to make workforce need predictions without taking into account children's surgeries that occur in ambulatory surgery centers (ASCs). The likelihood of ASC patients being cared for by non–pediatric anesthesiology subspecialists is much greater than it is for patients in children's hospitals.[12,13,26] As the ACS verification program for children's surgical centers grows, it may influence workforce trends in ambulatory surgery centers as well.

CURRENT EDUCATION REQUIREMENTS AND IDENTIFIED GAPS

It often is believed that graduates of anesthesiology residency programs are capable of caring for healthy, school-aged children and those who do a pediatric anesthesiology fellowship choose to specialize in the care of neonates and children 2 years of age and younger. This statement, frequently used as advice when anesthesiology residents consider a pediatric anesthesiology fellowship, appears to hold strong roots in the ACGME requirements for core residents to care for 20 patients 2 years of age and younger with a subset of 5 who must be less than 3 months old.[1] The question asked earlier is reiterated, "Is 2 months of experience in pediatric anesthesiology and a minimum of 80 anesthetics for children ages 3 years old to 12 years old enough to qualify someone to take care of these children?" Extending this critical look to the ACGME requirements for pediatric anesthesiology fellows,[4,6] "Are the numbers shown in **Table 1** enough to develop CA skills necessary to care for critically ill neonates and children?"

SIMULATION TRAINING

Children are more likely than adults to experience morbidity and mortality in the perioperative period.[29] Their care requires a high level of skill and knowledge of complex medical conditions.[29] The margin for error in pediatrics is very small, much smaller than for adults. Developing methods to assess and improve advanced skills in pediatric anesthesiology training is imperative. Simulation has been shown to be a valuable tool for accomplishing this necessary skill development.[30–32]

For teaching specific procedural skills and sequences, partial task trainers are excellent tools. These models typically represent a part of the body on which the procedure is performed. They often are paired with computers to increase fidelity and realism. Models exist for training on intubation, intravenous line placement, arterial line placement, cricothyrotomy, intraosseous access, bronchoscopy, ultrasound-guided versions of the aforementioned models, and ultrasound diagnostic examinations, among others. Task trainers permit trainees to develop the procedural knowledge and motor skills necessary to complete tasks without risking harm to patients.[33]

A training program at Cincinnati Children's Hospital using the phantom task trainer and real-time feedback to teach ultrasound-guided regional anesthesia skills was successful in improving the regional anesthesia skills of the residents and fellows.[33] The term, *deliberate practice*, applies to real-time feedback by an expert coach and intentional self-reflection by the learner.[34]

Simulation also is useful for teaching trainees to manage certain clinical scenarios. Multiple centers joined together to develop high-fidelity simulation boot camps in which residents engaged in a variety of activities that simulated high-risk, low-frequency cases.[35] For example, a simulation-based training program was effective at improving survival of children after cardiopulmonary resuscitation.[36]

Additionally, simulation has an emerging role as part of certification. Simulation-based stations are included in ABMS ABA primary anesthesiology board certification examinations[37] in the form of OSCEs. Other countries, such as Israel and the United Kingdom, utilize similar OSCEs for anesthesiology certification.[38]

COMPETENCY-BASED EDUCATION AND ASSESSMENT

One difficulty in transitioning to a competence-based education (CBE) in anesthesiology has been the lack of acceptance by both trainees and attending physicians.[39] This type of education necessitates an individualized approach to education, where some residents are able to learn and advance quickly whereas others require more educational opportunities and time.[39,40] Some critics of CBE purport there is an inherent amount of subjective bias because the tools used for competency verification are yet to be validated.[40] However, the assessment tools currently used for time-based progression suffer the same lack of validation. ACGME milestones are formative, expressly not to be used in a summative manner,[1,4,5] lengthy, and not mobile-friendly for smartphone on-the-fly use; and, although they were developed through expert consensus, they have not been studied with respect to reliability and validity. Design, development, and testing of entrustable professional activities (EPAs)[41] and aligned assessment instruments are ongoing educational research being conducted by a national consortium of core anesthesiology residency programs.[42] Fellowships subsequently may follow with EPA development and aligned assessments.[43]

Another difficulty is how to make it financially possible to graduate a resident or fellow early who is not on a time-based track. If a trainee is determined competent after only 2 years for residency or 6 months for pediatric anesthesiology fellowship, what happens to the federal Medicaid money that funds the training? Can it be used to enroll another trainee off-cycle? Can it be used to further support the education and development of this person in a different way, perhaps with time spent developing research and teaching potential, leadership, communication, or advocacy? How can trainees meet ACGME work-hour requirements and ABA minimum required days of work? These drivers are out of the scope of this discussion. Likely, advocates of CBE will need to devise innovative solutions within these limitations.

HAVE LIFELONG LEARNERS BEEN CREATED THROUGH PEDIATRIC ANESTHESIOLOGY FELLOWSHIPS AND MAINTENANCE OF CERTIFICATION IN PEDIATRIC ANESTHESIOLOGY?

Maintenance of Certification in Anesthesia (MOCA) by the ABA is somewhat controversial. Many ABA diplomates question the minimal or nonexistent proof that participation in MOCA, especially Part 4, improves patient outcomes and makes a clinically superior anesthesiologist. Amid national questioning about the American Board of Internal Medicine and its money management,[44,45] the ABA re-envisioned MOCA with the second iteration MOCA 2.0.[46] Diplomates of the ABA no longer have to recertify by taking a high-stakes pass/fail examination every 10 years.[46] Instead, they must complete 30 questions per quarter by using the MOCA Minute app or Web site Part 3 and must obtain 25 points from specified activities every 5 years for quality improvement or Part 4 credit.[46] Diplomates of the ABA spend thousands of dollars each year to meet the requirements of MOCA 2.0. The authors applaud the ABA and Foundation for Anesthesia Education and Research for funding a biannually distributed grant for prospective, hypothesis-driven research projects which evaluate, "the value of primary certification and the Maintenance of Certification in Anesthesiology program (MOCA) to clinicians and the public."[47] With the development of MOCA 2.0 and this grant, the ABA is signifying that they truly do exist "to advance the highest standards of the practice of anesthesiology."[47] Per the ABA, the MOCA program, which is designed to promote lifelong learning, also is a commitment to quality clinical outcomes and patient safety.[47] The authors anxiously await reliability and validity studies, which substantiate that participation in MOCA is equated with a clinically superior pediatric anesthesiologist.

CONCLUSIONS: LOOKING TOWARD THE FUTURE OF PEDIATRIC ANESTHESIA EDUCATION

Although it is agreed that medical education and assessment should move toward competency-based curriculum, the neophyte stage of educational research within US anesthesiology residency and fellowship programs is acknowledged. Continued, multi-institutional research and analysis will guide the development and implementation of EPAs for the specialty. Alliances among accreditation, certification, and professional organizations are necessary to affect these proposed changes and overcome barriers and challenges. The pediatric anesthesiology education community needs to work collaboratively at a national level to produce reliable and validated curricula for both residents and fellows. Quality programs and training opportunities must be ensured by incorporating validated didactics, simulation, and clinical experiences. It is owed to the specialty of pediatric anesthesiology, trainees, and most importantly, patients, to prevail.

Clinics Care Points

- Recently, there has been an increase in fellowship positions for pediatric anesthesiology, many recruitment challenges, and trends toward increasingly unfilled positions in the pediatric anesthesiology fellowship match.

- It is unclear if current training program positions in pediatric anesthesiology will meet future workforce needs; data collection and analysis on pediatric anesthesiology cases for outpatient surgeries is necessary to answer this question.

- A probable solution to mitigate the above pediatric anesthesiology fellowship challenges would be to increase the number of required cases during pediatric anesthesiology fellowship training. The pediatric anesthesiology education community would benefit from a study that examines required case numbers and actual cases numbers at all institutions which sponsor pediatric anesthesiology fellowships, as well as studies examining the development and achievement of clinical competency. Concordantly, if we expect all physician anesthesiologists to care for healthy school-aged children, then the ACGME should increase required case numbers for children under 12 years-old and number of weeks on pediatric anesthesiology rotations during core anesthesiology residency. This latter suggestion also lacks evidence in current literature to guide decision making.

- If the pediatric anesthesiology community seeks to develop academic leaders in the field, then a structured, validated faculty development curriculum should be developed in areas including: quality Improvement, leadership, communication, scholarship, dissemination strategies, etc. This program could also incorporate coaching, mentorship, and sponsorship from those currently in leadership positions at academic pediatric anesthesiology institutions. We must push our institutions and members to take seats at the negotiating table in order to ensure adequate department funding. Only this will allow pediatric anesthesiologists to meet the tripartite mission of clinical care, research, and education.

DISCLOSURE

The authors have no commercial or financial conflicts of interest. S.A. Mitchell and T.J. Boyer are both recipients of a Just in Time Training in Anesthesia Curriculum Enhancement Grant from Indiana University Purdue University of Indianapolis and an Indiana University Health Values Education Grant for Creation of a Nationally Recognized

Anesthesia POCUS Curriculum and Implementation for IU Health Department of Anesthesia.

REFERENCES

1. Accreditation Council for Graduate Medical Education. ACGME program requirements for graduate medical education in anesthesiology 2019. p. 1–66. Available at: https://www.acgme.org/Portals/0/PFAssets/ProgramRequirements/040_Anesthesiology_2019_TCC.pdf?ver=2019-03-21-161242-837. Accessed November 16, 2019.

2. Association of American Medical Colleges. Electronic residency application service. Available at: https://www.aamc.org/services/eras-for-institutions/program-staff/getting-started. Accessed November 16, 2019.

3. National Resident Matching Program. 2019. Available at: http://www.nrmp.org/. Accessed November 16, 2019.

4. Accreditation Council for Graduate Medical Education. ACGME program requirements for graduate medical education in pediatric anesthesiology (subspecialty of anesthesiology) 2019. p. 1–52. Available at: https://www.acgme.org/Portals/0/PFAssets/ProgramRequirements/042_PediatricAnesthesiology_2019.pdf?ver=2019-06-17-095425-273. Accessed November 16, 2019.

5. Accreditation Council for Graduate Medical Education, American Board of Anesthesiology. The Pediatric Anesthesiology Milestone Project. 2015:1-20. Available at: https://www.acgme.org/Portals/0/PDFs/Milestones/PediatricAnesthesiology.pdf. Accessed November 16, 2019.

6. Accreditation Council for Graduate Medical Education, Review Committee for Anesthesiology. Pediatric anesthesiology fellowship minimum case numbers. In: Program Requirements for Graduate Medical Education in Pediatric Anesthesiology (Subspecialty of Anesthesiology). 1-2. 2016. Available at: https://www.acgme.org/Portals/0/PFAssets/ProgramResources/042_Peds_AN_Minimums.pdf?ver=2016-01-07-124928-940. Accessed November 16, 2019.

7. American Board of Anesthesiology. Pediatric anesthesiology certification examination. Available at: http://www.theaba.org/Exams/Pediatric-Anesthesiology/Pediatric-Anesthesiology. Accessed November 16, 2019.

8. American Board of Anesthesiology. When is the last time I can register for the Pediatric Anesthesiology Examination with "grandfathering criteria"? In: Ask the ABA. 2014. Available at: http://www.theaba.org/Ask-the-ABA#collapseSix. Accessed November 16, 2019.

9. Ahmad M, Tariq R. History and evolution of anesthesia education in United States. J Anesth Clin Res 2017;8(6):1–9.

10. Cladis F, Yanofsky S. Education in pediatric anesthesiology: the evolution of a specialty. Int Anesthesiol Clin 2019;57(4):3–14.

11. The American Board of Pediatrics. Pediatric-anesthesiology training program. Available at: https://www.abp.org/content/pediatrics-anesthesiology-program. Accessed December 8, 2019.

12. Muffly M, Scheinker D, Muffly T, et al. Practice characteristics of board-certified pediatric anesthesiologists in the US: a nationwide survey. Cureus 2019;11(9):e5745.

13. Muffly MK, Muffly TM, Weterings R, et al. The current landscape of US pediatric anesthesiologists: demographic characteristics and geographic distribution. Anesth Analg 2016;123(1):179–85.

14. O'Leary JD, Crawford MW. Perspectives on Canadian core fellowship training in pediatric anesthesia: a survey of graduate fellows. Can J Anaesth 2015;62(10): 1071–81.

15. Dewyer NA, Kram YA, Long S, et al. Impact of a pediatric anesthesiologist on operating room efficiency during pediatric tonsillectomies and adenotonsillectomies. Ear Nose Throat J 2017;96(6):E24–8.

16. Andropoulos DB, Walker SG, Kurth CD, et al. Advanced second year fellowship training in pediatric anesthesiology in the United States. Anesth Analg 2014; 118(4):800–8.

17. DiNardo JA, Andropoulos DB, Baum VC. Special article: a proposal for training in pediatric cardiac anesthesia. Anesth Analg 2010;110(4):1121–5.

18. Nasr VG, Guzzetta NA, Miller-Hance WC, et al. Consensus statement by the congenital cardiac anesthesia society: milestones for the pediatric cardiac anesthesia fellowship. Anesth Analg 2019;126(1):198–207.

19. Benzon HA, De Oliveira GS Jr, Hardy CA, et al. Status of pediatric anesthesiology fellowship research education in the United States: a survey of fellowship program directors. Paediatr Anaesth 2014;24(3):327–31.

20. McGowan FX Jr, Davis PJ. The advanced pediatric anesthesiology fellowship: moving beyond a clinical apprenticeship. Anesth Analg 2014;118(4):701–3.

21. Cladis FP, Lockman JL, Lupa MC, et al. Pediatric anesthesiology fellowship positions: is there a mismatch? Anesth Analg 2019;129(6):1784–6.

22. National Resident Matching Program. Results and data: specialties matching service 2020 appointment year. Washington, DC: National Resident Matching Program; 2020. p. 1–158. Available at: https://mk0nrmp3oyqui6wqfm.kinstacdn.com/wp-content/uploads/2020/02/Results-and-Data-SMS-2020.pdf. Accessed March 5, 2020.

23. American Board of Anesthesiology. Pediatric Anesthesiology (PA) Certification Examination. 2016. Available at: http://www.theaba.org/Exams/Pediatric-Anesthesiology/Pediatric-Anesthesiology. Accessed March 5, 2020.

24. Association of American Medical Colleges [AAMC]. Statement for the record submitted by the Association of American Medical Colleges (AAMC) to the House of Representatives Committee on Small Business: The doctor is out. Rising student loan debt and the decline of the small medical practice. Submitted June 11, 2019:1-7. Available at: https://www.aamc.org/system/files/c/1/498034-aamcstatementtothehousesmallbusinesscommitteeregardingmedicaled.pdf. Accessed March 5, 2020.

25. Brock-Utne JG, Jaffe RA. Is the golden age of academic anesthesia over? Academic anesthesia: quo vadis? Anesthesiology News. 2020. Available at: https://www.anesthesiologynews.com/Correspondence/Article/02-20/Is-the-Golden-Age-of-Academic-Anesthesia-Over-/57173. Accessed May 10, 2017.

26. Muffly MK, Singleton M, Agarwal R, et al. The pediatric anesthesiology workforce: projecting supply and trends 2015–2035. Anesth Analg 2018;126(2):568–78.

27. American College of Surgeons. Optimal resources for children's surgical care v.1 released 2015. Available at: https://www.facs.org/-/media/files/quality-programs/csv/acs-csv_standardsmanual.ashx. Accessed May 10, 2017.

28. American College of Surgeons Children's Surgery Verification Program. 2017. Available at: https://www.facs.org/qualityprograms/childrens-surgery/childrens-surgery-verification; https://www.facs.org/quality-programs/childrens-surgery/childrens-surgery-verification. Accessed May 10, 2017.

29. Murat I, Constant I, Maud'huy H. Perioperative anaesthetic morbidity in children: a database of 24,165 anaesthetics over a 30-month period. Paediatr Anaesth 2004;14(2):158–66.

30. Fehr JJ, Boulet JR, Waldrop WB, et al. Simulation-based assessment of pediatric anesthesia skills. Anesthesiology 2011;115(6):1308–15.

31. Blum RH, Muret-Wagstaff SL, Boulet JR, et al. Simulation-based assessment to reliably identify key resident performance attributes. Anesthesiology 2018; 128(4):821–31.

32. Cooper JB, Taqueti V. A brief history of the development of mannequin simulators for clinical education and training. Postgrad Med J 2008;84(997):563–70.

33. Moore DL, Ding L, Sadhasivam S. Novel real-time feedback and integrated simulation model for teaching and evaluating ultrasound-guided regional anesthesia skills in pediatric anesthesia trainees. Paediatr Anaesth 2012;22(9):847–53.

34. Mitchell SA, Boyer TJ. Deliberate practice in medical simulation. StatPearls.. 2020. Available at: https://www.statpearls.com/kb/viewarticle/63806?utm_source=pubmed. Accessed May 10, 2020.

35. Ambardekar AP, Singh D, Lockman JL, et al. Pediatric anesthesiology fellow education: is a simulation-based boot camp feasible and valuable? Paediatr Anaesth 2016;26(5):481–7.

36. Andreatta P, Saxton E, Thompson M, et al. Simulation-based mock codes significantly correlate with improved pediatric patient cardiopulmonary arrest survival rates. Pediatr Crit Care Med 2011;12(1):33–8.

37. American Board of Anesthesiology. Anesthesiology certification examination. Available at: http://www.theaba.org/Exams/APPLIED-(Staged-Exam)/About-APPLIED-(Staged-Exam). Accessed November 16, 2019.

38. Hastie MJ, Spellman JL, Pagano PP, et al. Designing and implementing the objective structured clinical examination in anesthesiology. Anesthesiology 2014;120(1):196–203.

39. Chuan A, Wan AS, Royse CF, et al. Competency-based assessment tools for regional anaesthesia: a narrative review. Br J Anaesth 2018;120(2):264–73.

40. Ebert TJ, Fox CA. Competency-based education in anesthesiology: history and challenges. Anesthesiology 2014;120(1):24–31.

41. Cate OT. Entrustment as assessment: recognizing the ability, the right, and the duty to act. J Grad Med Educ 2016,8(2):261–2.

42. Maniker R, Ambardekar A, Chen F, et al. Defining entrustable professional activities for United States anesthesiology residency training. San Francisco, CA: Association of University Anesthesiologists annual meeting poster session; 2020. Available at: https://www.aievolution.com/ars2001/index.cfm?do=abs.viewAbs&abs=4698. Accessed May 20, 2020.

43. Viola L, Clay S, Samuels P. Education in pediatric anesthesiology: competency, innovation, and professionalism in the 21st century. Int Anesthesiol Clin 2012; 50(4):1–2.

44. Fisher WG. Opinion: time for an ABIM board review on maintenance of certification. Physician Sense. 2018. Available at: https://www.mdlinx.com/physiciansense/opinion-time-for-an-abim-board-review-on-maintenance-of-certification/. Accessed May 20, 2020.

45. Gallegos A. Class-action suit filed against ABIM over MOC. Internal Medicine News. 2018. Available at: https://www.mdedge.com/internalmedicine/article/191234/practice-management/class-action-suit-filed-against-abim-over-moc. Accessed May 20, 2020.

46. American Board of Anesthesiology. About MOCA 2.0. Available at: http://www.theaba.org/MOCA/About-MOCA-2-0. Accessed May 21, 2020.

47. American Board of Anesthesiology. FAER/ABA announce new co-sponsored Research in Education Grant 2018. Available at: http://www.theaba.org/ABOUT/News-Announcements/FAER-ABA-Announce-New-Co-Sponsored-Research-in-Edu. Accessed May 21, 2020.

Regional Anesthesia
Options for the Pediatric Patient

Nisha Pinto, MD*, Amod Sawardekar, MD, MBA,
Santhanam Suresh, MD, MBA

KEYWORDS

- Pediatric regional anesthesia ● Peripheral nerve block ● Peripheral nerve catheter
- Ultrasound-guided regional anesthesia

KEY POINTS

- Regional anesthesia is safe and effective in the pediatric population.
- Use of ultrasound guidance for peripheral nerve blocks is beneficial to be able to visualize needle advancement and local anesthetic deposition.
- For longer acting analgesia, continuous nerve catheters can be used.

INTRODUCTION

The use of regional anesthesia in the pediatric population has been increasing, especially with the introduction of ultrasound technology.[1] There have been multiple reviews addressing the safety and complication rates in this population, as a large percentage of these regional blocks are performed after the induction of general anesthesia.[1-3] Regional anesthesia is an important contributor of multimodal analgesia to improve patients' health care experience and reduce hospital length of stays.

The Pediatric Regional Anesthesia Network (PRAN) database is a multicenter, collaborative registry looking specifically at the safety of regional nerve blocks performed at numerous children's hospitals. The most recent analysis of these data includes a large data set, with more than 100,000 regional blocks, including both peripheral and neuraxial blocks.[4] The investigators concluded that the use of regional blockade in children was safe, with minor catheter-related failures being the most common adverse events.[4] There were no reported cases of permanent neurologic damage, and the rates of transient neurologic deficit and local anesthesia toxicity were low, at 2.4 and 0.76, respectively, per 10,000.[4] In addition to the low incidence

Department of Pediatric Anesthesiology, Ann & Robert H. Lurie Children's Hospital of Chicago, Feinberg School of Medicine, Northwestern University, 225 East Chicago Avenue, Box 19, Chicago, IL 60611, USA
* Corresponding author.
E-mail address: npinto@luriechildrens.org

Anesthesiology Clin 38 (2020) 559–575
https://doi.org/10.1016/j.anclin.2020.05.005
1932-2275/20/© 2020 Elsevier Inc. All rights reserved.
anesthesiology.theclinics.com

of complications, the use of ultrasound for regional anesthesia has allowed local anesthetic dosing to decrease. This is important in the neonatal and infant population and may increase effectiveness of blocks due to accurate localization.[5]

This review discusses the use of regional anesthesia through ultrasound guidance in the pediatric population, and this includes indications, anatomy, ultrasound techniques, and complications of peripheral nerve blocks of the extremities and trunk based on the current pediatric literature.

DISCUSSION
Upper Extremity Blocks

The brachial plexus can be blocked at several different locations to provide motor and sensory blocks for children undergoing surgical procedures of the upper extremity. Blockade of the brachial plexus can be completed at the axillary, interscalene, supraclavicular, and infraclavicular locations. The most common type of brachial plexus block performed is the supraclavicular block. With the increased use of ultrasound guidance, these blocks can be performed at any location safely and effectively. Regional anesthesia with the use of ultrasound guidance allows for better recognition of the anatomy of the brachial plexus and improved visualization of nearby structures during needle placement.

Axillary block
Indications, anatomy, and complications The axillary block provides analgesia to the elbow, forearm, and hand. The terminal branches of the brachial plexus, the median, radial, and ulnar nerves, lie superficially in the axilla where they can be blocked as they surround the axillary artery. Although anatomic variations exist, the ulnar nerve is most commonly located anterior and inferior to the artery, and the radial nerve lies posteriorly. The median nerve is usually located superior and anterior to the axillary artery (**Fig. 1**).[6] An important consideration to successfully perform this block is the location of the musculocutaneous nerve, as it lies outside the axillary neurovascular sheath and therefore must be blocked separately from the other nerves. This nerve provides sensation to the posterior aspect of the forearm and is located between the biceps brachii and coracobrachialis muscles.

Ultrasound-guided axillary blocks in the pediatric literature are not well described, but the techniques used in adults can be applied.[7,8] With the ultrasound probe placed transverse to the humerus, an out-of-plane technique may be used.[9] Circumferential spread of local anesthetic can be achieved with multiple injections while repositioning

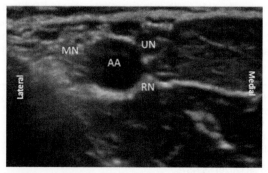

Fig. 1. Axillary approach to the brachial plexus block. AA, axillary artery; MN, median nerve; RN, radial nerve; UN, ulnar nerve.

the needle, which must be done carefully, given the axillary sheath's superficial depth.[10,11]

Complications of an axillary block include infection, intravascular injection, hematoma, and nerve injury. With ultrasound guidance, the risk of accidental intravascular injection into the axillary artery is likely reduced.

Interscalene block

Indications, anatomy, and complications The interscalene block provides analgesia to the shoulder and proximal humerus. This brachial plexus block is performed at the interscalene groove, where the trunks and roots lie posterior to the sternocleidomastoid muscle. The nerve roots, C5–C7, lie between the anterior and middle scalene muscles (**Fig. 2**). The C8 and T1 dermatomes are often spared, so this block may not adequately cover more distal procedures of the arm.

This block can be performed under ultrasound guidance by placing the probe in the transverse oblique plane at the lateral edge of the sternocleidomastoid muscle, at the level of the cricoid cartilage. The interscalene groove, which is located deep to the sternocleidomastoid muscle and lateral to the subclavian artery, contains the neurovascular bundle of the C5, C6, and C7 nerve roots.[12] The use of ultrasound to perform this block may decrease the volume of local anesthetic needed compared with using nerve stimulation.[13]

Side effects associated with the interscalene block include hemidiaphragmatic paralysis, recurrent laryngeal nerve block, and Horner syndrome.[13,14] If larger volumes of local anesthetic are used, there are risks of contralateral, epidural, or intrathecal spread, leading to respiratory depression and possible loss of consciousness. The use of ultrasound may decrease the amount of local anesthetic needed for this block.[15,16] Despite concern for performing this block under general anesthesia due to risk of neurologic complications, a joint committee practice advisory from the European Society of Regional Anesthesia and Pain Therapy and the American Society of Regional Anesthesia and Pain Medicine stated that performing regional anesthesia in the pediatric population under general anesthesia or deep sedation was safe.[17]

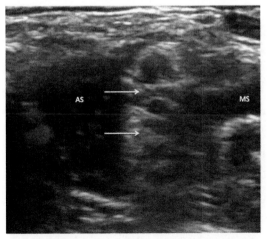

Fig. 2. Interscalene block. Arrows indicate the interscalene groove. AS, anterior scalene muscle; MS, middle scalene muscle.

Supraclavicular block

Indications, anatomy, and complications The supraclavicular block, which is performed at the level of the divisions, provides analgesia to the upper arm, elbow, and hand. The divisions of the brachial plexus are located superficial and lateral to the subclavian artery (**Fig. 3**). All roots of the brachial plexus are blocked at this location. However, the suprascapular nerve, which innervates the shoulder joint, may be spared.

Under ultrasound guidance, the probe is placed in the coronal-oblique plane just superior to the upper border of the midclavicle. The subclavian artery lies adjacent to the brachial plexus and appears hypoechoic and pulsatile. In an in-plane approach, the needle is directed medially toward the brachial plexus, which lies lateral and superior to the subclavian artery. This approach decreases the risk of intraneural injection as well as the risk of vascular injury.[8]

Complications of this block include intravascular injection, infection, hematoma, and pneumothorax. The risk of pneumothorax may be higher than other brachial plexus blocks due to the proximity of the apex of the lung, which lies just medial to the first rib. An in-plane approach with visualization of the entire needle while performing this block may help prevent this complication.

Infraclavicular block

Indications, anatomy, and complications The infraclavicular block, similar to the supraclavicular block, is used for surgeries of the elbow, forearm, and hand. At this level, the cords of the brachial plexus are blocked. The cords are superficial to the axillary artery and veins and medial and inferior to the coracoid process (**Fig. 4**). The pectoralis major and minor are located superficial to the brachial plexus. The medial cord can be difficult to visualize on ultrasound due to its location between the axillary artery and vein.[18] This location is well suited for placement of brachial plexus catheters in children for prolonged analgesia.[19,20]

In performing an ultrasound-guided infraclavicular block, the probe is placed inferior to the clavicle in a transverse orientation. The needle is directed laterally toward the cords and advanced using an out-of-plane technique. The local anesthetic is injected

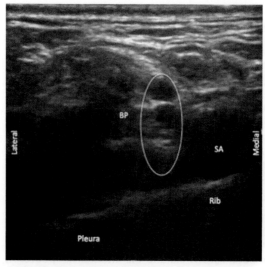

Fig. 3. Supraclavicular block. BP, brachial plexus; SA, subclavian artery.

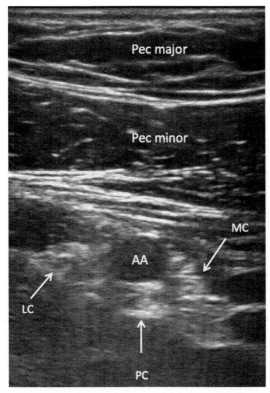

Fig. 4. Infraclavicular block. AA, axillary artery; LC, lateral cord; MC, medial cord; PC, posterior cord; Pec major, pectoralis major muscle; Pec minor, pectoralis minor muscle.

into the deep portion of the neurovascular sheath.[21] Another technique, described by De José María and colleagues,[18] places the probe parallel to the clavicle in a parasagittal plane, and the needle is directed toward the brachial plexus.

Complications related to infraclavicular blocks are similar to those of supraclavicular blocks.[22] Vascular injury is also possible, given the proximity of the axillary artery and vein.

Lower Extremity Blocks

Femoral and saphenous nerve blocks

Indications, anatomy, and complications The femoral nerve block is commonly used for surgeries of the knee. This block provides analgesia to the anterior thigh and knee and can be performed as a single-shot technique; a continuous catheter can be placed when longer-term pain relief is required.[23,24] The femoral nerve, originating from L2 to L4, is located deep to the fascia iliaca and lateral to the femoral artery and vein (**Fig. 5**). On ultrasound, the neurovascular bundle is visualized with the probe placed in the inguinal crease.[25] Given the risk of falls due to motor blockade, an alternative is to block the saphenous nerve, a branch of the femoral nerve, at the level of the adductor canal (**Fig. 6**). The saphenous block can be performed proximally to provide sensory analgesia to the anterior knee or more distally to block sensation to the medial aspect of the lower leg.[26]

For ultrasound-guided femoral nerve blocks, the probe is placed in the inguinal crease. The femoral artery is identified, and the nerve is visualized just lateral to the

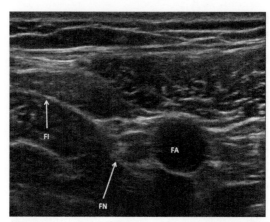

Fig. 5. Femoral nerve block. FA, femoral artery; FI, fascia iliaca; FN, femoral nerve.

pulsating artery. The femoral vein should be visualized just medial to the artery. In contrast to the artery, it does not appear pulsatile and should be compressible. The needle should be placed at the lateral portion of the femoral nerve, using an in-plane or out-of-plane approach, with local anesthetic deposited to surround the nerve.[23,26] The saphenous nerve block is performed with the probe placed on the medial aspect of the thigh while the leg is abducted and laterally rotated. In an in-plane approach, the sartorius muscle is identified, and the needle is directed toward the saphenous nerve where local anesthetic is injected.

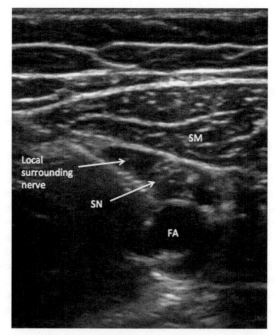

Fig. 6. Saphenous nerve block. FA, femoral artery; SM, sartorius muscle; SN, saphenous nerve.

Complications for the femoral and saphenous nerve blocks include hematoma from vascular puncture, nerve injury, and infection.

Sciatic block

Indications, anatomy, and complications The sciatic nerve is blocked via the subgluteal, popliteal fossa, or anterior approach in children.[26,27] The nerve roots of L4 to S3 comprise the sciatic nerve. This nerve provides sensation to the posterior thigh as well as the distal leg; the medial compartment receives innervation from the femoral nerve. The nerve courses and exits the pelvis through the greater sciatic foramen and then travels inferiorly to the gluteus maximus muscle (**Fig. 7**). It divides into the tibial and common peroneal nerves around the posterior popliteal fossa (**Fig. 8**). This block may be performed as a single-shot or continuous catheter technique in the pediatric population.[28,29]

The three different approaches to the sciatic nerve block can all be performed using ultrasound guidance. In the subgluteal approach, the patient lies in the prone or lateral decubitus position with the hip and knee flexed. The probe is placed between the greater trochanter and the ischial tuberosity, and the sciatic nerve is identified deep to the gluteus maximus muscle (see **Fig. 7**). The needle can be advanced in an in-plane or out-of-plane approach, with local anesthetic injected to surround the nerve.[30,31] The anterior approach allows the patient to remain supine. In this approach, the patient's leg is abducted and laterally rotated, and the ultrasound probe is placed just below the inguinal crease. Once the femur is identified, the nerve can be found

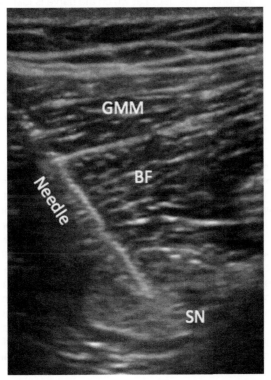

Fig. 7. Subgluteal approach to the sciatic nerve block. BF, biceps femoris muscle; GMM, gluteus maximus muscle; SN, sciatic nerve.

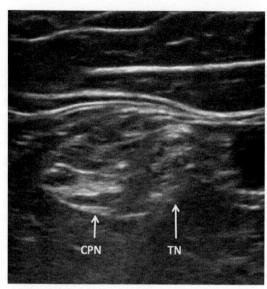

Fig. 8. Popliteal approach to the sciatic nerve block. CPN, common peroneal nerve; TN, tibial nerve.

deep and medial to the femur. The depth at which the nerve is identified in larger patients can be quite deep, making this approach challenging in the adolescent age group or in obese patients. Finally, the sciatic nerve can be blocked at the popliteal fossa.[32] The nerve splits into the common peroneal and tibial nerves in this location (see **Fig. 8**). The patient can remain supine, or be in a prone position, and the probe is placed in the popliteal crease to visualize the popliteal artery. The tibial nerve is located adjacent to the artery and can be traced proximally where it merges with the common peroneal nerve to make up the sciatic nerve.

Complications of this block include hematoma from vascular puncture, infection, and local anesthetic toxicity.

Lumbar plexus block

Indications, anatomy, and complications The lumbar plexus has branches that provide innervation to the lower abdomen and upper leg and lies deep to the paravertebral muscles within the psoas muscle. It originates from the nerve roots of T12 to L5, and its branches include the lateral femoral cutaneous, genitofemoral, femoral, and obturator nerves. To provide complete sensory analgesia to the lower extremity, a lumbar plexus block in combination with a sciatic nerve block can be performed.[33]

With the patient placed in the lateral decubitus position, the probe is placed lateral to midline, and the transverse processes of L4 or L5 are identified. The erector spinae and quadratus lumborum muscles are located deep to the transverse process, and deep to that, within the psoas major muscle, the plexus will be found. The plexus can be difficult to identify in this area solely with ultrasound guidance, as the plexus has similar echogenicity as the muscle. Therefore, to facilitate performance of this block, a nerve stimulator serves as a useful adjunct. Proximity to the plexus can be confirmed with twitches of the quadriceps muscles.

Complications include hematoma, infection, and retroperitoneal bleeding due to the anatomic location and depth of the lumbar plexus.

Truncal blocks

Truncal blocks, which include the rectus sheath block, transversus abdominis plane block, ilioinguinal/iliohypogastric block, paravertebral block, erector spinae plane block, and pudendal block have been used more frequently since the inception of widespread ultrasound use. They are a useful analgesic adjunct for a multitude of thoracic and abdominal surgeries.

Rectus sheath block

Indications, anatomy, and complications The rectus sheath block can be used for umbilical hernia and single-incision laparoscopic surgeries, as it provides analgesia to the midline, anterior abdominal wall.[34] The thoracolumbar nerves, T7 to T11, lie posterior to the abdominus muscle, which is located on the anterior abdominal wall (**Fig. 9**).

Using ultrasound guidance, the rectus abdominis muscle is identified when the probe is placed lateral to the umbilicus. The rectus abdominis is the only muscle layer at this level, and the posterior sheath is found just deep to this muscle and above the peritoneum. The needle is visualized using an in-plane technique and advanced medially between the rectus abdominis muscle and the posterior sheath. Local anesthetic is injected between the muscle and this sheath.[35] This block may fail if local anesthetic is deposited between the two layers of the posterior rectus sheath.

Complications of this block include intravascular injection, infection, and possible bowel injury.

Ilioinguinal/iliohypogastric block

Indications, anatomy, and complications The ilioinguinal/iliohypogastric (IL/IH) block can be used to provide analgesia for surgeries to the inguinal area and anterior scrotum, including repair of an inguinal hernia and cryptorchidism. The nerves

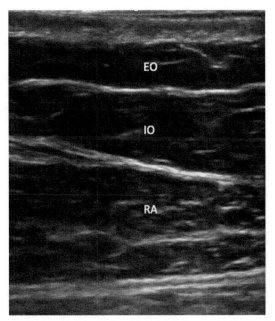

Fig. 9. Rectus sheath block. EO, external oblique muscle; IO, internal oblique muscle; RA, rectus abdominis muscle.

originate from the T12 and L1 roots of the lumbar plexus. Because these nerves travel across the internal oblique aponeurosis, they can be blocked medial to the anterior superior iliac spine. This block has been shown to be equivalent in terms of pain relief compared with caudal blocks for inguinal surgeries, with a lower volume of local anesthetic needed and a longer block duration.[36,37]

For ultrasound-guided IL/IH blocks, the probe is placed medial to the anterior superior iliac spine, in line with the umbilicus. The three muscle layers are visualized: the external oblique, internal oblique, and transversus abdominus. At this level, however, the external oblique muscle may be aponeurotic (**Fig. 10**).[38] The needle is advanced, in-plane, toward the IL/IH nerves, which lie between the internal oblique and transversus abdominal muscle layers. The nerves seem ovular.

Complications of this block include bowel injury, infection at the injection site, intravascular injection, femoral nerve injury, and pelvic hematoma.

Transversus abdominis plane block

Indications, anatomy, and complications The transversus abdominis plane (TAP) block provides analgesia to the anterior abdominal wall by blocking nerves that innervate the skin, muscles, and parietal peritoneum. This block is a useful adjunct in abdominal, gynecologic, and laparoscopic surgeries. However, it does not provide a surgical level of analgesia.[39] Lateral to the rectus abdominis, there are three abdominal muscle layers: the external oblique, internal oblique, and transverse abdominus. The plane between the internal oblique and transverse abdominis layer is where the thoracolumbar nerve roots, from T8 to L1, are located (**Fig. 11**). To provide a longer duration of analgesia, a continuous TAP catheter is placed to help avoid neuraxial analgesia.[40,41]

Under ultrasound guidance, the probe is placed near the umbilicus and then moved laterally away from the rectus abdominus until the three muscle layers are identified.[42] The needle is inserted in an in-plane technique into the TAP plane, which lies between the internal oblique and transverse abdominus layers; local anesthetic is deposited and causes separation of the two layers along the fascial plane.[39]

Complications include infection, bowel puncture, and intravascular injection.

Paravertebral nerve block

Indications, anatomy, and complications The paravertebral nerve block (PVNB) is a useful analgesic adjunct in thoracic and upper abdominal procedures. The spinal nerves are blocked in the paravertebral space, which is an area bordered by the

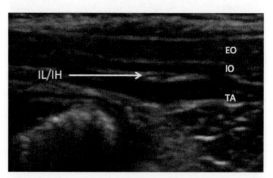

Fig. 10. Ilioinguinal/iliohypogastric nerve block. EO, external oblique muscle; IL/IH, ilioinguinal/iliohypogastric nerves; IO, internal oblique muscle; transversus abdominis (TA) muscle.

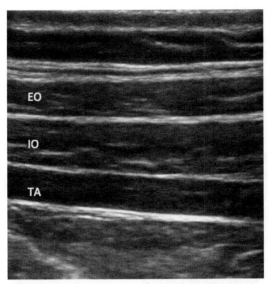

Fig. 11. Transversus abdominis plane block. EO, external oblique muscle; IO, internal oblique muscle; TA, transversus abdominis muscle.

vertebral body medially, by the costotransverse ligament and transverse process posteriorly, and by the parietal pleura anterolaterally (**Fig. 12**).[43] This block provides a unilateral sympathetic and somatic nerve blockade. PVNB has been shown to be a viable alternative to thoracic epidurals in the pediatric population, particularly in patients undergoing Nuss repair of pectus excavatum.[44] Previously, a landmark technique or direct placement by the surgeon was used in the pediatric population. However, because ultrasound use has increased, more anesthesia providers are performing these blocks under ultrasound guidance.

The patient is placed in either a lateral position, if doing a unilateral block, or prone, if bilateral blocks are being performed. Once the appropriate vertebral level is identified by landmarks, the probe is placed midline and the spinous process is identified. To obtain a view with both the transverse process and parietal pleura, the probe should be moved lateral and rotated slightly oblique.[45] The internal intercostal membrane (IICM), when seen, is a hyperechoic structure that connects the internal intercostal muscle to the edge of the transverse process. The needle is advanced from lateral to medial, using an in-plane technique, until the tip is through the IICM, in the space between the pleura and shadow of the transverse process.[45] Local anesthetic is injected, and, if the needle is in the correct position, the parietal pleura should be displaced anteriorly.

Overall, the complication rate of the PVNB is low. However, complications include infection, pleural puncture, and hematoma.

Erector spinae plane block
Indications, anatomy, and complications The erector spinae plane (ESP) block is a novel block that can be used to provide thoracic and abdominal analgesia. Its mechanism of action is believed to be a result of local anesthetic blockade of the dorsal and ventral rami of the spinal nerves.[46,47] The erector spinae muscle is composed

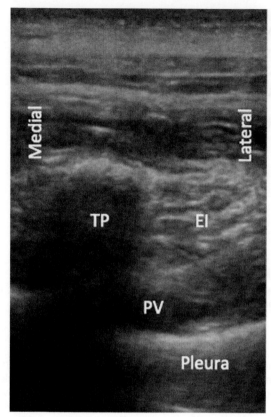

Fig. 12. Paravertebral nerve block. EI, external intercostal muscle; PV, paravertebral space; TP, transverse process.

of three muscles: the iliocostalis, longissimus, and spinalis. This muscle group is covered in a retinaculum, which extends from the sacrum to the skull base. This anatomic arrangement allows for local anesthetic that is injected in the ESP to spread in a cephalad-caudal direction.[47] Although there are significantly more case reports in the adult literature for the ESP block, this block has demonstrated to be a useful analgesic adjunct for both abdominal and thoracic surgeries in the pediatric population.[48–50]

Once the level at which the block is being performed is identified, the probe is placed lateral to the spinous process and then oriented in a longitudinal plane. With the probe centered on the transverse process, the trapezius, rhomboid, and erector spinae muscles should be identifiable, depending on which level this block is being done. The needle is advanced caudally, in-plane, until contact is made with the transverse process. Local anesthetic is then injected deep to the erector spinae muscle layer (**Fig. 13**).[47,51] The erector spinae muscles should be seen lifting off the transverse process once the local anesthetic has been deposited. This block can be performed in either a lateral decubitus or prone position, depending on whether it is unilateral or bilateral, and can be done as a single-shot or continuous catheter technique.[51]

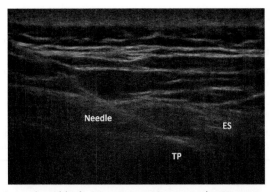

Fig. 13. Erector spinae plane block. ES, erector spinae muscle; TP, transverse process.

Given this is a novel block, there are limited pediatric studies. Reported complications for this block seem to be rare. Local anesthetic is injected deep to the erector spinae muscles but superficial to the paravertebral and epidural spaces giving some laxity to its use in patients with coagulopathies. ESP blocks carry the risk of infection and hematoma.

Pudendal block
Indications, anatomy, and complications The pudendal nerve originates from S2–S4 and enters the perineum through the lesser sciatic foramen and then traverses the pudendal canal before splitting into the perineal nerve and inferior rectal nerve. It provides motor and sensory innervation to the genital, perineal, and surrounding areas. It provides analgesia for urogenital procedures, such as circumcision and hypospadias repair, and can confer the benefits of longer analgesia when compared with caudal blockade.[52] It is commonly blocked as it exits the lesser sciatic foramen just medial and inferior to the ischial spine using a landmark technique with the patient in the lithotomy or frog leg position. Ultrasound guidance has been successfully used to visualize the neurovascular bundle in this area using an out-of-plane technique in this position.[53] Care should be taken to visualize the ischial tuberosity and the pudendal artery adjacent to the pudendal nerve. Because of the proximity of the pudendal artery, bleeding, as well as infection, are possible complications of this block.

SUMMARY

The field of pediatric regional anesthesia has been growing extensively in the past decade. With ultrasound technology becoming more commonplace and anesthesiologists gaining familiarity and experience with it, peripheral nerve blocks and neuraxial techniques are being performed more frequently with few reported adverse events. Because more studies are being conducted in the adult regional population, new and improved techniques are being adopted safely for pediatric patients. Peripheral nerve blocks such as the PVNB and ESP are being used, with applications to a wider array of surgical procedures. Safety and efficacy have been well documented, especially for the more common regional techniques. As we move toward fast-tracking patients and enhanced recovery protocols, the role for pediatric regional anesthesia will only continue to expand.

Clinics Care Points

- The use of regional anesthesia in the pediatric population is safe, even under heavy sedation or general anesthesia.

- The rates of transient neurologic deficits and local anesthetic toxicity are low, based on data from the PRAN database.

- Local anesthetic dosing can be decreased with the use of ultrasound technology, which is important in the neonatal and infant population.

- Proper ultrasound and needle technique, with consideration to adjacent anatomic structures, is key in avoiding complications such as vascular and nerve injury.

DISCLOSURE

The authors have nothing to disclose.

REFERENCES

1. Lam DK, Corry GN, Tsui BC. Evidence for the use of ultra- sound imaging in pediatric regional anesthesia: A systematic review. Reg Anesth Pain Med 2016;41: 229–41.

2. Tsui BC, Pillay JJ. Evidence-based medicine: assessment of ultrasound imaging for regional anesthesia in infants, children, and adolescents. Reg Anesth Pain Med 2010;35:S47–54.

3. Guay J, Suresh S, Kopp S. The use of ultrasound guidance for perioperative neuraxial and peripheral nerve blocks in children: a cochrane review. Anesth Analg 2017;24(3):948–58.

4. Walker BJ, Long JB, Sathyamoorthy M, et al. Complications in pediatric regional anesthesia: an analysis of more than 100,000 blocks from the Pediatric Regional Anesthesia Network. Anesthesiology 2018;129(4):721–32.

5. Marhofer P, Ivani G, Suresh S, et al. Everyday regional anesthesia in children. Pediatr Anesth 2012;22(10):995–1001.

6. Rapp H, Grau T. Ultrasound-guided regional anesthesia in pediatric patients. Reg Anesth Pain Manag 2004;8:179–98.

7. Roberts S. Ultrasonographic guidance in pediatric regional anesthesia. Part 2: Techniques. Pediatr Anesth 2006;16:1112–24.

8. Marhofer P. Upper extremity peripheral blocks. Tech Reg Anesth Pain Manag 2007;11:215–21.

9. O'Donnell BD, Iohom G. An estimation of the minimum effective anesthetic volume of 2% lidocaine in ultrasound-guided axillary brachial plexus block. Anesthesiology 2009;111:25–9.

10. Diwan R, Lakshmi V, Shah T, et al. Continuous axillary block for upper limb surgery in a patient with epidermolysis bullosa simplex. Pediatr Anesth 2001;11: 603–6.

11. Dadure C, Motais F, Ricard C, et al. Continuous peripheral nerve blocks at home in the treatment of complex regional pain syndrome in children. Anesthesiology 2005;102:387–91.

12. Van Geffen GJ, Tielens L, Gielen M. Ultrasound-guided interscalene brachial plexus block in a child with femur fibula ulna syndrome. Pediatr Anesth 2006; 16:330–2.

13. McNaught A, Shastri U, Carmichael N, et al. Ultrasound reduces the minimum effective local anesthetic volume compared with peripheral nerve stimulation for interscalene block. Br J Anaesth 2010;06:124–30.
14. Fredrickson MJ. Ultrasound-assisted interscalene catheter placement in a child. Anaesth Intensive Care 2007;35:807–8.
15. Renes SH, Retting HC, Gielen MJ, et al. Ultrasound-guided low-dose interscalene brachial plexus block reduced the incidence of hemidiaphragmatic paresis. Reg Anesth Pain Med 2009;34:498–502.
16. Ilfeld BM, Morey TE, Wright TW, et al. Interscalene perineural ropivicaine infusion: a comparison of two dosing regimens for postoperative analgesia. Reg Anesth Pain Med 2004;29:9–16.
17. Ivani G, Suresh S, Ecoffey C, et al. The European Society of Regional Anaesthesia and Pain Therapy and the American Society of Regional Anesthesia and Pain Medicine Joint Committee Practice Advisory on Controversial Topics in Pediatric Regional Anesthesia. Reg Anesth Pain Med 2015;40(5):526–32.
18. De José María B, Banus E, Navarro EM, et al. Ultrasound-guided supraclavicular vs infraclavicular brachial plexus blocks in children. Pediatr Anesth 2008;18: 838–44.
19. Mariano ER, Ilfeld BM, Cheng GS, et al. Feasibility of ultrasound-guided peripheral nerve block catheters for pain control on pediatric medical missions in developing countries. Pediatr Anesth 2008;18:598–601.
20. Ponde VC. Continuous infraclavicular brachial plexus block: a modified technique to better secure catheter position in infants and children. Anesth Analg 2008;106:94–6.
21. Diwan R, Raux O, Troncin R, et al. Continuous infraclavicular brachial plexus block for acute pain management in children. Anesth Analg 2003;97:691–3.
22. Ilfeld BM, Morey TE, Enneking FK. Infraclavicular perineural local anesthetic infusion: a comparison of three dosing regimens for postoperative analgesia. Anesthesiology 2004;100:395–402.
23. Casati A, Baciarello M, Di Cianni S, et al. Effects of ultrasound guidance on the minimum effective anaesthetic volume required to block the femoral nerve. Br J Anaesth 2007;98:823–7.
24. Johnson CM. Continuous femoral nerve blockade for analgesia in children with femoral fractures. Anaesth Intensive Care 1994;22:281–3.
25. Oberndorfer U, Marhofer P, Bösenberg A, et al. Ultrasonographic guidance for sciatic and femoral nerve blocks in children. Br J Anaesth 2007;98(6):797–801.
26. Simion C, Suresh S. Lower extremity peripheral nerve blocks in children. Tech Reg Anesth Pain Manag 2007;11:222–8.
27. van Geffen GJ, Scheuer M, Muller A, et al. Ultrasound-guided bilateral continuous sciatic nerve blocks with stimulating catheters for postoperative pain relief after bilateral lower limb amputations. Anaesthesia 2006;61:1204–7.
28. Ganesh A, Rose J, Wells L, et al. Continuous peripheral nerve blockade for inpatient and outpatient postoperative analgesia in children. Anesth Analg 2007; 105(5):1234–42.
29. Ilfeld BM, Morey TE, Wang RD, et al. Continuous popliteal sciatic nerve block for postoperative pain control at home: a randomized, double-blinded, placebo-controlled study. Anesthesiology 2002;97:959–65.
30. Chelly JE, Greger J, Casati A, et al. Continuous lateral sciatic blocks for acute postoperative pain management after major ankle and foot surgery. Foot Ankle Int 2002;23:749–52.

31. Dadure C, Bringuier S, Nicolas F, et al. Continuous epidural block versus continuous popliteal nerve block for postoperative pain relief after major podiatric surgery in children: a prospective comparative randomized study. Anesth Analg 2006;102:744–9.

32. Schwemmer U, Markus CK, Greim CA, et al. Sonographic imaging of the sciatic nerve and its division in the popliteal fossa in children. Pediatr Anesth 2004;14: 1005–8.

33. Johr M. The right thing in the right place: Lumbar plexus block in children. Anesthesiology 2005;102:865–6.

34. Ferguson S, Thomas V, Lewis I. The rectus sheath block in paediatric anaesthesia: new indications for an old technique? Pediatr Anesth 1996;6:463–6.

35. Willschke H, Bosenberg A, Marhofer P, et al. Ultrasonography-guided rectus sheath block in paediatric anaesthesia: a new approach to an old technique. Br J Anaesth 2006;97:244–9.

36. Jagannathan N, Sohn L, Sawardekar A, et al. Unilateral groin surgery in children: will the addition of an ultrasound-guided ilioinguinal nerve block enhance the duration of analgesia of a single-shot caudal block? Pediatr Anesth 2009;19(1): 892–8.

37. Hannallah RS, Broadman LM, Belman AB, et al. Comparison of caudal and ilioinguinal/iliohypogastric nerve blocks for control of post-orchiopexy pain in pediatric ambulatory surgery. Anesthesiology 1987;66:832–4.

38. Markham SJ, Tomlinson J, Hain WR. Ilioinguinal nerve block in children. A comparison with caudal block for intra and postoperative analgesia. Anaesthesia 1986;41:1098–103.

39. Suresh S, Chan VW. Ultrasound guided transversus abdominis plane block in infants, children and adolescents: a simple procedural guidance for their performance. Pediatr Anesth 2009;19(1):296–9.

40. Visoiu M, Boretsky KR, Goyal G, et al. Postoperative analgesia via transversus abdominis plane (TAP) catheter for small weight children - our initial experience. Pediatr Anesth 2012;22:281–4.

41. Taylor L, Birmingham P, Yerkes E, et al. Children with spinal dysraphism: transversus abdominis plane (TAP) catheters to the rescue! Pediatr Anesth 2010;20: 951–4.

42. Pak T, Mickelson J, Yerkes E, et al. Transverse abdominis plane block: a new approach to the management of secondary hyperalgesia following major abdominal surgery. Pediatr Anesth 2009;19(1):54–6.

43. Page EA, Taylor KL. Paravertebral block in paediatric abdominal surgery—a systematic review and meta-analysis of randomized trials. Br J Anaesth 2017;118(2): 159–66.

44. Hall Burton DM, Boretsky K. Paravertebral vs epidural for Nuss procedures. Pediatr Anesth 2014;24:516–20.

45. Boretsky1 K, Visoiu M, Bigeleisen P. Ultrasound-guided approach to the paravertebral space for catheter insertion in infants and children. Pediatr Anesth 2013; 23:1193–8.

46. Forero M, Adhikary SD, Lopez H, et al. The erector spinae plane block: a novel analgesic technique in thoracic neuropathic pain. Reg Anesth Pain Med 2016; 41:621–7.

47. Chin KJ, Adhikary S, Sarwani N, et al. The analgesic efficacy of pre-operative bilateral erector spinae plane (ESP) blocks in patients having ventral hernia repair. Anaesthesia 2017;72:452–60.

48. Ueshima H, Otake H. Clinical experiences of erector spinae plane block for children. J Clin Anesth 2017;44:41.

49. Aksu C, Gürkan Y. Ultrasound guided erector spinae block for postoperative analgesia in pediatric nephrectomy surgeries. J Clin Anesth 2018;45:35–6.

50. Aksu C, Gürkan Y. Opioid sparing effect of Erector Spinae Plane block for pediatric bilateral inguinal hernia surgeries. J Clin Anesth 2018;50:62–3.

51. Tsui BCH, Fonseca A, Munshey F, et al. The erector spinae plane (ESP) block: A pooled review of 242 cases. J Clin Anesth 2019;53:29–34.

52. Zoher N, Fouad Z, Raymond K, et al. The effectiveness of pudendal nerve block versus caudal block anesthesia for hypospadias in children. Anesth Analg 2013; 117:1401–7.

53. Gaudet-Ferrand I, De La Arena P, Bringuier S, et al. Ultrasound guided pudendal nerve block in children: A new technique of ultrasound guided transperineal approach. Pediatr Anesth 2018;28(1):53–8.

Pediatric Anesthesia Outside the Operating Room

Safety and Systems

Mary Landrigan-Ossar, MD, PhD[a,b,*], Christopher Tan Setiawan, MD[c,d]

KEYWORDS

- Offsite anesthesia • Nonoperating room anesthesia • Cardiac catheterization
- Interventional radiology • Radiation therapy • Magnetoencephalogram

KEY POINTS

- Offsite anesthesia comprises one-third of anesthesia volume and continues to grow, requiring increasing anesthesia resources to meet this demand.
- Large registry datasets show that although radiology locations and the cardiac catheterization suite demonstrated elevated anesthesia risk, nonoperating room anesthesia risk is generally on par with that in the operating room.
- Each area where anesthesia is delivered has unique environmental and patient care challenges which must be understood and mitigated to ensure patient and staff safety.
- Standardization of patient assessment, room setup, and monitoring are recommended.
- Internal and hospital-based responses to emergencies in the outfield must be explicitly delineated. Simulation can play an important role in education around crisis response, especially in the most remote of locations.

INTRODUCTION

Anesthesia care outside the operating room, or nonoperating room anesthesia (NORA), is an expanding area of pediatric anesthesia practice. Locations include diagnostic and interventional radiology, dental clinics, gastroenterology and pulmonary suites, radiation oncology locations, and the cardiac catheterization laboratory, among others. The trend toward more outfield procedures, which is seen in both adult and pediatric anesthesia, is driven by many factors. These include evolving technology

[a] Department of Anesthesiology, Critical Care and Pain Medicine, Boston Children's Hospital, 300 Longwood Avenue, Boston, MA 02115, USA; [b] Harvard Medical School, Boston, MA, USA; [c] Department of Anesthesiology and Pain Management, University of Texas Southwestern Medical Center, Dallas, TX, USA; [d] Department of Anesthesiology, Children's Medical Center, 1935 Medical District Drive, Dallas, TX 75235, USA
* Corresponding author. Department of Anesthesiology, Critical Care and Pain Medicine, Boston Children's Hospital, 300 Longwood Avenue, Boston, MA 02115.
E-mail address: mary.landrigan-ossar@childrens.harvard.edu
Twitter: @MaryLandrigan (M.L.-O.)

Anesthesiology Clin 38 (2020) 577–586
https://doi.org/10.1016/j.anclin.2020.06.001
1932-2275/20/© 2020 Elsevier Inc. All rights reserved.
anesthesiology.theclinics.com

with an increasing range of treatment options, nonportable equipment such as MRI scanners, linear accelerators, and radiation sources, as well as caseload in the operating rooms, which has not decreased despite increases in NORA cases. The anesthesiologist working in these offsite locations must understand the unique environmental, logistical, and perioperative considerations to minimize risk in each remote location. With an integrative approach that focuses on these challenges, anesthesia and procedural teams can coordinate to deliver consistent, safe, high-quality care.

DEMOGRAPHIC TRENDS

There has been steady growth in the number of anesthesia cases outside the operating room. From 2010 to 2014, a review of the National Anesthesia Outcomes Registry (NACOR) revealed an increase from 28% to 36% of all anesthesia cases being classified as NORA.[1] Should current trends continue, within the next decade, NORA will constitute 50% of all anesthesia encounters.[2,3] Although adults require anesthesia primarily for painful invasive procedures, such as cardiac catheterization and endoscopy, the largest category of cases for which children require anesthesia is diagnostic radiologic imaging, illustrating that many children cannot cooperate with procedures tolerated by awake adults.[4,5] There is also an increasing expectation from parents that children in the outfield receive anesthesia or sedation care for procedures that were historically done on unsedated children.[6]

Technologic advances have allowed increasingly complex cases to be performed in a minimally invasive manner, often on patients who would be considered a higher perioperative risk for operating room procedures. This transition has increased the demand for anesthesia coverage involving cases that cannot be accommodated in the operating rooms, either due to physical limitations of equipment (ie, MRI or radiation therapy) or scheduling in operating rooms that are already fully booked. NACOR data have shown that although the number of offsite anesthetics increased, there was no decrease in the same time interval in operating room anesthetics.[1]

PREANESTHETIC ASSESSMENT, PATIENT SELECTION, AND RISK STRATIFICATION

Regardless of the anesthetizing location, the goals of the preanesthesia evaluation remain the same: to identify the high-risk patient and evaluate the safety of a proposed anesthetic and intervention in a particular location.[7] The anesthesiologist has a key role in determining with proceduralists and ordering physicians the risks versus indications of a particular procedure. Collaborations between anesthesiologists and radiologists to weigh the relative radiation risk of computed tomography (CT) versus the anesthesia risk of MRI, for example, describe a way forward for such conversations.[8,9] As the perioperative physician-expert in the perioperative surgical home, the anesthesiologist must similarly embrace this role for offsite cases to ensure patient safety.[10,11]

Preanesthesia evaluation for outfield and operating room procedures must be held to the same standard as the operating room. For scheduled cases, all patients receiving anesthesia regardless of anesthesia location should have standardized triage and assessment performed ideally by the same trained personnel. Emergency procedures or add-on cases occurring outside working hours, which are more common in NORA, present a significant assessment challenge.[12] An additional obstacle is the potential lack of immediately available patient records (ie, pediatric case occurring at an adult facility with a different medical record system), which may limit timely knowledge of pertinent patient concerns. Substandard preanesthesia assessment has been implicated as contributory to poor patient outcomes in the Anesthesia Closed Claims database.[13] Centralization of the preanesthesia evaluation as well as patient and staff scheduling has proved to be helpful at many institutions[14,15]; this system allows for early anesthesiologist involvement and streamlined communication as to the need for timely preoperative testing, specialist consultation, or medical optimization in complex patients with multiple comorbidities. Several institutions have demonstrated a reduction in case delays and cancellations after adopting such a system.[16,17]

MONITORING AND EQUIPMENT

Over the past half century, safety in anesthesia has improved with the development of monitoring technology and adherence to accepted standards for appropriate monitoring and care in the operating room. The American Society of Anesthesiologists (ASA) as well as United States regulatory bodies, such as Centers for Medicare and Medicaid Services and the Joint Commission, have specified the requirements for room setup, monitoring, and staffing for anesthesia and sedation locations.[18,19] These standards require the continuous assessment of oxygenation, ventilation, circulation, and temperature as well as requirements for pediatric-specific airway supplies, suction, oxygen and power supply, and emergency carts. The Anesthesia Closed Claims database has shown that most of the NORA claims were paid out due to substandard care, with one-third of claims attributed to inadequate ventilation monitoring.[13,20]

Offsite environments are extremely variable and are primarily designed to accommodate a procedure or technology rather than the administration of anesthesia. In the United States, operating rooms are planned according to standards outlined by the Facility Guidelines Institute, used as a reference by various federal and state regulatory oversight agencies,[21] but these standards may not have been followed in designing outfield locations, which have only recently begun to request pediatric anesthesia service in significant numbers. For example, a multiinstitution survey of pediatric proton therapy facilities showed that 21% did not have recovery rooms and 43% did not have gas evacuation outlets.[22] Space and ergonomic constraints resulting from high-dose radiation, magnetic fields, bulky imaging equipment, and robotic delivery devices can interfere with access to patients and essential equipment, potentially impeding immediate patient access in emergent situations (**Fig. 1**). In some environments, the anesthesia team must be reliant on remote patient monitoring with audiovisual equipment to assess the clinical scenario in another room, while further complicated by radiofrequency interference, noise pollution, and blind spots. All of these factors may delay early recognition and treatment of acute changes in a patient's clinical condition. A review of the Wake Up Safe database for adverse events in radiation oncology underscores that deficiencies in monitoring with subsequent failure to respond promptly to physiologic deterioration can result in patient harm.[23] This problem is accentuated when pediatric anesthesia services are requested at an adjoining adult-centered facility or a site completely detached from any neighboring hospital. Anesthesia events may be rare in these areas, and pediatric emergency response teams may not exist or have significantly delayed response times.

RISK OF PEDIATRIC NONOPERATING ROOM ANESTHESIA

The trend in nonoperating room cases toward minimally invasive procedures may result in a decrease in procedure-related risk compared with an open surgical procedure.[24,25] Anesthetic risk, however, does not necessarily decrease; in some cases, this risk may be potentially greater than that of the indicated procedure, such as a patient with a compressing anterior mediastinal mass for biopsy or a child with uncompensated congenital heart disease for central venous access.

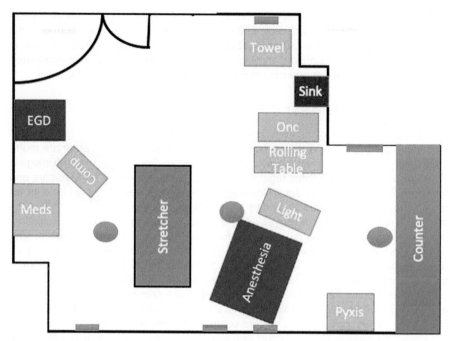

Fig. 1. Procedure room setup. Note difficult access to head of bed from room entrance.

Conventional understanding has held that NORA cases involve higher risk. Contributory factors included variable locations with limited resources, unfamiliar or outdated equipment, constrained work environments, and procedural staff with minimal clinical training to assist in emergencies.[26] The Anesthesia Closed Claims database reinforced this belief by showing that patients suffering harm during offsite procedures were more likely to be at extremes of age and have a higher ASA physical status classification than patients in the operating room and that adverse outfield events were twice as likely to result in serious injury or death.[13,27] Studies involving closed claim analyses, however, are limited by lack of incidence data and by the fact that minor or major adverse events that do not result in litigation are not represented.

Since 2008, the ASA Anesthesia Quality Institute's NACOR database has allowed researchers to more completely examine incidence data for adverse anesthesia events. Data compiled from more than 3 million cases in the NACOR database confirms Closed Claims data that offsite anesthesia locations involved older patients, a higher proportion of patients who were ASA physical class III and higher, a higher rate of emergent procedures, and more anesthetics that were started after working hours.[1,28] Despite these potentially negative factors, NACOR data do not show that offsite anesthesia as a whole is associated with increased morbidity and mortality compared with operating-room-based anesthesia. In addition to NACOR, the Pediatric Sedation Research Consortium (PSRC) and the Wake Up Safe project, focused on pediatric anesthesia adverse events, have shown similar results. These latter sources find an increased risk in radiology and cardiac catheterization areas.[1,5,29] The most recent analysis of the Closed Claims data supports the findings of these databases that cardiac catheterization and radiology suites are areas of increased risk.[13] Further analysis of these higher-risk subgroups is certainly warranted to identify what factors or system failures are responsible so that they can be mitigated. A risk stratification for pediatric cardiac catheterization has been described, with consideration of patient and procedure factors.[30] The anesthesia team must recognize the higher preexisting potential for risk in these patients and mitigate that risk whenever possible. Vigilant anticipation, prompt recognition, and swift management of minor adverse events before they escalate in severity is key to safe practice both in and outside the operating rooms.

RESPONDING TO EMERGENCIES

One factor that must be considered in risk mitigation is the response to inevitable emergencies. The distance from operating room support, relative frequency of after-hours NORA cases, and higher likelihood of complicated rescue in offsite locations require anesthesiologists to rely on procedural staff for immediate assistance during emergencies.[23] The approach to critical events has 2 components: the actions and responsibilities of staff in the immediate area and the additional support from emergency response teams. Staff with training and competencies to assist in routine clinical care as well as pediatric emergencies are essential to a remote anesthesia site. However, staff in outlying areas may have little experience with anesthesia and sedation, particularly for pediatric patients, and may not know how to prioritize an anesthesiologist's concerns in a crisis. Ongoing education and training around emergency response is critical in overcoming this gap. Nurses assisting with patient care and recovery should be Pediatric Advanced Life Support certified and technologists can have Basic Life Support certification.[31] Cultivating an atmosphere of mutual respect is essential to the development of a highly functional team who will respond seamlessly in a crisis. Daily multidisciplinary rounds can play a valuable role, allowing information sharing and discussion of responses to anticipated complications before the start of cases.[32] Simulation can be useful in helping staff practice the technical and communication-based skills necessary in an emergency.[33–35] The improved portability of simulation mannequins allows for more practical simulation exercises in the procedure area itself (**Fig. 2**).

The response by outside emergency responders must be codified and evaluated. Some institutions have "anesthesia stat" responses, which summon help from the main operating room, whereas others may activate the hospital code team for

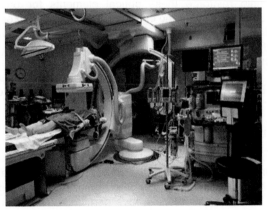

Fig. 2. Interventional radiology suite setup with portable simulation manikin. Control tower for simulation is placed behind anesthesia machine.

outfield assistance. Whichever mechanism is chosen, it is essential that these lines of communication are worked out in advance. Staff in outfield locations should be familiar with whom to call in the event of an emergency, and responding teams should understand their role on arrival. Testing the availability, proficiency, and timeliness of emergency responses by regular review and simulation ahead of their need is crucial.[36]

PERSONAL AND PATIENT SAFETY

Some environmental hazards are unique or more prevalent in offsite locations, and attention must be paid to safeguard patients as well as staff. Ionizing radiation in the cardiac catheterization and interventional radiology (IR) suites, the areas of highest occupational exposure, may be underappreciated by anesthesiologists.[37,38] There are no immediate physical signs to indicate exposure, and effects of radiation are removed in time from exposure. The IR suite is designed in such a way that the anesthesiologist working across the table from the radiologist is exposed to 4 times more radiation.[39,40] For radiation oncology interventions, the risk and degree of radiation exposure to staff is so great that they are excluded from the procedure room during treatments, requiring remote patient monitoring. In nuclear medicine and some radiation oncology procedures, such as interstitial or intraoperative brachytherapy, the patient becomes the source of radiation. Care must be taken to limit time in close proximity to the patient; in some procedures, waste products must be treated as radioactive waste, particularly urine.[41] The age-old safety triad of "distance, shielding, and time" mandates the routine use of standing lead shields, lead aprons, and glasses. Staff exposed regularly should wear personal dosimeters monitored by their institution's radiation safety office.[42] The Environmental Protection Agency has detailed information about radiation exposure, appropriate shielding, and dose monitoring.[43]

The risk of a ferromagnetic projectile in the MRI room (ie, Zone IV) is constant, as the magnet is always on. Anesthesiology providers should always be cognizant of the fact that ferromagnetic items in a scanner room are pulled into the magnet bore, harming or killing patients or staff in the process.[44,45] These "never" events can only be avoided through a collaborative approach to rigorous screening of staff and patients before entering Zone IV to ensure that unsafe items are excluded.[46] Institutional magnet safety training with continuing education and certification requirements can help reinforce these critical elements for providers routinely involved in these environments. In the event of an emergency in Zone IV, the patient must be moved from the scanner to an appropriately prepared area in a ferromagnetic-safe zone (Zone II or III), so that additional support staff and resuscitation equipment may be used. Other anesthetic considerations include the potential for burns from monitoring wires or medication patches in contact with skin; in addition, both hypothermia and hyperthermia have been described in children during MRI.[47]

PEDIATRIC PROCEDURAL SEDATION BY NONANESTHESIOLOGISTS

The incidence of pediatric procedural sedation administered by nonanesthesiologist physicians has mirrored the growth in nonoperating room anesthesia, for many of the same reasons.[6] The increasing number of publications on the topic is an indicator of this progression.[48] Large-scale studies have demonstrated safe pediatric procedural sedation of appropriately selected patients by emergency physicians, intensivists, hospitalists, and advanced practice nurses, using a variety of medication regimens.[49–53] Data from sedation programs contributing to the Pediatric Sedation Research Consortium indicate that in organized programs with well-established rescue capacity and ongoing quality improvement, there have been no deaths, and the incidence of serious adverse events is on par with anesthesia care.[54] There is sparse data showing the rate of adverse events for smaller, less-organized sedation practices or for dental practices, particularly freestanding offices.[55] Regulatory bodies in the United States have placed all sedation in hospitals under the ultimate oversight of anesthesiologists, and it is important that anesthesiologists working in the outfield be aware of the state of procedural sedation in their institution.[18,56] High-quality sedation must be safe, effective, efficient, timely, and equitable and is best achieved when anesthesiologists and sedationists work together to develop protocols for training, care delivery, oversight, and quality improvement.[57] This effort will ensure that patients continue to receive high-quality care regardless of location or provider.

SUMMARY

Nonoperating room anesthesia will continue to be a significant part of pediatric anesthesia practice in the years to come. Anesthesia and procedural teams have successfully moved the care of complex patients for challenging procedures out of the operating room with a model of safety that compares favorably to the operating room. In order to achieve this, anesthesiologists serve a crucial role in evaluating the safety of an anesthetic in a specific patient for a particular procedure and in a location with increased potential for risk with less rescue support. This role in these environments extends from being an unyielding advocate for patient safety to acting as an educator in clinical training and emergency preparedness simulation, as well as a potential consultant for the design and construction of these locations. Safe care is possible in NORA environments only as a cooperative effort between anesthesia and procedural teams, so that risks may be recognized and responses to anticipated adverse events can be optimized.

Clinics Care Points

- Anesthesia outside the operating room is increasingly common. Trends indicate that in another ten years, half of all anesthetics will be delivered in the outfield.

- Consistency of processes for the outfield is crucial for safe care. Preanesthetic assessment, patient selection, and risk stratification should be handled in the same manner used for patients going to the operating room.

- Monitoring and equipment should be standardized when possible to that used in the main operating room. In some locations, physical constraints such as magnetic fields or the need for remote monitoring may require modifications.

- Recent information from large databases indicates that risk for pediatric non-operating room anesthesia is generally similar to the risk for anesthesia in the operating room. Anesthesia in radiology and the cardiac catheterization lab may incur higher risk.

- The appropriate response to emergencies in the outfield environment is crucial to patient safety. In-room staff and outside responders must all know their role in the case of emergency. Simulation has an important role in the development of these safety protocols.

DISCLOSURE

The authors have nothing to disclose.

REFERENCES

1. Chang B, Kaye AD, Diaz JH, et al. Interventional procedures outside of the operating room: results from the national anesthesia clinical outcomes registry. J Patient Saf 2018;14(1):9–16.
2. Boggs SD, Barnett SR, Urman RD. The future of nonoperating room anesthesia in the 21st century: emphasis on quality and safety. Curr Opin Anaesthesiol 2017; 30(6):644–51.
3. Warner ME, Martin DP. Scheduling the nonoperating room anesthesia suite. Curr Opin Anaesthesiol 2018;31(4):492–7.
4. Nagrebetsky A, Gabriel RA, Dutton RP, et al. Growth of nonoperating room anesthesia care in the united states: a contemporary trends analysis. Anesth Analg 2017;124(4):1261–7.
5. Couloures KG, Beach M, Cravero JP, et al. Impact of provider specialty on pediatric procedural sedation complication rates. Pediatrics 2011;127(5):e1154–60.
6. Cravero JP, Blike GT. Pediatric anesthesia in the nonoperating room setting. Curr Opin Anaesthesiol 2006;19(4):443–9.
7. Tobias JD. Preoperative anesthesia evaluation. Semin Pediatr Surg 2018;27(2): 67–74.
8. Callahan MJ, MacDougall RD, Bixby SD, et al. Ionizing radiation from computed tomography versus anesthesia for magnetic resonance imaging in infants and children: patient safety considerations. Pediatr Radiol 2018;48(1):21–30.
9. Masaracchia MM, Tsapakos MJ, McNulty NJ, et al. Changing the paradigm for diagnostic MRI in pediatrics: Don't hold your breath. Paediatr Anaesth 2017; 27(9):880–4.
10. Ferrari LR. How can the Perioperative Surgical Home be applied to pediatric anesthesia practice? Paediatr Anaesth 2017;27(10):982–3.
11. Cravero JP, Callahan MJ. The radiological home: Pediatric anesthesiologist's role in risk assessment for imaging procedures. Paediatr Anaesth 2017;27(9):878–9.
12. Chang B, Urman RD. Non-operating room anesthesia: the principles of patient assessment and preparation. Anesthesiol Clin 2016;34(1):223–40.
13. Woodward ZG, Urman RD, Domino KB. Safety of non-operating room anesthesia: a closed claims update. Anesthesiol Clin 2017;35(4):569–81.
14. Chow VW, Hepner DL, Bader AM. Electronic care coordination from the preoperative clinic. Anesth Analg 2016;123(6):1458–62.
15. Edwards AF, Slawski B. Preoperative Clinics. Anesthesiol Clin 2016;34(1):1–15.
16. Ferschl MB, Tung A, Sweitzer B, et al. Preoperative clinic visits reduce operating room cancellations and delays. Anesthesiology 2005;103(4):855–9.
17. Varughese AM, Hagerman N, Townsend ME. Using quality improvement methods to optimize resources and maximize productivity in an anesthesia screening and consultation clinic. Paediatr Anaesth 2013;23(7):597–606.
18. The Joint Commission. 2020 Comprehensive Accreditation Manual for Hospitals. Oak Brook (IL): The Joint Commisssion; 2019.
19. Anesthesiologists ASo. Statement on Nonoperating Room Anesthetizing Locations. 2018. Available at: https://www.asahq.org/standards-and-guidelines/statement-on-nonoperating-room-anesthetizing-locations?&ct=53bfdddfbe8ebd3302 72f059e48ea7b64e4b23a79ffb61b1cc70742477d3ed3ab08c9d8d2b547f92938 6ba946da8f8767adf087e141dc8019106ab5b16852f6a. Accessed May 1, 2020.
20. Metzner J, Posner KL, Domino KB. The risk and safety of anesthesia at remote locations: the US closed claims analysis. Curr Opin Anaesthesiol 2009;22(4): 502–8.

21. Facilities ASoACoEa. Operating Room Design Manual. 2011. Available at: https://www.asahq.org/about-asa/governance-and-committees/asa-committees/commi ttee-on-equipment-and-facilities/operating-room-design-manual. Accessed January 5, 2020.

22. Owusu-Agyemang P, Grosshans D, Arunkumar R, et al. Non-invasive anesthesia for children undergoing proton radiation therapy. Radiother Oncol 2014; 111(1):30–4.

23. Christensen RE, Nause-Osthoff RC, Waldman JC, et al. Adverse events in radiation oncology: A case series from wake up safe, the pediatric anesthesia quality improvement initiative. Paediatr Anaesth 2019;29(3):265–70.

24. Bang JY, Arnoletti JP, Holt BA, et al. An endoscopic transluminal approach, compared with minimally invasive surgery, reduces complications and costs for patients with necrotizing pancreatitis. Gastroenterology 2019;156(4):1027–40.e3.

25. Katsanos K, Mailli L, Krokidis M, et al. Systematic review and meta-analysis of thermal ablation versus surgical nephrectomy for small renal tumours. Cardiovasc Intervent Radiol 2014;37(2):427–37.

26. Van De Velde M, Kuypers M, Teunkens A, et al. Risk and safety of anesthesia outside the operating room. Minerva Anestesiol 2009;75(5):345–8.

27. Robbertze R, Posner KL, Domino KB. Closed claims review of anesthesia for procedures outside the operating room. Curr Opin Anaesthesiol 2006;19(4):436–42.

28. Gabriel RA, Burton BN, Tsai MH, et al. After-hour versus daytime shifts in non-operating room anesthesia environments: national distribution of case volume, patient characteristics, and procedures. J Med Syst 2017;41(9):140.

29. Uffman JC, Tumin D, Beltran RJ, et al. Severe outcomes of pediatric perioperative adverse events occurring in operating rooms compared to off-site anesthetizing locations in the Wake Up Safe Database. Paediatr Anaesth 2019;29(1):38–43.

30. Odegard KC, Vincent R, Baijal RG, et al. SCAI/CCAS/SPA expert consensus statement for anesthesia and sedation practice: recommendations for patients undergoing diagnostic and therapeutic procedures in the pediatric and congenital cardiac catheterization laboratory. Anesth Analg 2016;123(5):1201–9.

31. Landrigan-Ossar M, McClain CD. Anesthesia for interventional radiology. Paediatr Anaesth 2014;24(7):698–702.

32. Chau A, Vijjeswarapu MA, Hickey M, et al. Cross-disciplinary perceptions of structured interprofessional rounds in promoting teamwork within an academic tertiary care obstetric unit. Anesth Analg 2017;124(6):1968–77.

33. Cumin D, Boyd MJ, Webster CS, et al. A systematic review of simulation for multidisciplinary team training in operating rooms. Simul Healthc 2013;8(3):171–9.

34. Armenia S, Thangamathesvaran L, Caine AD, et al. The role of high-fidelity team-based simulation in acute care settings: a systematic review. Surg J (N Y) 2018; 4(3):e136–51.

35. Flin R, Maran N. Basic concepts for crew resource management and non-technical skills. Best Pract Res Clin Anaesthesiol 2015;29(1):27–39.

36. Blike GT, Christoffersen K, Cravero JP, et al. A method for measuring system safety and latent errors associated with pediatric procedural sedation. Anesth Analg 2005;101(1):48–58 [table of contents].

37. Sensakovic WF, Flores M, Hough M. Occupational Dose and Dose Limits: Experience in a Large Multisite Hospital System. J Am Coll Radiol 2016;13(6):649–55.

38. Whitney GM, Thomas JJ, Austin TM, et al. Radiation safety perceptions and practices among pediatric anesthesiologists: a survey of the physician membership of the Society for Pediatric Anesthesia. Anesth Analg 2019;128(6):1242–8.

39. Anastasian ZH, Strozyk D, Meyers PM, et al. Radiation exposure of the anesthesiologist in the neurointerventional suite. Anesthesiology 2011;114(3):512–20.
40. Dagal A. Radiation safety for anesthesiologists. Curr Opin Anaesthesiol 2011; 24(4):445–50.
41. Committee RH. Radiation Protection in nuclear medicine. Australian radiation Protection and nuclear safety agency. Radiation Protection Series Web site 2008. Available at: https://www.arpansa.gov.au/regulation-and-licensing/regulatory-publications/radiation-protection-series. Accessed February 10 2020.
42. Kim JH. Three principles for radiation safety: time, distance, and shielding. Korean J Pain 2018;31(3):145–6.
43. Radiation IWGoM. Radiation Protection guidance for diagnostic and interventional X-ray procedures: federal guidance report #14. Washington, DC: Agency EP; 2014.
44. News A. Boy, 6, killed in freak MRI accident. ABC News 2006.
45. Gilk T, Latino RJ. MRI Safety 10 Years Later. Patient Safety and Quality Healthcare; 2011. Available at: https://www.psqh.com/analysis/mri-safety-10-years-later/. Accessed July 6, 2020.
46. Cross NM, Hoff MN, Kanal KM. Avoiding MRI-related accidents: a practical approach to implementing MR safety. J Am Coll Radiol 2018;15(12):1738–44.
47. Salerno S, Granata C, Trapenese M, et al. Is MRI imaging in pediatric age totally safe? A critical reprisal. Radiol Med 2018;123(9):695–702.
48. Havidich JE, Cravero JP. The current status of procedural sedation for pediatric patients in out-of-operating room locations. Curr Opin Anaesthesiol 2012;25(4): 453–60.
49. Miller AF, Monuteaux MC, Bourgeois FT, et al. Variation in Pediatric Procedural Sedations Across Children's Hospital Emergency Departments. Hosp Pediatr 2018;8(1):36–43.
50. Beach ML, Cohen DM, Gallagher SM, et al. Major adverse events and relationship to nil per os status in pediatric sedation/anesthesia outside the operating room: a report of the pediatric sedation research consortium. Anesthesiology 2016;124(1):80–8.
51. Grunwell JR, Travers C, Stormorken AG, et al. Pediatric procedural sedation using the combination of ketamine and propofol outside of the emergency department: a report from the pediatric sedation research consortium. Pediatr Crit Care Med 2017;18(8):e356–63.
52. Sulton C, McCracken C, Simon HK, et al. Pediatric procedural sedation using dexmedetomidine: a report from the pediatric sedation research consortium. Hosp Pediatr 2016;6(9):536–44.
53. Kamat PP, McCracken CE, Simon HK, et al. Trends in Outpatient Procedural Sedation: 2007-2018. Pediatrics 2020;145(5):e20193559.
54. Cravero JP, Blike GT, Beach M, et al. Incidence and nature of adverse events during pediatric sedation/anesthesia for procedures outside the operating room: report from the Pediatric Sedation Research Consortium. Pediatrics 2006; 118(3):1087–96.
55. Lee HH, Milgrom P, Starks H, et al. Trends in death associated with pediatric dental sedation and general anesthesia. Paediatr Anaesth 2013;23(8):741–6.
56. Centers for Medicare and Medicaid Services. Conditions for Coverage and Conditions of Participations. 1993. Available at: https://www.cms.gov/Regulations-and-Guidance/Legislation/CFCsAndCoPs/Hospitals. Accessed July 6, 2020.
57. Connors JM, Cravero JP, Kost S, et al. Great expectations-defining quality in pediatric sedation: outcomes of a multidisciplinary consensus conference. J Healthc Qual 2015;37(2):139–54.

Pediatric Anesthesia Outside the Operating Room

Case Management

Christopher Tan Setiawan, MD[a,b],
Mary Landrigan-Ossar, MD, PhD[c,d],*

KEYWORDS

- Pediatric non–operating room anesthesia • Off-site anesthesia • Remote
- Cardiac catheterization • Interventional radiology • Radiation oncology
- Brachytherapy • Magnetoencephalography

KEY POINTS

- Each location in which anesthesia may be provided outside the operating room has specific procedural and logistical challenges. These challenges must be accounted for in making a plan for safe, high-quality anesthesia.
- Monitored anesthesia care or anesthesia with a natural airway is more likely to be administered in a non–operating room environment compared with an operating room.
- Procedures requiring anesthesia outside the operating room vary in their length, need for immobility, presence of painful stimuli, and procedural risk; anesthetic plans need to vary to accommodate these differences.
- In some remote locations, risk stratification regarding patient selection, planned intervention, involved staff or resources, and postoperative disposition must be considered.
- Patient monitoring is more likely to be remote, which may involve the potential for delay in recognition of and intervention for adverse events, placing the patient at increased risk of harm.

ANESTHETIC MANAGEMENT IN OFF-SITE LOCATIONS

When planning an anesthetic for a non–operating room procedure, several factors should be considered. Procedures can vary in length and may require patient

[a] Department of Anesthesiology and Pain Management, University of Texas Southwestern Medical Center, Dallas, TX, USA; [b] Department of Anesthesiology, Children's Medical Center, 1935 Medical District Drive, Dallas, TX 75235, USA; [c] Department of Anesthesiology, Critical Care and Pain Medicine, Boston Children's Hospital, 300 Longwood Avenue, Boston, MA 02115, USA; [d] Harvard Medical School, Boston, MA, USA
* Corresponding author. Department of Anesthesiology, Critical Care and Pain Medicine, Boston Children's Hospital, 300 Longwood Avenue, Boston, MA 02115.
E-mail address: mary.landrigan-ossar@childrens.harvard.edu
Twitter: @MaryLandrigan (M.L.-O.)

Anesthesiology Clin 38 (2020) 587–604
https://doi.org/10.1016/j.anclin.2020.06.003   **anesthesiology.theclinics.com**
1932-2275/20/© 2020 Elsevier Inc. All rights reserved.

immobility and perhaps intervals of apnea. Painful stimuli may or may not be expected, and access to the patient may be limited. Anesthetic considerations may vary depending on these features. **Table 1** lists several types of procedures and these characteristics. Other considerations include patient comorbidities and their relative severity and stability, the skill and comfort level of the anesthesia providers, distance from the operating room, available emergency response systems, and whether it will be necessary to transport the patient under anesthesia from one location to another or even from one facility to another.[1,2] National Anesthesia Clinical Outcomes Registry data show that monitored anesthesia care and general anesthesia with an unsecured airway are more common in non–operating room anesthesia compared with the main operating room.[3] The most important aspect of choosing an anesthetic is a collegial discussion with the proceduralist to ensure that the planned anesthetic is safe for the patient and compatible with procedural goals.

DIAGNOSTIC RADIOLOGY

Diagnostic radiology, consisting of radiography, fluoroscopy, MRI, computed tomography (CT), and nuclear medicine scans, comprises the largest proportion of pediatric outfield anesthesia.[4] These painless scans require a motionless patient for acceptable image quality. Radiology departments have made great progress in helping patients avoid sedation for diagnostic scans. The technique of feed and wrap allows many neonates to avoid anesthesia for scans, reducing both the immediate sedation risk and the potential for anesthetic neurotoxicity.[5] The important role Child Life specialists and prescan patient preparation in helping children successfully complete scans without sedation cannot be overemphasized.[6]

When anesthesia is required, procedures can often be performed while the child is deeply sedated with propofol, dexmedetomidine, or a medication combination.[7,8] Apnea is occasionally required, necessitating intubation. If the anesthesiologist is concerned about anesthetic risk when a long scan is requested in a child with medical comorbidities, a conversation between the radiologist and anesthesiologist can clarify the relative risks of radiation and anesthesia and the need for a particular imaging modality; it is possible that a shorter nonsedated scan, such as CT, may be used, or that the MRI sequences can be decreased.[9,10] Overall, anesthesia and sedation for diagnostic radiology is very safe. The Wake Up Safe database focusing on pediatric

Table 1
Types of non–operating room procedures

Procedure Type	Procedure Length[a]	Painful	Need for Immobility	Access to Patient During Procedure
Diagnostic radiology; ie, CT scan	Short	−	+	+/−
Diagnostic radiology; ie, MRI, nuclear medicine	Long	−	+	−
Interventional radiology	Variable	+	+/−	Limited
Cardiac catheterization	Variable	+/−	+	Limited
GI procedures	Short	+	+/−	+
Radiation oncology	Short but frequent repeats	−	+	−

Abbreviations: CT, computed tomography; GI, gastrointestinal.
[a] Short, less than 1 hour; long, greater than 1 hour.

anesthesia shows a 0.05% incidence of adverse events (**Table 2**).[11] The Pediatric Sedation Research Consortium, which reports sedation data from multiple physician specialties, reports a serious adverse event rate of 0.3% to 0.9% for diagnostic radiology.[12,13] It is common to combine several diagnostic scans or minor procedures into 1 anesthetic. Wake Up Safe data show that transport of patients under anesthesia increases risk[2]; this risk must be carefully considered when planning a combination procedure.

ADVANCED DIAGNOSTIC IMAGING
PET/MRI and PET/Computed Tomography

PET/MRI in the pediatric setting is an emerging modality that has seen increasing investigation and clinical application; at this point, initial operational and logistical costs limit this modality mainly to tertiary care hospitals. Oncologic investigations remain one of the most common applications of PET/MRI, and reports have shown favorable application for staging and treatment planning in many cancer types.[14–17] PET/MRI combines the excellent soft tissue contrast of MRI with complementary physiologic information supplied by PET. When paired with MRI, PET/MRI yields certain advantages compared with conventional PET/CT, which include superior soft tissue imaging and the potential decreased need for multiple anesthetics if both PET/CT and MRI are required.[18] Another major advantage of PET/MRI in the pediatric population is a 70% to 80% dose reduction in radiation exposure compared with PET/CT[15,19,20]; this may have a significant impact on total cumulative radiation exposure associated with serial imaging to monitor disease progression. In general, PET/MRI in the pediatric population is clinically indicated whenever a PET scan is required.[14] Although combined scans have required prolonged time under anesthesia, improvements in imaging are reducing scan and anesthesia time for these procedures.[18]

Table 2		
Location of perioperative adverse events from the Wake Up Safe database		
Location	**Severe AEs[a] (n = 819)**	**Less Severe AEs (n = 775)**
Operating room	610 (74%)	622 (80%)
Off-site location[b]	209 (26%)	153 (20%)
CT scan	12 (1%)	5 (0.7%)
Cardiac catheterization	118 (14%)	80 (10%)
Endoscopy suite	17 (2%)	4 (0.5%)
Interventional radiology	26 (3%)	25 (3%)
MRI	30 (4%)	33 (4%)
Nuclear medicine	1 (0.1%)	1 (0.1%)
PET scan	0	2 (0.3%)
Radiation oncology	1 (0.1%)	2 (0.3%)
Sedation unit	2 (0.2%)	1 (0.1%)
Treatment room	2 (0.2%)	0

Abbreviation: AEs, adverse events.
[a] AEs resulting in temporary, severe, or permanent severe harm, death, or escalation of care.
[b] Percentages of specific out of operating room (OOR) locations listed here add up to total percentage of all OOR locations shown in this row.
From Uffman JC, Tumin D, Beltran RJ, Tobias JD. Severe outcomes of pediatric perioperative adverse events occurring in operating rooms compared to off-site anesthetizing locations in the Wake Up Safe Database. *Paediatr Anaesth.* 2019;29(1):38-43; with permission.

Because it brings significant research interest, PET/MRI units may be located in proximity to a research and cyclotron center (ie, investigation of radionuclide tracers), which may require significant anesthesia planning and logistical coordination.

Magnetoencephalography

Magnetoencephalography (MEG) has played an increasing role in the management of medically intractable epilepsy. MEG records magnetic fields generated by passive or provoked synchronized neuronal activity.[21] MEG's clinical advantages include (1) the ability to localize foci in patients with MRI-negative epilepsy, (2) the capacity to differentiate between focal and multifocal disease, (3) the potential to avoid the risks of invasive phase 2 confirmation (ie, subdural grid placement), and (4) the ability to localize seizure foci with respect to eloquent areas of the brain (ie, motor cortex, areas for expressive language), which could potentially alter surgical approach.[21–24] When coregistered with MRI, termed magnetic source imaging, the stereotactic data obtained can provide three-dimensional information crucial to presurgical epilepsy evaluation.[25]

Sedation or general anesthesia for adequate clinical MEG-electroencephalography recording has been suggested by the America Clinical MEG Society's Clinical Practice Guidelines.[26] Because the postsynaptic potential of neurons is measured in the femtotesla range, MEG is performed in a magnetically shielded room (MSR), composed of mu-metal and aluminum, which diverts lower and higher frequencies, respectively.[27] Anesthesia equipment and monitors create additional electromagnetic interference, so extensions of breathing circuits, monitoring lines, and infusion tubing are fed into the MSR via portholes and patient monitoring occurs remotely. Because MRI may also be required in sequence with MEG, transport concerns and magnetic field precautions should be anticipated. The anesthesia team should be prepared to manage the high likelihood of seizures encountered in this remote location.[28]

There are limited data regarding the ideal anesthetic management for MEG. Anesthetic regimens that excessively induce or suppress interictal epileptiform activity or expand the region of epileptiform foci should be avoided.[29] For example, Szmuk and colleagues[30] reported that midazolam as premedication was associated with a high MEG failure rate versus chloral hydrate (73% vs 5.8%). Despite potential anticonvulsant properties at higher concentrations, propofol-based anesthesia for successful MEG recording has been described,[28–32] with fewer artifacts reported when using lower infusion rates (ie, <100–$150 \ \mu g \cdot kg^{-1} \cdot min^{-1}$) supplemented by opiates or other adjuncts.[28,32] Case reports also describe etomidate infusions for successful MEG sedation.[29] Dexmedetomidine has shown promise as an effective anesthetic in MEG sedation with no reported effect on interictal activity and is used in many centers.[12,32–35] Larger, prospective controlled studies examining a variety of anesthetic protocols may better identify the ideal anesthetic management for pediatric MEG patients in an outpatient setting.

INTERVENTIONAL RADIOLOGY

Interventional radiology (IR) procedures for children can range from short procedures such as biopsies and drain placements to interventional or neurointerventional treatment of complex vascular anomalies lasting up to 12 hours.[36,37] In trauma and CF-associated hemoptysis, IR is used for rapid control of hemorrhage.[38,39] Catheter-delivered chemotherapy as well as cryoablation and radiofrequency ablations are being used in oncology patients.[40,41] IR physicians are also consulted for the placement of challenging long-term venous access.[42] In the authors' experience, up to 50% of procedures in IR are same-day add-ons, and these tend to involve patients with American Society of Anesthesiologists (ASA) physical status III or higher, limiting the time available for preoperative assessment. Safety data specific to pediatric IR are sparse. The Wake Up Safe database shows that 3% of severe adverse events were occurring in IR, although incidence data are lacking in this analysis (see **Table 2**).

A small amount of patient movement may be tolerable for short procedures away from vital structures, whereas more complex procedures generally require intubation and prolonged immobility. With the exception of trauma, blood loss is unlikely, although adequate intravenous access for hydration to offset the diuretic effect of contrast and sclerosant-associated hemoglobinuria is necessary.[43] Reactions to contrast are anaphylactoid and require treatment similar to that for true anaphylaxis.[44] Patients who have previously reacted to contrast require pretreatment with antihistamines and steroid before repeat exposure.[45] Postoperative care of IR patients should include consideration of whether the patient needs to remain supine in the recovery room after solid organ biopsy or femoral artery access; if distraction does not suffice, supplementation with benzodiazepines or alpha-2 agonists such as dexmedetomidine may be helpful.[46,47] Postprocedure disposition should be discussed between the IR physician and the anesthesiologist to determine the appropriate level of care. Similarly, some procedures may be considered to be too high risk for off-site care (eg, patients with a difficult airway or mediastinal mass), and it may be necessary to move a procedure to the operating room for better access to support and emergency resources.

RADIATION ONCOLOGY
Radiation Therapy: Photons and Protons

Fractionated radiotherapy plays an essential role in multimodal management of early-stage or late-stage malignancy. Ionizing radiation is delivered in the form of photons (x-rays, γ-rays) or particle radiation (ie, proton therapy) using precise targeting systems.[48,49] Treatments are typically divided into 20 to 33 short sessions or fractions, which occur daily or twice daily over 4 to 6.5 weeks; the protracted course allows healthy cells to repair inadvertent DNA breaks and minimize radiation toxicity.[50] Treatments are painless, but children must lie completely motionless alone in a vault, sometimes confined by a mask or restraint. Despite methods to avoid sedation through Child Life specialists, toys or award systems, or distraction devices such as the AVATAR (audiovisual-assisted therapeutic ambience in radiation therapy [RT]) system, anesthesia may still be required.[51–53]

The initial encounter is focused on creation of immobilization devices (ie, thermoplastic mask, vacuum-formed cushion) for daily positioning, placement of reference markers (often small tattoos), and CT imaging in the immobilization device for treatment planning. Because head and neck treatments typically require a mask, vigilance to ensure proper head position during mask creation is critical, because this fixed airway position will be encountered during subsequent procedures. Sometimes, positioning for treatment makes spontaneous ventilation difficult, as in head flexion for craniospinal treatment. At 1 author's (C.T.S.) institution, holes are cut to allow for airway access and the cut end of a laryngeal mask airway is placed between the teeth during CT simulation to replicate use of an advanced airway for future treatments if needed. Mask fit may become difficult over time because of weight gain from steroid treatment, and repeat simulation with mask creation may ultimately be required.

Anesthetic management for these procedures has evolved. Ketamine sedations were associated with a 23% to 24% incidence of complications and included uncontrolled patient movement, sialorrhea, hallucinations, and slow recovery. As propofol sedation has been adopted, review of safety data has revealed a trend toward fewer complications.[54] An international, multi-institutional survey of 15,000 proton therapy anesthetics per year revealed that 72% of children less than 4 years of age received general anesthesia, with intravenous propofol used in 57% of procedures, and sevoflurane with a laryngeal mask airway used in 36% of procedures.[55]

Safety data for pediatric sedation in RT are limited to individual institutions or smaller numbers of patients. Complication rates of 0.01% to 3.5%[54,56,57] have been reported, with airway complications being most prevalent.[57,58] Anghelescu and colleagues'[57] retrospective review of 3833 anesthetics in 177 patients reported an increased incidence of complications during simulation sessions, suggesting that the required head manipulation, repositioning, and need for additional transport could be contributory. Christensen and colleagues'[59] evaluation of the Wake Up Safe database identified 6 major adverse events. In 1 procedure, the process of mask molding was complicated by laryngospasm. In 3 cases of medication errors (ie, incorrect infusion pump programming), remote monitoring of equipment in poor lighting conditions may have prevented earlier recognition.[59] Indwelling central venous access devices are common and can be accessed for daily treatments, but they must be treated with care whenever accessed. Line-related complications, including sepsis, thrombosis, infiltration, and dislodgement, were found in 15% to 23% of patients in early studies, with ports being less problematic than peripherally inserted central catheter lines.[55,58,60] Collisions and clearance issues between patient, gantry, or couch are commonly reported in RT and stereotactic radiation surgery,[61,62] despite standard collision safety mechanisms, such as closed-circuit television, touch-guard sensors, and infrared detection. One study found that the use of 3 additional cameras resulted in a blind-spot reduction of up to 87% and 10-fold reduction in vault reentry.[61] The use of multiple adjustable pan-tilt-zoom network cameras may increase sensitivity of patient monitoring in these environments and should be considered when assessing a new location that involves similar remote monitoring (**Fig. 1**).

In some cases of neuro-oncologic malignancy, craniospinal irradiation (CSI) is used to treat subarachnoid disease spread.[63] CSI's target volume encompasses the calvarium and spinal canal, resulting in exit-dose irradiation of multiple tissues anterior to the spinal canal. Acute and late toxicities are correlated with the radiation sensitivity of tissue affected, target volume, and the treatment time course.[64,65] These conditions include pneumonitis and pulmonary fibrosis, neurocognitive defects, ototoxicity, impaired vertebral bone growth, cardiac damage, vascular disease, endocrine dysfunction, and late-onset secondary malignancies.[63,64,66,67] Pediatric patients are particularly susceptible to long-term toxicity compared with adults because of higher numbers of susceptible proliferating cells and a longer life expectancy at time of exposure. Although there is debate regarding the advantages of proton therapy, which may include reduction of secondary damage in CSI treatments, and the financial, logistic, and ethical issues associated with the transition from conventional photon therapy, the use of proton therapy has become a standard at some centers.[48,49]

Palliative Radiation Interventions

RT is occasionally used to alleviate the symptoms of advanced or metastatic disease, such as pain, dyspnea, bleeding, spinal cord compression or other neurologic sequelae, bowel or bladder dysfunction, or inability to eat.[68,69] Representing approximately 11% of RT procedures,[70] these treatments are typically limited in terms of duration, field extent, and cumulative dose.[68] Benefits of palliative RT include

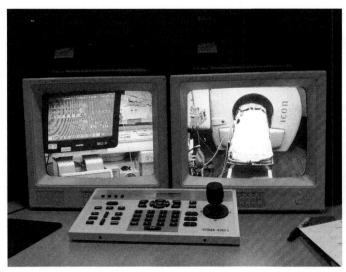

Fig. 1. Patient and monitors seen on closed-circuit television in the Gamma Knife radiosurgery suite.

decreased medication side effects (ie, narcotics), reduced overall hospital stay, minimized need for invasive procedures, and improved routine life at home.

These cases present challenges to the anesthesia team, from a logistical as well as a clinical standpoint. Palliative patients can present with debilitating symptoms, such as intractable vomiting, respiratory compromise, coagulopathy, and unstable neurologic symptoms, which all create additional anesthetic risk and necessitate a higher level of postoperative care. It is important for providers to specify the intent of these treatments to parents,[68] and this indication must similarly be considered in the anesthetic plan when weighing the utility and inherent risks of sedation.

Stereotactic Radiosurgery

Stereotactic radiosurgery (SRS) is used for the treatment of various benign (ie, arteriovenous malformations) and malignant intracranial lesions.[71–73] SRS is indicated for treating unresectable tumors (ie, located deep in eloquent areas), tumors with recurrence after prior radiotherapy, or residual disease.[74] In contrast with fractionated radiotherapy, which uses repeated small doses of radiation, SRS relies on the delivery of a single or limited number of large doses of radiation to a precisely localized target.[75] Although data are limited, newer technologies in frameless SRS have shown precision similar to conventional frame-based radiosurgery, and may have applications to pediatric patients, especially patients for palliation.[76,77]

Frame-based SRS poses unique anesthetic challenges (**Fig. 2**).[78] Imaging, planning, and SRS treatment all occur during 1 session, requiring immobility and often prolonged wait times; general anesthesia is often required in young or uncooperative patients. Anesthetic considerations include multiple locations with their associated risks (ie, radiation and magnetic fields), frequent transfers, and possible intrafacility transport of the anesthetized patient in a bulky head frame, remote patient monitoring, unpredictable duration of treatment, and increased risk of positioning injury or hypothermia. Each site in the process (angiography and/or MRI suite, SRS procedure room, holding area) must be fully set up and prepared for pediatric anesthesia. A

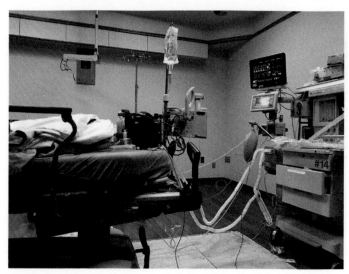

Fig. 2. Patient in head frame for stereotactic radiosurgery.

preinduction time-out with all involved members to discuss the sequence of diagnostic and interventional procedures, assess readiness of each location, and anticipate potential obstacles is essential for safety. Propofol-based intravenous anesthesia has the advantage of allowing transport while maintaining a titratable depth of anesthesia in variable locations.[79] Use of portable monitors can expedite seamless monitoring and portable infusion pumps allow reliable delivery of intravenous anesthetic agents and carrier fluids.

Frame-based stereotactic radiosurgery in children has been associated with complications such as loosening and dislodgment of pins, skull fractures, and penetration of the skull and associated sequelae.[80–82] Special head frame posts can conform to the curvature of the smaller pediatric skull, but particular care must be directed at patients less than 2 years old who are at increased risk for complications.[71] Frame placement, positioning, and transfer of anesthetized pediatric patients must be done in a coordinated manner with an emphasis on clear communication, because there is potential for trauma to the patient's face, skull, or cervical spine, risk of accidental extubation, and potential for difficult emergent airway intervention. In their Wake Up Safe review of adverse events in radiation oncology, Christensen and colleagues[59] reported bronchospasm and unintended extubation in a frame-based SRS patient, which resulted in a bradycardic arrest; direct laryngoscopy attempts were complicated by the frame, which ultimately required removal. In addition to standard emergency supplies, hardware for emergent frame removal must accompany anesthetized patients throughout the SRS workflow.

Brachytherapy

In contrast with external beam radiotherapy (EBRT), brachytherapy places the radiation source in proximity to the treatment site, increasing local control and decreasing the probability of long-term complications.[83] Brachytherapy has been described for many pediatric tumors.[84] The use of brachytherapy for multimodal management of craniopharyngiomas, for example, is well established; by stereotactically accessing the cystic component, often through a cyst puncture catheter connected to a subcutaneous reservoir, phosphorus-32 (P^{32}, a B-emitter) can be injected directly into the cyst.[85–87] In the operating room, interstitial or intracavity applicators are surgically implanted for subsequent radiation loading procedures if necessary, or intraoperative high-dose-rate (HDR) brachytherapy is performed after gross surgical resection.[88] Intrafacility transport of the anesthetized patient between the operating room, imaging areas (ie, CT, MRI), and the dedicated radiation room may be required, and the anesthetic should be planned to minimize transport-associated complications. High-risk patients or procedures, such as patients with tumor involvement of the oropharynx or treatments to the tracheobronchial tree, may entail difficult airway management or need for postoperative intubation or intensive care admission.[89] The anticipated risks of the intended procedure should be discussed regarding the ideal location for treatment (eg, pediatric hospital), necessary equipment, and postoperative management plans.

Conventional low-dose-rate brachytherapy delivers therapy while minimizing surrounding tissue damage. A course of therapy may take several days and sedation or general anesthesia for prolonged immobility of pediatric patients to prevent dislodgement of implants is often required.[89–91] Despite historical caution regarding the use of HDR for pediatric brachytherapy and concern for excessive morbidity, several institutions have shown successful application in pediatric patients.[84,92,93] HDR has the advantage of minimizing radiation exposure to staff and patients' families, and treatments last on the order of minutes instead of days. Treatments are frequent, generally twice daily over the course of 12 treatments, instead of 1 single prolonged treatment.[83] Although there is limited literature regarding the use of regional anesthesia for pediatric brachytherapy,[94] such applications could potentially minimize excessive anesthetics in cooperative children and adolescents. Depending on institutional and geographic factors, brachytherapy procedures may be performed in locations remote from the pediatric hospital, such as at a cancer hospital or RT center. Because it avoids the need for prolonged sedation, HDR (and EBRT) has the logistic advantage in these situations, because it can potentially be used on an outpatient basis after surgical implantation of after-loading catheters.

GASTROENTEROLOGY PROCEDURE UNIT

Gastrointestinal (GI) endoscopy procedures in pediatric patients range from diagnostic upper or lower endoscopies to interventions, including retrograde cholangiograms and stenting, varicosity banding, and sclerotherapy. Over time, there has been a shift from sedation primarily administered by gastroenterologists to care by anesthesiologists in the gastroenterology procedure unit, with sedation by dedicated nonanesthesiologist physicians also described.[95–97] Despite the airway being shared in these procedures, a common practice is for deep sedation/anesthesia without an artificial airway, with the exception of certain interventions and very young or critically ill children.[98] Risk stratification is essential for determining the anesthetic plan and location of the procedure. GI risk factors such as achalasia, GI motility issues, food impaction, and reflux must be considered,[98] and young age has been shown to be an independent risk factor for sedation events.[97]

The rate of adverse events in this setting is low, with Wake Up Safe data showing a rate comparable with other lower-risk off-site environments (**Table 2**).[99] A single-institution report of 454 pediatric patients had an adverse event rate of 2.6%,[100] and the Pediatric Sedation Research Consortium database of 12,000 procedures showed an adverse event rate of 4.8%, with no deaths or resuscitations recorded.[97]

CARDIAC CATHETERIZATION LABORATORY

Intravascular device technologies and imaging advances in the cardiac catheterization laboratory, such as three-dimensional rotational angiography, MRI guidance, and multimodal image fusion, have paved the way to new interventional and hybrid surgical approaches in the youngest and most critically ill patients. In contrast with diagnostic examinations, interventions have been reported to increase the risk of morbidity and mortality.[101–108] Wake Up Safe data show an increased likelihood of severe outcomes in cardiac catheterization suites, implicating the greater complexity of patients and interventions, rather than the remote location (see **Table 2**).[99] A review of anesthesia-related cardiac arrests in the Pediatric Perioperative Cardiac Arrest (POCA) Registry reported that 34% of events occurred in patients with cardiac disease, showing the higher anesthesia risk for these patients.[104]

Risk stratification for cardiac catheterization should focus on the patient's congenital or acquired cardiac disorder, accompanying patient comorbidities, the risks of the intended intervention, availability of resources, and the expertise of the providers. The Society for Cardiovascular Angiography and Interventions (SCAI), Society for Pediatric Anesthesia (SPA), and Congenital Cardiac Anesthesia Society (CCAS) consensus recommendations identified the cardiac lesions associated with increased risk to be hypoplastic left heart syndrome, pulmonary arterial hypertension, and left ventricular outlet obstruction.[102] POCA Registry data confirm that patients with uncorrected (59%) and palliated (26%) single-ventricle physiology had the highest risk of cardiac arrest, whereas patients with cardiomyopathy (50%) or aortic stenosis (62%) had the highest risk of mortality.[104]

Several risk-standardization models have been developed. The Congenital Cardiac Catheterization Project on Outcomes (C3PO) developed the CHARM (Catheterization for Congenital Heart Disease Adjustment for Risk Method) model for risk assessment.[103,109] The multicenter Congenital Cardiac Interventional Study Consortium (CCISC) developed and refined the CRISP (Catheterization Risk Score for Pediatrics) score based on diagnostic, procedural, and physiologic risk categories to aid in preprocedural risk stratification for serious adverse events.[110,111] The NCDR (National Cardiovascular Data Registry) IMPACT (Improving Pediatric and Congenital Treatment) recently reported a model based on evaluation of 39,725 catheterizations at 74 United States centers, which included procedure-type risk; hemodynamic indicators; and medical comorbidities such as single-ventricle physiology, coagulation disorders, and renal insufficiency.[112]

Anesthesia providers in this setting must understand the impact of a particular anesthetic and procedure on a particular cardiac physiology and have the ability to anticipate, identify, and promptly treat any significant hemodynamic or physiologic deterioration. This ability may require advanced diagnosis (ie, transesophageal echocardiogram), pharmacologic management, cardiopulmonary resuscitation, initiation of massive transfusion, or emergent cannulation and extracorporeal mechanical oxygenation support. Precatheterization diagnostic procedures (ie, transthoracic or transesophageal echocardiogram) and postoperative concerns (postoperative intensive care unit, delayed complications such as reperfusion injury) must be anticipated and optimized.[101] In the United States, pediatric cardiac anesthesiology fellowship training programs are in their infancy; the CCAS recently published milestones based on those of the Accreditation Council on Graduate Medical Education that may aid in standardizing subspecialty training.[113]

As with other non–operating room locations, a team environment creating an avenue for open communication aids all providers in the preparation and management of these complicated procedures and patients. A gatekeeper provider (ie, cardiac board runner) can optimize communication by assisting in multispecialty planning for an intervention and allocating resources, especially during emergencies. Periodic multidisciplinary huddles between cardiologists, anesthesiologists, cardiac surgeons, perfusionists, and cardiac intensivists can help address safety concerns of a high-risk patient or procedure and any anticipated complication or major adverse event.

SUMMARY

Non–operating room anesthesia will continue to be a significant part of pediatric anesthesia practice in the years to come. Anesthesia and procedural teams have successfully moved the care of complex patients for challenging procedures out of the operating room with a model of safety that compares largely favorably with the operating room. Off-site locations that are still at increased risk, such as radiology and the cardiac catheterization laboratory, must be studied so that risk may be mitigated wherever possible. Other areas with infrequent, low anesthetic volume, or locations far removed from immediate rescue teams should be approached with caution and careful planning. The anesthesiologist must understand each unique environment, pertinent patient-related factors, and anesthetic requirements to ensure a safe approach to each anesthetic encounter. Safe care is possible in these environments with open communication between anesthesia and procedural teams as well as careful logistical planning and resource management, so that risks may be recognized and responses to anticipated adverse events can be optimized.

Clinics Care Points

- Diagnostic Radiology case are painless, of variable length, and require a motionless patient. Sedation with propofol, dexmedetomidine, or a combination is a common anesthetic choice. Collaboration with radiology and ordering services is essential.

- Interventional Radiology cases are of varying length and are generally painful. Patient motion may be tolerable. Natural airway sedation and endotracheal anesthesia are used depending on case and patient factors.

- Radiation Oncology cases are short but frequent, and require a motionless patient completely remote from the care team. Changes in the patient's physical condition over the course of treatment may impact safe airway management.

- Stereotactic Radiosurgery may require prolonged periods under anesthesia, and in some cases require transport under anesthesia. Preparation of all locations is essential, as is team time-out prior to transport.

- The challenge in the gastroenterology procedure suite is that of sharing the airway of a sedated patient with the proceduralist. Nevertheless, many cases are accomplished with natural airway sedation.

- The cardiac catheterization lab is one of the highest-risk outfield locations. The anesthesia team must coordinate closely with the interventional cardiology team to ensure safe patient care.

DISCLOSURE

The authors have nothing to disclose.

REFERENCES

1. Miketic RM, Uffman J, Tumin D, et al. Experience with combining pediatric procedures into a single anesthetic. Pediatr Qual Saf 2019;4(5):e207.

2. Haydar B, Baetzel A, Stewart M, et al. Complications associated with the anesthesia transport of pediatric patients: an analysis of the wake up safe database. Anesth Analg 2020;131(1):245–54.

3. Chang B, Kaye AD, Diaz JH, et al. Interventional Procedures Outside of the Operating Room: Results From the National Anesthesia Clinical Outcomes Registry. J Patient Saf 2018;14(1):9–16.

4. Couloures KG, Beach M, Cravero JP, et al. Impact of provider specialty on pediatric procedural sedation complication rates. Pediatrics 2011;127(5): e1154–60.

5. Bilotta F, Evered LA, Gruenbaum SE. Neurotoxicity of anesthetic drugs: an update. Curr Opin Anaesthesiol 2017;30(4):452–7.

6. Durand DJ, Young M, Nagy P, et al. Mandatory Child Life Consultation and Its Impact on Pediatric MRI Workflow in an Academic Medical Center. J Am Coll Radiol 2015;12(6):594–8.

7. Boriosi JP, Eickhoff JC, Klein KB, et al. A retrospective comparison of propofol alone to propofol in combination with dexmedetomidine for pediatric 3T MRI sedation. Paediatr Anaesth 2017;27(1):52–9.

8. Nagoshi M, Reddy S, Bell M, et al. Low-dose dexmedetomidine as an adjuvant to propofol infusion for children in MRI: A double-cohort study. Paediatr Anaesth 2018;28(7):639–46.

9. Callahan MJ, MacDougall RD, Bixby SD, et al. Ionizing radiation from computed tomography versus anesthesia for magnetic resonance imaging in infants and children: patient safety considerations. Pediatr Radiol 2018;48(1):21–30.

10. Masaracchia MM, Tsapakos MJ, McNulty NJ, et al. Changing the paradigm for diagnostic MRI in pediatrics: Don't hold your breath. Paediatr Anaesth 2017; 27(9):880–4.

11. Khawaja AA, Tumin D, Beltran RJ, et al. Incidence and causes of adverse events in diagnostic radiological studies requiring anesthesia in the wake-up safe registry. J Patient Safety 2018;14(1).

12. Sulton C, McCracken C, Simon HK, et al. Pediatric Procedural Sedation Using Dexmedetomidine: A Report From the Pediatric Sedation Research Consortium. Hosp Pediatr 2016;6(9):536–44.

13. Beach ML, Cohen DM, Gallagher SM, et al. Major Adverse Events and Relationship to Nil per Os Status in Pediatric Sedation/Anesthesia Outside the Operating Room: A Report of the Pediatric Sedation Research Consortium. Anesthesiology 2016;124(1):80–8.

14. Kwatra NS, Lim R, Gee MS, et al. PET/MR Imaging:: Current Updates on Pediatric Applications. Magn Reson Imaging Clin N Am 2019;27(2):387–407.

15. Schafer JF, Gatidis S, Schmidt H, et al. Simultaneous whole-body PET/MR imaging in comparison to PET/CT in pediatric oncology: initial results. Radiology 2014;273(1):220–31.

16. Gatidis S, Schmidt H, Gucke B, et al. Comprehensive Oncologic Imaging in Infants and Preschool Children With Substantially Reduced Radiation Exposure Using Combined Simultaneous (1)(8)F-Fluorodeoxyglucose Positron Emission Tomography/Magnetic Resonance Imaging: A Direct Comparison to (1)(8)F-Fluorodeoxyglucose Positron Emission Tomography/Computed Tomography. Invest Radiol 2016;51(1):7–14.

17. Sher AC, Seghers V, Paldino MJ, et al. Assessment of Sequential PET/MRI in Comparison With PET/CT of Pediatric Lymphoma: A Prospective Study. AJR Am J Roentgenol 2016;206(3):623–31.

18. Vogelius ESS. Pediatric PET/MRI: A Review. J Am Osteopath Coll Radiol 2017; 6(1):15–27.
19. Chawla SC, Federman N, Zhang D, et al. Estimated cumulative radiation dose from PET/CT in children with malignancies: a 5-year retrospective review. Pediatr Radiol 2010;40(5):681–6.
20. Hirsch FW, Sattler B, Sorge I, et al. PET/MR in children. Initial clinical experience in paediatric oncology using an integrated PET/MR scanner. Pediatr Radiol 2013;43(7):860–75.
21. Gofshteyn JS, Le T, Kessler S, et al. Synthetic aperture magnetometry and excess kurtosis mapping of Magnetoencephalography (MEG) is predictive of epilepsy surgical outcome in a large pediatric cohort. Epilepsy Res 2019;155: 106151.
22. Sutherling WW, Mamelak AN, Thyerlei D, et al. Influence of magnetic source imaging for planning intracranial EEG in epilepsy. Neurology 2008;71(13):990–6.
23. Onal C, Otsubo H, Araki T, et al. Complications of invasive subdural grid monitoring in children with epilepsy. J Neurosurg 2003;98(5):1017–26.
24. Schwartz ES, Dlugos DJ, Storm PB, et al. Magnetoencephalography for pediatric epilepsy: how we do it. AJNR Am J Neuroradiol 2008;29(5):832–7.
25. Stefan H, Trinka E. Magnetoencephalography (MEG): Past, current and future perspectives for improved differentiation and treatment of epilepsies. Seizure 2017;44:121–4.
26. Bagic AI, Knowlton RC, Rose DF, et al. American Clinical Magnetoencephalography Society Clinical Practice Guideline 1: recording and analysis of spontaneous cerebral activity. J Clin Neurophysiol 2011;28(4):348–54.
27. Hari R, Baillet S, Barnes G, et al. IFCN-endorsed practical guidelines for clinical magnetoencephalography (MEG). Clin Neurophysiol 2018;129(8):1720–47.
28. Hanaya R, Okamoto H, Fujimoto A, et al. Total intravenous anesthesia affecting spike sources of magnetoencephalography in pediatric epilepsy patients: focal seizures vs. non-focal seizures. Epilepsy Res 2013;105(3):326–36.
29. Balakrishnan G, Grover KM, Mason K, et al. A retrospective analysis of the effect of general anesthetics on the successful detection of interictal epileptiform activity in magnetoencephalography. Anesth Analg 2007;104(6):1493–7, table of contents.
30. Szmuk P, Kee S, Pivalizza EG, et al. Anaesthesia for magnetoencephalography in children with intractable seizures. Paediatr Anaesth 2003;13(9):811–7.
31. Fujimoto A, Ochi A, Imai K, et al. Magnetoencephalography using total intravenous anesthesia in pediatric patients with intractable epilepsy: lesional vs non-lesional epilepsy. Brain Dev 2009;31(1):34–41.
32. Konig MW, Mahmoud MA, Fujiwara H, et al. Influence of anesthetic management on quality of magnetoencephalography scan data in pediatric patients: a case series. Paediatr Anaesth 2009;19(5):507–12.
33. Tenney JR, Miller JW, Rose DF. Intranasal Dexmedetomidine for Sedation During Magnetoencephalography. J Clin Neurophysiol 2019;36(5):371–4.
34. Talke P, Stapelfeldt C, Garcia P. Dexmedetomidine does not reduce epileptiform discharges in adults with epilepsy. J Neurosurg Anesthesiol 2007;19(3):195–9.
35. Mason KP, O'Mahony E, Zurakowski D, et al. Effects of dexmedetomidine sedation on the EEG in children. Paediatr Anaesth 2009;19(12):1175–83.
36. Landrigan-Ossar M. Common procedures and strategies for anaesthesia in interventional radiology. Curr Opin Anaesthesiol 2015;28(4):458–63.

37. Brinjikji W, Krings T, Murad MH, et al. Endovascular Treatment of Vein of Galen Malformations: A Systematic Review and Meta-Analysis. AJNR Am J Neuroradiol 2017;38(12):2308–14.

38. Bize PE, Duran R, Madoff DC, et al. Embolization for multicompartmental bleeding in patients in hemodynamically unstable condition: prognostic factors and outcome. J Vasc Interv Radiol 2012;23(6):751–60.e4.

39. Flight WG, Barry PJ, Bright-Thomas RJ, et al. Outcomes Following Bronchial Artery Embolisation for Haemoptysis in Cystic Fibrosis. Cardiovasc Intervent Radiol 2017;40(8):1164–8.

40. Adam A, Kenny LM. Interventional oncology in multidisciplinary cancer treatment in the 21(st) century. Nat Rev Clin Oncol 2015;12(2):105–13.

41. Ravindran K, Dalvin LA, Pulido JS, et al. Intra-arterial chemotherapy for retinoblastoma: an updated systematic review and meta-analysis. J Neurointerv Surg 2019;11(12):1266–72.

42. Duszak R Jr, Bilal N, Picus D, et al. Central venous access: evolving roles of radiology and other specialties nationally over two decades. J Am Coll Radiol 2013;10(8):603–12.

43. Barranco-Pons R, Burrows PE, Landrigan-Ossar M, et al. Gross hemoglobinuria and oliguria are common transient complications of sclerotherapy for venous malformations: review of 475 procedures. AJR Am J Roentgenol 2012;199(3):691–4.

44. Cochran ST. Anaphylactoid reactions to radiocontrast media. Curr Allergy Asthma Rep 2005;5(1):28–31.

45. Schopp JG, Iyer RS, Wang CL, et al. Allergic reactions to iodinated contrast media: premedication considerations for patients at risk. Emerg Radiol 2013;20(4):299–306.

46. Mohammady M, Atoof F, Sari AA, et al. Bed rest duration after sheath removal following percutaneous coronary interventions: a systematic review and meta-analysis. J Clin Nurs 2014;23(11–12):1476–85.

47. Govender P, Jonas MM, Alomari AI, et al. Sonography-guided percutaneous liver biopsies in children. AJR Am J Roentgenol 2013;201(3):645–50.

48. Berrington de Gonzalez A, Vikram B, Buchsbaum JC, et al. A Clarion Call for Large-Scale Collaborative Studies of Pediatric Proton Therapy. Int J Radiat Oncol Biol Phys 2017;98(5):980–1.

49. Kirsch DG, Tarbell NJ. New technologies in radiation therapy for pediatric brain tumors: the rationale for proton radiation therapy. Pediatr Blood Cancer 2004;42(5):461–4.

50. Tobin CD, Clark CA, McEvoy MD, et al. An approach to moderate sedation simulation training. Simul Healthc 2013;8(2):114–23.

51. Scott MT, Todd KE, Oakley H, et al. Reducing Anesthesia and Health Care Cost Through Utilization of Child Life Specialists in Pediatric Radiation Oncology. Int J Radiat Oncol Biol Phys 2016;96(2):401–5.

52. Hiniker SM, Bush K, Fowler T, et al. Initial clinical outcomes of audiovisual-assisted therapeutic ambience in radiation therapy (AVATAR). Pract Radiat Oncol 2017;7(5):311–8.

53. Haeberli S, Grotzer MA, Niggli FK, et al. A psychoeducational intervention reduces the need for anesthesia during radiotherapy for young childhood cancer patients. Radiat Oncol 2008;3:17.

54. Verma V, Beethe AB, LeRiger M, et al. Anesthesia complications of pediatric radiation therapy. Pract Radiat Oncol 2016;6(3):143–54.

55. Fortney JT, Halperin EC, Hertz CM, et al. Anesthesia for pediatric external beam radiation therapy. Int J Radiat Oncol Biol Phys 1999;44(3):587–91.
56. Owusu-Agyemang P, Grosshans D, Arunkumar R, et al. Non-invasive anesthesia for children undergoing proton radiation therapy. Radiother Oncol 2014; 111(1):30–4.
57. Anghelescu DL, Burgoyne LL, Liu W, et al. Safe anesthesia for radiotherapy in pediatric oncology: St. Jude Children's Research Hospital Experience, 2004-2006. Int J Radiat Oncol Biol Phys 2008;71(2):491–7.
58. Seiler G, De Vol E, Khafaga Y, et al. Evaluation of the safety and efficacy of repeated sedations for the radiotherapy of young children with cancer: a prospective study of 1033 consecutive sedations. Int J Radiat Oncol Biol Phys 2001;49(3):771–83.
59. Christensen RE, Nause-Osthoff RC, Waldman JC, et al. Adverse events in radiation oncology: A case series from wake up safe, the pediatric anesthesia quality improvement initiative. Paediatr Anaesth 2019;29(3):265–70.
60. Bratton J, Johnstone PA, McMullen KP. Outpatient management of vascular access devices in children receiving radiotherapy: complications and morbidity. Pediatr Blood Cancer 2014;61(3):499–501.
61. Nguyen SM, Chlebik AA, Olch AJ, et al. Collision Risk Mitigation of Varian True-Beam Linear Accelerator With Supplemental Live-View Cameras. Pract Radiat Oncol 2019;9(1):e103–9.
62. Spraker MB, Fain R 3rd, Gopan O, et al. Evaluation of near-miss and adverse events in radiation oncology using a comprehensive causal factor taxonomy. Pract Radiat Oncol 2017;7(5):346–53.
63. Holmes JA, Chera BS, Brenner DJ, et al. Estimating the excess lifetime risk of radiation induced secondary malignancy (SMN) in pediatric patients treated with craniospinal irradiation (CSI): Conventional radiation therapy versus helical intensity modulated radiation therapy. Pract Radiat Oncol 2017;7(1):35–41.
64. Goodman TR, Mustafa A, Rowe E. Pediatric CT radiation exposure: where we were, and where we are now. Pediatr Radiol 2019;49(4):469–78.
65. Oeffinger KC, Hudson MM. Long-term complications following childhood and adolescent cancer: foundations for providing risk-based health care for survivors. CA Cancer J Clin 2004;54(4):208–36.
66. Grant EJ, Brenner A, Sugiyama H, et al. Solid Cancer Incidence among the Life Span Study of Atomic Bomb Survivors: 1958-2009. Radiat Res 2017;187(5): 513–37.
67. Medek S, De B, Pater L, et al. Practice Patterns Among Radiation Oncologists Treating Pediatric Patients With Proton Craniospinal Irradiation. Pract Radiat Oncol 2019;9(6):441–7.
68. Stachelek GC, Terezakis SA, Ermoian R. Palliative radiation oncology in pediatric patients. Ann Palliat Med 2019;8(3):285–92.
69. Rao AD, Chen Q, Ermoian RP, et al. Practice patterns of palliative radiation therapy in pediatric oncology patients in an international pediatric research consortium. Pediatr Blood Cancer 2017;64(11).
70. Holzman RS, Yoo L, Fox VL, et al. Air embolism during intraoperative endoscopic localization and surgical resection for blue rubber bleb nevus syndrome. Anesthesiology 2005;102(6):1279–80.
71. Murphy ES, Chao ST, Angelov L, et al. Radiosurgery for Pediatric Brain Tumors. Pediatr Blood Cancer 2016;63(3):398–405.

72. Bir SC, Konar SK, Patra DP, et al. Management of a complex intracranial arteriovenous malformation with gamma knife radiosurgery: A case report with review of literature. J Clin Neurosci 2018;49:26–31.

73. Jung EW, Murphy ES, Jung DL, et al. Pediatric radiosurgery: a review. Appl Radiol Oncol 2015;4(2):6–13.

74. Gailloud P, O'Riordan DP, Burger I, et al. Diagnosis and management of vein of galen aneurysmal malformations. J Perinatol 2005;25(8):542–51.

75. Regis J, Tamura M, Guillot C, et al. Radiosurgery with the world's first fully robotized Leksell Gamma Knife PerfeXion in clinical use: a 200-patient prospective, randomized, controlled comparison with the Gamma Knife 4C. Neurosurgery 2009;64(2):346–55 [discussion: 355–46].

76. Keshavarzi S, Meltzer H, Ben-Haim S, et al. Initial clinical experience with frameless optically guided stereotactic radiosurgery/radiotherapy in pediatric patients. Childs Nerv Syst 2009;25(7):837–44.

77. Nanda R, Dhabbaan A, Janss A, et al. The feasibility of frameless stereotactic radiosurgery in the management of pediatric central nervous system tumors. J Neurooncol 2014;117(2):329–35.

78. Bauman GS, Brett CM, Ciricillo SF, et al. Anesthesia for pediatric stereotactic radiosurgery. Anesthesiology 1998;89(1):255–7.

79. White PF. Propofol: its role in changing the practice of anesthesia. Anesthesiology 2008;109(6):1132–6.

80. Furlanetti LL, Monaco BA, Cordeiro JG, et al. Frame-based stereotactic neurosurgery in children under the age of seven: Freiburg University's experience from 99 consecutive cases. Clin Neurol Neurosurg 2015;130:42–7.

81. Berry C, Sandberg DI, Hoh DJ, et al. Use of cranial fixation pins in pediatric neurosurgery. Neurosurgery 2008;62(4):913–8 [discussion: 918–9].

82. Baerts WD, de Lange JJ, Booij LH, et al. Complications of the Mayfield skull clamp. Anesthesiology 1984;61(4):460–1.

83. Nag S, Tippin DB. Brachytherapy for pediatric tumors. Brachytherapy 2003; 2(3):131–8.

84. Nag S, Tippin D, Ruymann FB. Long-term morbidity in children treated with fractionated high-dose-rate brachytherapy for soft tissue sarcomas. J Pediatr Hematol Oncol 2003;25(6):448–52.

85. Liu Z, Tian Z, Yu X, et al. Stereotactic intratumour irradiation with nuclide for craniopharyngiomas. Chin Med J (Engl) 1996;109(3):219–22.

86. Zhao R, Deng J, Liang X, et al. Treatment of cystic craniopharyngioma with phosphorus-32 intracavitary irradiation. Childs Nerv Syst 2010;26(5):669–74.

87. Ansari SF, Moore RJ, Boaz JC, et al. Efficacy of phosphorus-32 brachytherapy without external-beam radiation for long-term tumor control in patients with craniopharyngioma. J Neurosurg Pediatr 2016;17(4):439–45.

88. Nag S, Tippin D, Ruymann FB. Intraoperative high-dose-rate brachytherapy for the treatment of pediatric tumors: the Ohio State University experience. Int J Radiat Oncol Biol Phys 2001;51(3):729–35.

89. Benrath J, Kozek-Langenecker S, Hupfl M, et al. Anaesthesia for brachytherapy–51/2 yr of experience in 1622 procedures. Br J Anaesth 2006;96(2): 195–200.

90. Kozek-Langenecker SA, Marhofer P, Sator-Katzenschlager SM, et al. (+)-ketamine for long-term sedation in a child with retinoblastoma undergoing interstitial brachytherapy. Paediatr Anaesth 2005;15(3):248–50.

91. Roessler B, Six LM, Gustorff B. Anaesthesia for brachytherapy. Curr Opin Anaesthesiol 2008;21(4):514–8.

92. Potter R, Knocke TH, Kovacs G, et al. Brachytherapy in the combined modality treatment of pediatric malignancies. Principles and preliminary experience with treatment of soft tissue sarcoma (recurrence) and Ewing's sarcoma. Klin Padiatr 1995;207(4):164–73.
93. Laskar S, Pilar A, Khanna N, et al. Interstitial brachytherapy for pediatric soft tissue sarcoma: Evolving practice over three decades and long-term outcomes. Pediatr Blood Cancer 2018;65(9):e27112.
94. Gustorff B, Lierz P, Felleiter P, et al. Ropivacaine and bupivacaine for long-term epidural infusion in a small child. Br J Anaesth 1999;83(4):673–4.
95. van Beek EJ, Leroy PL. Safe and effective procedural sedation for gastrointestinal endoscopy in children. J Pediatr Gastroenterol Nutr 2012;54(2):171–85.
96. Lightdale JR, Acosta R, Shergill AK, et al. Modifications in endoscopic practice for pediatric patients. Gastrointest Endosc 2014;79(5):699–710.
97. Biber JL, Allareddy V, Allareddy V, et al. Prevalence and Predictors of Adverse Events during Procedural Sedation Anesthesia-Outside the Operating Room for Esophagogastroduodenoscopy and Colonoscopy in Children: Age Is an Independent Predictor of Outcomes. Pediatr Crit Care Med 2015;16(8):e251–9.
98. Chung HK, Lightdale JR. Sedation and Monitoring in the Pediatric Patient during Gastrointestinal Endoscopy. Gastrointest Endosc Clin N Am 2016;26(3):507–25.
99. Uffman JC, Tumin D, Beltran RJ, et al. Severe outcomes of pediatric perioperative adverse events occurring in operating rooms compared to off-site anesthetizing locations in the Wake Up Safe Database. Paediatr Anaesth 2019;29(1): 38–43.
100. Agostoni M, Fanti L, Gemma M, et al. Adverse events during monitored anesthesia care for GI endoscopy: an 8-year experience. Gastrointest Endosc 2011;74(2):266–75.
101. Odegard KC, Bergersen L, Thiagarajan R, et al. The frequency of cardiac arrests in patients with congenital heart disease undergoing cardiac catheterization. Anesth Analg 2014;118(1):175–82.
102. Odegard KC, Vincent R, Baijal RG, et al. SCAI/CCAS/SPA Expert Consensus Statement for Anesthesia and Sedation Practice: Recommendations for Patients Undergoing Diagnostic and Therapeutic Procedures in the Pediatric and Congenital Cardiac Catheterization Laboratory. Anesth Analg 2016;123(5): 1201–9.
103. Lin CH, Hegde S, Marshall AC, et al. Incidence and management of life-threatening adverse events during cardiac catheterization for congenital heart disease. Pediatr Cardiol 2014;35(1):140–8.
104. Ramamoorthy C, Haberkern CM, Bhananker SM, et al. Anesthesia-related cardiac arrest in children with heart disease: data from the Pediatric Perioperative Cardiac Arrest (POCA) registry. Anesth Analg 2010;110(5):1376–82.
105. Vincent RN, Moore J, Beekman RH, et al. Procedural characteristics and adverse events in diagnostic and interventional catheterisations in paediatric and adult CHD: initial report from the IMPACT Registry. Cardiol Young 2016; 26(1):70–8.
106. Bennett D, Marcus R, Stokes M. Incidents and complications during pediatric cardiac catheterization. Paediatr Anaesth 2005;15(12):1083–8.
107. Braz LG, Modolo NS, do Nascimento P Jr, et al. Perioperative cardiac arrest: a study of 53,718 anaesthetics over 9 yr from a Brazilian teaching hospital. Br J Anaesth 2006;96(5):569–75.
108. Vitiello R, McCrindle BW, Nykanen D, et al. Complications associated with pediatric cardiac catheterization. J Am Coll Cardiol 1998;32(5):1433–40.

109. Bergersen L, Gauvreau K, Foerster SR, et al. Catheterization for Congenital Heart Disease Adjustment for Risk Method (CHARM). JACC Cardiovasc Interv 2011;4(9):1037–46.

110. Nykanen DG, Forbes TJ, Du W, et al. CRISP: Catheterization RISk score for Pediatrics: A Report from the Congenital Cardiac Interventional Study Consortium (CCISC). Catheter Cardiovasc Interv 2016;87(2):302–9.

111. Hill KD, Du W, Fleming GA, et al. Validation and refinement of the catheterization RISk score for pediatrics (CRISP score): An analysis from the congenital cardiac interventional study consortium. Catheter Cardiovasc Interv 2019;93(1):97–104.

112. Jayaram N, Spertus JA, Kennedy KF, et al. Modeling Major Adverse Outcomes of Pediatric and Adult Patients With Congenital Heart Disease Undergoing Cardiac Catheterization: Observations From the NCDR IMPACT Registry (National Cardiovascular Data Registry Improving Pediatric and Adult Congenital Treatment). Circulation 2017;136(21):2009–19.

113. Nasr VG, Guzzetta NA, Miller-Hance WC, et al. Consensus Statement by the Congenital Cardiac Anesthesia Society: Milestones for the Pediatric Cardiac Anesthesia Fellowship. Anesth Analg 2018;126(1):198–207.

New Trends in Fetal Anesthesia

Kha M. Tran, MD[a],*, Debnath Chatterjee, MD[b]

KEYWORDS

- Fetal anesthesia • Fetal surgery • EXIT • PRESTO

KEY POINTS

- Minimally invasive procedures typically are performed with moderate sedation, but neuraxial or general anesthetics may be used. These procedures typically are done for complicated multiple gestations but also may be done to treat cardiac abnormalities, cystic lung lesions, diaphragmatic hernia, lower urinary tract obstruction, and sacrococcygeal teratoma.
- Open mid-gestation fetal surgery is performed most commonly to repair fetal myelomeningocele. These cases typically require maternal general anesthesia with additional measures to optimize fetal cardiac function, uterine relaxation, and maternal and fetal perfusion. The fetus is returned to the uterus to continue growth and development.
- Ex utero intrapartum therapy is performed for fetuses that need help transitioning to extrauterine life. The anesthetic is similar to that for mid-gestation surgery, but the uterine relaxation must be reversed promptly after the baby is delivered. A second team must be prepared to receive the newborn after the procedure is completed.

INTRODUCTION

Fetal therapy is a new field that is beginning to mature as more fetal treatment centers are being established and collaborative efforts are undertaken to improve the care of the mother and fetus.

Anesthetic management should be grounded in an understanding of the pathophysiology of the underlying fetal anomaly, the rationale, and the technical details of the fetal intervention. Practical considerations also include the preferences and philosophies of the practitioners and the infrastructure, staffing models, and characteristics of the patient population.

A discussion of the physiology of pregnancy, the fetus, and the placenta can be found in other resources.[1] What follows is an overview of the diseases that are

[a] University of Pennsylvania Perelman School of Medicine, Center for Fetal Diagnosis and Treatment, Children's Hospital of Philadelphia, 3401 Civic Center Boulevard, Philadelphia, PA 19104, USA; [b] Children's Hospital Colorado, Anschutz Medical Campus, 13123 East 16th Avenue, Aurora, CO 80045, USA
* Corresponding author.
E-mail address: trank@email.chop.edu

Anesthesiology Clin 38 (2020) 605–619
https://doi.org/10.1016/j.anclin.2020.05.006   anesthesiology.theclinics.com
1932-2275/20/© 2020 Elsevier Inc. All rights reserved.

diagnosed more commonly and treated in the prenatal or immediate postnatal periods. The rationale and approach to treatment are presented. A common endpoint of many fetal disease processes is hydrops fetalis, which often is the symptom that prompts a fetal intervention. If the fetus develops hydrops, the mother also is at risk of developing pulmonary edema from maternal mirror syndrome.[2] Supportive therapy for the mother and treatment of the fetal disease process will treat the maternal mirror syndrome. Detailed discussion of the outcomes of the various inventions is beyond the scope of this review. The anesthetic management is broken down into minimally invasive, open mid-gestation, and ex utero intrapartum therapy (EXIT) procedures.

DISEASES AND TREATMENTS
Complicated Multiple Gestation

Twin-twin transfusion syndrome (TTTS) is a complication of monochorionic twin pregnancy, where one twin (the recipient) becomes hyperdynamic and hypervolemic. Polyuria, polyhydramnios, and cardiac changes, such as ventricular hypertrophy and dilation, may develop. The other twin (the donor) becomes hypovolemic, with ensuing oliguria and oligohydramnios. Both twins are at risk for death, preterm delivery, and periventricular leukomalacia. A similar situation may develop where there is a discrepancy in the hemoglobin concentration between the twins in the absence of a discrepancy in amniotic fluid volume. This condition is known as twin anemia-polycythemia sequence.[3] In some cases, one or both twins may have other concomitant congenital abnormalities. In some cases, twin reversed arterial perfusion (TRAP) sequence may develop. One twin may not develop a heart, and the normal pump twin provides perfusion to the acardiac twin.[4]

The treatment of complicated multiple gestations depends on the therapeutic goals. If the goal is for both twins to survive, fetoscopic ablation of the problematic vascular anastomoses is undertaken with laser energy, which should result in more balanced blood flow to both twins. In some cases, the family and surgical team may opt to maximize the chances for only one twin's survival.[5,6] In these cases, radiofrequency ablation (RFA) of the umbilical cord of the other twin is performed. If the twins happen to be both monochorionic and monoamniotic, the umbilical cord that has been treated with RFA also must be divided to prevent a cord accident from the entanglement of the twins and their umbilical vessels.[6]

Airway Obstruction

Fetal airway obstruction can be divided into extrinsic and intrinsic causes. A majority of fetuses with extrinsic airway obstruction due to a mass or micrognathia do not require therapy in the middle of gestation because they are on placental circulatory support. The problems arise at birth, because the airway obstruction impedes the newborn's first breath. Intrinsic obstruction from a laryngeal web or atresia may require therapy in the middle of gestation if the airway obstruction is so severe that lung fluid cannot escape to the amniotic fluid.[7] If the trapped lung fluid causes overdistension of the fetal lungs, the fetal heart is compressed and hydrops fetalis may develop.[8] Mid-gestation therapy only attenuates the causes of the hydrops, and further measures still are required to ensure a secure airway at birth.

The treatment of fetal airway obstruction at birth requires risk stratification.[9,10] If there is little to no chance a secure airway can be established expeditiously immediately after birth, EXIT delivery is undertaken, which involves actions to secure the airway before the umbilical cord is clamped. Because the umbilical cord is patent, the fetal airway may be secured in a controlled manner over the course of an hour or more, as long as the uteroplacental interface is intact. The airway may be secured by direct laryngoscopy, rigid bronchoscopy, or tracheostomy, and mass debulking or resection also may occur.

If there is a reasonable chance the newborn airway can be secured after birth, or if the mother is not a candidate for an EXIT delivery, arrangements are made to have a second full team, including nursing, neonatal, anesthesia, and surgical providers present for the birth of the child.[11] These teams assess the neonate at birth and act according to clinical needs. This may involve no intervention, application of continuous positive airway pressure, intubation with direct or video laryngoscopy, fiberoptic or rigid bronchoscopy, or tracheostomy. Appropriate nomenclature, communication, booking of cases, and organizing of teams can be unwieldy in these situations, so the phrase, Procedure REquiring Second Team in the Operating room (PRESTO), was developed to facilitate communication between all the involved teams. At the Children's Hospital of Philadelphia, this type of case is denoted by PRESTO for airway.

Treatment of intrinsic airway obstruction in the middle of gestation is undertaken less commonly. This may involve using a fetoscope and laser to create a defect in a tracheal web.[12] As the lung fluid escapes through the new defect, the lungs and heart decompress. Even if the airway decompression is successful, and the hydrops resolves, the fetus still may require an EXIT delivery. The defect created by the laser only allows decompression of the airway and lungs, but the defect is likely not large enough to allow adequate ventilation with a natural airway or easy passage of an endotracheal tube.

Lung Masses

Lung masses, such as congenital pulmonary airway malformation, bronchopulmonary sequestration, and hybrid lesions, threaten the fetus in a variety of ways. Mass effect causes mediastinal shift and cardiac tamponade physiology, which may cause nonimmune hydrops. A large lesion also prevents the growth of normal lung tissue.[13]

Treatment of lung lesions varies depending on the symptomatology and characteristics of the lesion. In many cases, no fetal intervention is required, the pregnancy may be carried to term, and the child can be scheduled for an elective lobectomy. If the lung lesion is large, with evidence of mediastinal shift, radiographic evidence of significant hypoplasia, or other concerning factors, the surgical and obstetric teams may consider a cesarean delivery, with a PRESTO thoracotomy or an EXIT procedure with a fetal thoracotomy.[14] Even larger lesions may cause hydrops in the middle of gestation and prompt the surgical teams to intervene earlier. If the lesion has macrocysts, serial aspirations or continuous drainage with a shunt alleviates cardiac compression.[15] If the lesion is solid or otherwise not amenable to minimally invasive approaches to decompression, open fetal surgery with fetal thoracotomy and resection of the lesion is performed. The fetus then is placed back in the uterus to continue gestation.

Heart Defects

Catheter-based cardiac interventions are performed for various indications.[16] The more common indications include fetuses with (1) severe aortic stenosis and evolving hypoplastic left heart syndrome (HLHS); (2) pulmonary valve atresia, intact atrial septum, and evolving hypoplastic right heart syndrome; or (3) HLHS with an intact or highly restrictive atrial septum. In the first 2 cases, the catheter-based intervention consists of an aortic or pulmonary balloon valvuloplasty, with the hope of improving blood flow through the hypoplastic ventricle and promoting the development of a biventricular circulation. In the third case, the treatment consists of a fetal atrial septoplasty, with either a balloon or stent. The goal is simply to improve survival at birth because a newborn with HLHS and an intact atrial septum does not have any pathway for blood to travel from the lungs to the systemic circulation. The cardiac interventions often are carried out percutaneously by placing a catheter system across the maternal abdominal wall, uterus, and fetal chest wall into the heart. In some cases, the surgical and cardiac team may opt to perform a laparotomy to access the uterus and fetal heart more easily.[17–19]

Open fetal surgery to resect fetal pericardial teratomas with mass effect on the heart has been performed.[20] This therapy involves a maternal laparotomy and hysterotomy, followed by a fetal sternotomy and resection of the teratoma. After fetal chest closure, the fetus is returned to the uterus.

Congenital Diaphragmatic Hernia

Congenital diaphragmatic hernia (CDH) has been a target of fetal therapy for decades.[21] Various attempts at primary fetal repair or tracheal occlusion to allow lung growth were studied, but these strategies required at least 1 if not 2 major surgical procedures on the mother, and neonatal outcomes after these fetal interventions were equivalent to standard postnatal CDH repair.[22] Open fetal therapy for CDH, therefore, currently is not performed.

Newer minimally invasive, fetoscopic endoluminal tracheal occlusion involves placing a balloon in the fetal trachea between 27 weeks' and 31 weeks' gestation. These balloons are removed fetoscopically after 4 weeks to 6 weeks. The balloon promotes lung growth while in place, and, after the balloon is removed, the mother may deliver vaginally. European results have been promising, but these studies were not randomized.[23] The Tracheal Occlusion To Accelerate Lung Growth trial is under way at multiple institutions around the world.[24,25]

Myelomeningocele

Prenatal repair of myelomeningocele (MMC) has been shown to improve motor and sensory function and reduces the need for shunting of cerebrospinal fluid after birth.[26,27] As with any open mid-gestation fetal surgery, the treatment involves performing a maternal laparotomy and hysterotomy to access the fetal MMC. The MMC is repaired with various surgical techniques, and the fetus is replaced in the uterus.

In efforts to further decrease maternal morbidity from major surgery and even allow vaginal delivery, some fetal surgical teams are performing fetoscopic MMC repair. This fetoscopic approach still requires a maternal laparotomy, but the uterus is not opened. The risk of preterm labor is attenuated, and vaginal delivery is an option if no other maternal contraindications exist.[28–30] These advantages, however, come with the cost of longer surgical time and less clear neonatal outcomes. The specific surgical techniques have varied over time and between institutions. The techniques have ranged from single-layer to 3-layer closures of the MMC, with occasional use of patches.[31–33]

Lower Urinary Tract Obstruction

Lower urinary tract obstruction (LUTO) leads to renal damage and pulmonary hypoplasia. Posterior urethral valves are the most common cause of LUTO.[34] Decompression of the urinary tract is the goal of the prenatal intervention. If fetal imaging suggests a prenatal intervention may be helpful, serial samples of fetal urine are collected and analyzed to guide decision making for invasive fetal intervention. Therapeutic decisions are challenging in cases of LUTO, because the prognosis must be grim enough to warrant an intervention, although not so grim that the renal system is not salvageable. Interventions have included open fetal surgery, but most interventions are minimally invasive, such as serial vesicocentesis, placement of a vesicoamniotic shunt, and fetal cystoscopic procedures.[35–37]

Sacrococcygeal Teratoma

A large sacrococcygeal teratoma (SCT) imposes a great metabolic burden on the fetus that can cause high-output heart failure.[38] Although the fetal decompensation may be rapid, heart failure occurs more typically in a time frame that allows monitoring of the heart, tumor, and fetal growth.[39] The treatment of fetal SCT is individualized and depends on the fetal physiology, tumor morphology, and expertise of the fetal treatment center.

Interventions for prenatally diagnosed SCT include minimally invasive tumor ablation, open fetal debulking, EXIT procedure, and early delivery with debulking or complete resection immediately at birth.[40–44]

TYPES OF FETAL INTERVENTIONS

Fetal interventions can be divided into minimally invasive, open mid-gestation, and EXIT procedures.[1,45] Minimally invasive fetal interventions are the most common and typically are performed in early gestation or mid-gestation. Using ultrasound guidance, needles or trocars are inserted into the amniotic cavity, without the need for a hysterotomy.[46,47] During needle-based procedures, needles are inserted percutaneously under ultrasound guidance. During fetoscopic interventions, a 2.3-mm to 4.0-mm (7F to 12F) trocar that accommodates a 1.2-mm to 3-mm endoscope is placed percutaneously into the amniotic cavity with ultrasound guidance. Occasionally, a laparotomy may be necessary to exteriorize the uterus for complex fetoscopic repairs or when an anterior placenta precludes a percutaneous approach.[46,47] Common indications for minimally invasive fetal interventions and their pathophysiology are listed in **Table 1**.

Open fetal surgeries typically are performed in mid-gestation. After inducing maternal general anesthesia, the uterus is exposed via laparotomy, and then a hysterotomy is performed to obtain surgical access to the fetus. Profound uterine relaxation is achieved prior to hysterotomy and maintained until uterine closure. After fetal surgery, the uterus is closed, and the pregnancy is continued.

EXIT procedures are performed closer to term and allow life-saving fetal interventions to be performed while the fetus remains on placental circulatory support. Common indications for an EXIT procedure are listed in **Table 2**. Similar to open fetal surgeries, a hysterotomy is performed, and the fetus is partially delivered. Fetal direct laryngoscopy and endotracheal intubation typically are attempted first, and additional airway interventions, such as rigid bronchoscopy, fiberoptic intubation, elevating the mass off the airway, release of neck strap muscles, or partial excision of the mass, may be necessary for securing the fetal airway.[48–52] After completing the planned fetal intervention, the umbilical cord is clamped, and the newborn is delivered.

Anesthetic Management

The anesthesiologist plays an integral role in the multidisciplinary approach to fetal interventions. At the multidisciplinary team meeting with the mother and family, informed consent should include a discussion of the planned fetal intervention, surgical and anesthetic risks, benefits to the fetus, expected outcomes, and alternative treatment options.[1,45] If the fetus is viable (usually >24 weeks' gestational age) and the mother desires full fetal resuscitation, a plan should be made for emergent cesarean delivery and neonatal resuscitation in the event of intraoperative fetal distress that is not responsive to standard fetal resuscitative measures.[1,45] A preanesthetic evaluation also should be performed, focusing on maternal comorbidities, obstetric history, previous anesthetics, airway evaluation, and cardiopulmonary evaluation. Preoperative

Table 1
Common indications for minimally invasive interventions and open fetal surgery

Fetal Malformation	Pathophysiology	Fetal Intervention
Fetal anemia	Causes include Rh isoimmunization, parvovirus B19 infection, twin anemia-polycythemia sequence, etc; results in fetal heart failure and hydrops	Intrauterine blood transfusion
TTTS	Monochorionic-diamniotic twin pregnancy with unbalanced flow across placental intertwin vascular anastomoses. Donor twin develops oligohydramnios and growth restriction. Recipient twin develops polyhydramnios, cardiomyopathy, and hydrops. High risk of fetal demise and adverse neurologic outcomes	Serial amnioreduction Selective fetoscopic laser photocoagulation Selective fetal reduction via RFA
TRAP sequence	Monochorionic twin pregnancy with 1 acardiac twin. Normal (pump) twin provides retrograde perfusion to the acardiac twin, resulting in congestive heart failure, polyhydramnios, and preterm delivery	RFA of acardiac twin
LUTO	Dilated thick-walled bladder, renal dysplasia, and severe oligohydramnios; neonatal renal and respiratory failure	Vesicoamniotic shunt placement Fetal cystoscopy and ablation of posterior urethral valves
Congenital cystic lung lesions	Congenital pulmonary airway malformation or pleural effusion causing pulmonary hypoplasia, mediastinal shift, hydrops, and polyhydramnios	Serial thoracentesis Thoracoamniotic shunt placement Open fetal lobectomy
CDH	Herniated abdominal viscera and lung compression results in pulmonary hypoplasia and pulmonary hypertension	FETO, followed by the reversal of tracheal occlusion
Amniotic band syndrome	Constrictive amniotic bands with entanglement of fetal parts, leading to limb amputation, syndactyly, craniofacial or body wall defects	Fetoscopic laser release of amniotic bands

(continued on next page)

Table 1
(*continued*)

Fetal Malformation	Pathophysiology	Fetal Intervention
Aortic stenosis with evolving HLHS	Progressive left ventricular dysfunction and arrested growth of left-sided heart structures	Fetal aortic valvuloplasty with balloon dilation of aortic valve
HLHS with intact atrial septum	Absent or restricted left-to-right flow across foramen ovale leads to pulmonary venous hypertension; if present at birth, results in cyanosis, acidosis, and death	Fetal atrial septostomy
MMC	Damage to exposed spinal cord and Chiari II malformation leads to lower extremity paralysis and obstructive hydrocephalus	Open fetal MMC repair Fetoscopic MMC repair
SCT	Arteriovenous shunting, high-output cardiac failure, hydrops, and placentomegaly	Fetoscopic laser ablation Laser RFA Open fetal surgery

laboratory testing should include a complete blood cell count, a type and screen for minimally invasive fetal interventions, and a type and crossmatch for open fetal surgery and EXIT procedures. In addition, leukocyte-reduced, irradiated, O-negative blood that is crossmatched to the mother should be available for the fetus during open fetal surgery and EXIT procedures. Pertinent information for the anesthesiologist includes gestational age, estimated fetal weight for drug dosing, baseline fetal heart rate, the severity of fetal anomaly, and the location of the placenta, which determines maternal positioning during the fetal intervention.

Anesthesia for Minimally Invasive Fetal Interventions

The anesthetic technique for minimally invasive fetal interventions depends on the planned surgical approach, degree of invasiveness, duration of the procedure, patient

Table 2
Common indications for ex utero intrapartum therapy procedures or procedures requiring second team in the operating room

Type	Fetal Malformation
EXIT to airway	External obstruction—cervical teratoma, lymphatic/vascular malformation, severe micrognathia, oropharyngeal teratoma Intrinsic obstruction—congenital high airway obstruction syndrome, laryngeal or tracheal atresia, laryngeal web Iatrogenic—prior tracheal occlusion for congenital diaphragmatic hernia that has not been decompressed
EXIT to resection	Congenital pulmonary airway malformation Bronchopulmonary sequestration SCT Thoracic or mediastinal tumors

positioning, and preferences of the patient and surgeon. Currently, most minimally invasive fetal interventions are performed with local anesthetic infiltration or neuraxial anesthesia with or without intravenous sedation.[1,45] For interventions that require a laparotomy to exteriorize the uterus, maternal general endotracheal anesthesia typically is chosen.[47] When compared with spinal anesthesia, monitored anesthesia care with local anesthetic infiltration for minimally invasive fetal interventions was associated with less presurgical operating room time, vasopressor use, and intraoperative fluid administration.[53]

Preoperatively, standard fasting guidelines should apply, and aspiration prophylaxis medications should be administered. Intraoperatively, standard American Society of Anesthesiologists (ASA) monitors should be used. Maintaining adequate uteroplacental blood flow is critical, and vasopressors commonly are used to maintain maternal hemodynamics.[1,45] Intraoperative fluid administration was restricted in the past secondary to concerns of postoperative pulmonary edema.[54] Careful accounting of uterine irrigation fluids, however, has minimized the risks and lifted the restriction on intraoperative fluids. Maternal administration of sedatives and analgesics provides limited fetal analgesia via transplacental transfer. A randomized trial comparing remifentanil and diazepam for maternal sedation during fetoscopic interventions showed that remifentanil provided adequate fetal immobilization and improved operating conditions.[55] Fetal interventions on noninnervated tissues, such as the placenta (laser for TTTS), do not require additional fetal drug administration. For procedures, such as intrauterine transfusion or cordocentesis, fetal immobilization is ensured by fetal intramuscular or umbilical venous administration of a muscle relaxant to prevent fetal movement and dislodgement of the needle. For more invasive fetal procedures, such as fetal aortic balloon valvuloplasty or fetoscopic endoluminal tracheal occlusion, a fetal intramuscular cocktail of an opioid (fentanyl, 20 μg/kg), muscle relaxant (rocuronium, 2 mg/kg, or vecuronium, 0.2 mg/kg) and atropine, 20 μg/kg, commonly is administered using ultrasound guidance to ensure fetal analgesia and immobilization. Unlike open fetal surgeries and EXIT procedures, profound uterine relaxation typically is not necessary. Fetal monitoring involves measuring the fetal heart rate using Doppler ultrasonography at the beginning and end of the procedure. During fetal cardiac interventions, continuous fetal echocardiography is performed to monitor cardiac function.[1,45]

Postoperative complications after minimally invasive interventions depend on the complexity of the procedure. Obstetric complications include preterm premature rupture of membranes (PPROM), chorioamniotic membrane separation, chorioamnionitis, oligohydramnios, and preterm labor.[46,56] A recent meta-analysis found an overall maternal complication rate of approximately 6% for fetoscopic interventions and 21% for open fetal surgery.[57] Maternal complications include hemorrhage, surgical site infection, sepsis, and pulmonary edema. Unlike open fetal surgeries, minimally invasive fetal interventions do not preclude vaginal delivery in the index and subsequent pregnancies.[46,56] Similar to open fetal surgeries, fetoscopic interventions also do not affect subsequent fertility or reproductive potential.[58]

Anesthesia for Open Fetal Surgeries

Open mid-gestation fetal surgeries typically are performed under maternal general anesthesia.[1,45] Preoperative preparation on the day of surgery includes fasting; peripheral intravenous (PIV) catheter insertion; administration of antibiotics, aspiration, and venous thromboembolism prophylaxis medications; and indomethacin for tocolysis. For postoperative analgesia, a high lumbar epidural catheter is inserted, which is not bolused until the end of the surgery, secondary to concerns of intraoperative hemodynamic instability. In the operating room, the patient is positioned supine with uterine displacement. A rapid sequence induction is performed to facilitate endotracheal intubation. In addition to standard ASA monitors, an arterial catheter for close hemodynamic monitoring, a second PIV catheter, and a Foley catheter are inserted. General anesthesia typically is maintained with either an inhalational agent or a combination of inhalational and intravenous anesthetic agents.

The main anesthetic considerations during open fetal surgeries include maintaining uteroplacental blood flow, achieving profound uterine relaxation, and minimizing fetal cardiac dysfunction.[1,45,59] The uteroplacental circulation is a low-resistance vascular bed with limited ability for autoregulation. It is critical to maintain uteroplacental blood flow by avoiding hypotension, aortocaval compression, and uterine contractions. Vasopressors commonly are used to maintain maternal hemodynamics. Achieving profound uterine relaxation just prior to hysterotomy and maintaining it until uterine closure are paramount. Originally, high doses of inhalational agents were used for uterine relaxation, and this resulted in significant fetal cardiac dysfunction.[60] An alternative anesthetic protocol, supplemental intravenous anesthesia (SIVA), has been described, which includes anesthetic maintenance with propofol and remifentanil infusions until uterine hysterotomy and adding desflurane just prior to hysterotomy.[61] SIVA has allowed adequate uterine relaxation at a lower desflurane concentration (1–1.5 Minimum Alveolar Concentration) and is associated with a decreased incidence of fetal cardiac dysfunction. A similar anesthetic protocol, which includes anesthesia maintenance with desflurane, and a supplemental remifentanil infusion are being used at a major fetal care center to achieve adequate uterine relaxation at a lower desflurane concentration (DC Mark Rollins, personal communication, 2020). Traditionally, a magnesium sulfate bolus followed by an infusion is administered after uterine closure for postoperative tocolysis. Early administration of magnesium sulfate, after induction, has reduced the amount of inhalational anesthetic agent for uterine relaxation during open fetal surgery.[62] Intraoperative fluid administration typically is restricted to reduce the risk of postoperative maternal pulmonary edema.

After uterine exposure, the placental borders are mapped, and a hysterotomy is performed. Warm isotonic crystalloid is infused into the amniotic cavity to maintain uterine volume. The fetus is positioned within the uterus such that the desired fetal part is exposed through the hysterotomy. To ensure fetal analgesia and immobilization, a fetal intramuscular cocktail is administered. In cases of more potential for bleeding, such as thoracotomy or SCT debulking, a fetal PIV catheter is placed. The surgical repair is undertaken. Fetal echocardiography using a sterile probe allows the monitoring of fetal heart rate, filling, and function. Umbilical artery Dopplers also can be measured. After the repair, the hysterotomy is closed in multiple layers. The epidural catheter is bolused with a local anesthetic. After reversing neuromuscular blockade and administering prophylactic antiemetics, the patient is extubated awake.

Postoperative tocolysis is maintained with a magnesium sulfate infusion. In addition, indomethacin is continued for 48 to 72 hours postoperatively, with serial fetal echocardiography to detect premature closure of the ductus arteriosus.[63] Nifedipine usually is continued for the remainder of the pregnancy.[26] Plans for continuous fetal heart rate monitoring depend on the gestational age of the fetus and the predetermined plan for fetal distress. Postoperative multimodal analgesia is achieved using the epidural catheter, acetaminophen, and ketorolac administration. Maternal complications occur in approximately 21% of open fetal surgeries and include PPROM, preterm labor, oligohydramnios, pulmonary edema, placental abruption, chorioamnionitis, and uterine scar thinning.[56,57] An evaluation of the obstetric outcomes in patients from the Management of Myelomeningocele Study who underwent prenatal repair revealed that chorioamniotic membrane separation was associated with an increased risk of spontaneous rupture of membranes and oligohydramnios was a risk factor for preterm delivery.[64] At the time of cesarean delivery, 65% of the patients in the prenatal repair group had an intact, well-healed hysterotomy scar, and 11% of the patients had partial uterine dehiscence. For patients undergoing open fetal surgery, a cesarean delivery must be performed for the index pregnancy as well as future pregnancies.[47,56]

Anesthesia for Ex Utero Intrapartum Therapy Procedures

The anesthetic management of an EXIT procedure is similar to open fetal surgery, with a major difference that the fetus is delivered at the end of the procedure.[42,65] Most EXIT procedures are performed under maternal general anesthesia. Procedures have been performed, however, under neuraxial anesthesia with a nitroglycerin infusion for tocolysis and remifentanil infusion for fetal immobilization.[66,67] Fetal monitoring during an EXIT procedure may include intermittent fetal echocardiography. In addition, a pulse oximeter may be placed on a fetal hand or foot. Regardless of the indication for the EXIT procedure, securing the fetal airway should be the first step should the EXIT procedure be abandoned early secondary to placental abruption or severe fetal distress.[1,45]

If additional fetal interventions, such as resection of a thoracic or mediastinal mass, are planned, a fetal PIV is inserted for the administration of fluids and packed red blood cells. Upon completion of the fetal procedure, the fetus is ventilated, surfactant may be given, and the umbilical cord is cut. Rapid reversal of uterine tone after umbilical cord clamping is critical. In addition to turning off the volatile anesthetic agent, starting an oxytocin infusion, and manual uterine massage by the surgeons, other uterotonic drugs may be necessary. The newborn is transferred to an adjoining operating room for further resuscitation, as indicated. A second operating room team should be readily available for completion of surgery on the newborn, should the EXIT procedure be abandoned early. The epidural catheter is bolused, and the patient is extubated when awake. Because postoperative tocolysis is not necessary, magnesium sulfate is not used intraoperatively or continued postoperatively. Fluid restriction is not necessary. In a retrospective review of 65 EXIT cases at a single institution, the overall fetal/neonatal mortality rate was 15%, with only 1 fetal demise occurring intraoperatively. Seven mothers were transfused, and the estimated blood loss was 900 mL $\pm$ 300 mL for mothers who were not transfused.[42]

Procedure Requiring Second Team in the Operating Room

As discussed previously, some mothers and fetuses may not be candidates for an EXIT procedure, and some fetal disease processes may not be quite so severe as to warrant an EXIT procedure. Additionally, increasing focus on preventing maternal morbidity has led some teams to take a path that involves a planned cesarean section for the mother and a PRESTO for the newborn. All PRESTOs require close communication because the teams involved make treatment decisions in real time as the newborn is resuscitated. The anesthetic management of a PRESTO depends on the procedure performed. For airway cases, the anesthesia team may obtain vascular access and administer medications while the otolaryngology team performs rigid bronchoscopy or tracheostomy. For lung masses, the anesthesia team may secure the airway while the neonatal team obtains umbilical venous and arterial access, and the surgical team is preparing for thoracotomy. Needs, such as portable radiography, point-of-care laboratory testing, surfactant, inhaled nitric oxide, advanced ventilators, and possible extracorporeal life support, are considered and organized as appropriate. Roles in a PRESTO for SCT are similar to those for a lung lesion, with additional preparation for the management of massive hemorrhage. Detailed planning and open communication, with clear delineation of responsibilities amongst the team members, are critical.

SUMMARY

Fetal therapy is an exciting and dynamic field. The fetal anesthesia team works at the intersection of obstetric and pediatric anesthesia, and the team members must stay informed of developments in each field. The fetal anesthesiologist also must work in collaboration with the surgical, perinatal, and neonatal teams to understand developments in surgical techniques and postoperative medical management. Mutual respect, knowledge sharing, and understanding from all team members are vital components of a successful fetal therapy program.

Clinics Care Points

- For laser cases, mild airway obstruction in a mother can make operating conditions extremely challenging for the team. A lighter plane of anesthesia minimizes obstruction, but the anesthesiologist must manage maternal and surgical expectations appropriately.

- The anesthesia team should watch the surgical field closely when the uterine incision is first made. If amniotic fluid is ejected from the uterus under pressure, the patient may need more tocolysis.

- Unit doses of emergency fetal medications should be drawn up and available to give in the sterile field.

- If the fetus is decompensating during any procedure, optimize maternal ventilation and hemodynamics. Empiric vasopressor therapy may help. Rapidly assess the patency of the umbilical cord and integrity of the uteroplacental interface.

DISCLOSURE

None.

REFERENCES

1. Lin EE, Tran KM. Anesthesia for fetal surgery. Semin Pediatr Surg 2013; 22(1):50–5.
2. van Selm M, Kanhai HH, Gravenhorst JB. Maternal hydrops syndrome: a review. Obstet Gynecol Surv 1991;46(12):785–8.
3. Slaghekke F, Kist WJ, Oepkes D, et al. TAPS and TOPS: two distinct forms of feto-fetal transfusion in monochorionic twins. Z Geburtshilfe Neonatol 2009;213(6): 248–54.
4. Lewi L, Jani J, Deprest J. Invasive antenatal interventions in complicated multiple pregnancies. Obstet Gynecol Clin North Am 2005;32(1):105–26.
5. Djaafri F, Stirnemann J, Mediouni I, et al. Twin-twin transfusion syndrome - What we have learned from clinical trials. Semin Fetal Neonatal Med 2017;22(6): 367–75.
6. Moldenhauer JS, Johnson MP. Diagnosis and management of complicated monochorionic twins. Clin Obstet Gynecol 2015;58(3):632–42.
7. Lim F-Y, Crombleholme TM, Hedrick HL, et al. Congenital high airway obstruction syndrome: natural history and management. J Pediatr Surg 2003;38(6):940–5.

8. Mong A, Johnson AM, Kramer SS, et al. Congenital high airway obstruction syndrome: MR/US findings, effect on management, and outcome. Pediatr Radiol 2008;38(11):1171–9.

9. Laje P, Tharakan SJ, Hedrick HL. Immediate operative management of the fetus with airway anomalies resulting from congenital malformations. Semin Fetal Neonatal Med 2016;21(4):240–5.

10. Laje P, Peranteau WH, Hedrick HL, et al. Ex utero intrapartum treatment (EXIT) in the management of cervical lymphatic malformation. J Pediatr Surg 2015;50(2): 311–4.

11. Prickett K, Javia L. Fetal evaluation and airway management. Clin Perinatol 2018; 45(4):609–28.

12. Kohl T, Van de Vondel P, Stressig R, et al. Percutaneous fetoscopic laser decompression of congenital high airway obstruction syndrome (CHAOS) from laryngeal atresia via a single trocar–current technical constraints and potential solutions for future interventions. Fetal Diagn Ther 2009;25(1):67–71.

13. Adzick NS, Harrison MR, Crombleholme TM, et al. Fetal lung lesions: management and outcome. Am J Obstet Gynecol 1998;179(4):884–9.

14. Hedrick HL, Flake AW, Crombleholme TM, et al. The ex utero intrapartum therapy procedure for high-risk fetal lung lesions. J Pediatr Surg 2005;40(6):1038–44.

15. Peranteau WH, Adzick NS, Boelig MM, et al. Thoracoamniotic shunts for the management of fetal lung lesions and pleural effusions: a single-institution review and predictors of survival in 75 cases. J Pediatr Surg 2015;50(2):301–5.

16. McElhinney DB, Tworetzky W, Lock JE. Current status of fetal cardiac intervention. Circulation 2010;121(10):1256–63.

17. Barry OM, Friedman KG, Bergersen L, et al. Clinical and hemodynamic results after conversion from single to biventricular circulation after fetal aortic stenosis intervention. Am J Cardiol 2018;122(3):511–6.

18. Friedman KG, Sleeper LA, Freud LR, et al. Improved technical success, postnatal outcome and refined predictors of outcome for fetal aortic valvuloplasty. Ultrasound Obstet Gynecol 2018;52(2):212–20.

19. Gellis L, Tworetzky W. The boundaries of fetal cardiac intervention: Expand or tighten? Semin Fetal Neonatal Med 2017;22(6):399–403.

20. Rychik J, Khalek N, Gaynor JW, et al. Fetal intrapericardial teratoma: natural history and management including successful in utero surgery. Am J Obstet Gynecol 2016;215(6):780.e1-e7.

21. Harrison MR. Surgically correctable fetal disease. Am J Surg 2000;180(5): 335–42.

22. Harrison MR, Keller RL, Hawgood SB, et al. A randomized trial of fetal endoscopic tracheal occlusion for severe fetal congenital diaphragmatic hernia. N Engl J Med 2003;349(20):1916–24.

23. Jani JC, Nicolaides KH, Gratacos E, et al. Severe diaphragmatic hernia treated by fetal endoscopic tracheal occlusion. Ultrasound Obstet Gynecol 2009;34(3): 304–10.

24. Deprest J, Brady P, Nicolaides K, et al. Prenatal management of the fetus with isolated congenital diaphragmatic hernia in the era of the TOTAL trial. Semin Fetal Neonatal Med 2014;19(6):338–48.

25. Kovler ML, Jelin EB. Fetal intervention for congenital diaphragmatic hernia. Semin Pediatr Surg 2019;28(4):150818.

26. Adzick NS, Thom EA, Spong CY, et al. A Randomized Trial of Prenatal versus Postnatal Repair of Myelomeningocele. N Engl J Med 2011;364(11):993–1004.

27. Houtrow AJ, Thom EA, Fletcher JM, et al. Prenatal repair of myelomeningocele and school-age functional outcomes. Pediatrics 2020;145(2):e20191544.
28. Belfort MA, Whitehead WE, Shamshirsaz AA, et al. Fetoscopic repair of meningomyelocele. Obstet Gynecol 2015;126(4):881–4. https://doi.org/10.1097/AOG.0000000000000835.
29. Kabagambe SK, Chen YJ, Vanover MA, et al. New directions in fetal surgery for myelomeningocele. Childs Nerv Syst 2017;33(7):1–6.
30. Kohn JR, Rao V, Sellner AA, et al. Management of labor and delivery after fetoscopic repair of an open neural tube defect. Obstet Gynecol 2018;131(6):1062–8.
31. Belfort MA, Whitehead WE, Shamshirsaz AA, et al. Comparison of two fetoscopic open neural tube defect (ONTD) repair techniques: Single-layer vs three-layer closure. Ultrasound Obstet Gynecol 2019. https://doi.org/10.1002/uog.21915.
32. Flanders TM, Madsen PJ, Pisapia JM, et al. Improved postoperative metrics with modified myofascial closure in fetal myelomeningocele repair. Oper Neurosurg (Hagerstown) 2019;364(11):993.
33. Flanders TM, Heuer GG, Madsen PJ, et al. Detailed analysis of hydrocephalus and hindbrain herniation after prenatal and postnatal myelomeningocele closure: report from a single institution. Neurosurgery 2019;100(8):563.
34. Clayton DB, Brock JW. Current state of fetal intervention for lower urinary tract obstruction. Curr Urol Rep 2018;19(1):12.
35. Johnson MP, Wilson RD. Shunt-based interventions: Why, how, and when to place a shunt. Semin Fetal Neonatal Med 2017;22(6):391–8.
36. Vinit N, Gueneuc A, Bessières B, et al. Fetal cystoscopy and vesicoamniotic shunting in lower urinary tract obstruction: long-term outcome and current technical limitations. Fetal Diagn Ther 2020;47(1):74–83.
37. Saccone G, D'Alessandro P, Escolino M, et al. Antenatal intervention for congenital fetal lower urinary tract obstruction (LUTO): a systematic review and meta-analysis. J Matern Fetal Neonatal Med 2018;1–161. https://doi.org/10.1080/14767058.2018.1555704.
38. Flake AW, Harrison MR, Adzick NS, et al. Fetal sacrococcygeal teratoma. J Pediatr Surg 1986;21(7):563–6.
39. Wilson RD, Hedrick H, Flake AW, et al. Sacrococcygeal teratomas: prenatal surveillance, growth and pregnancy outcome. Fetal Diagn Ther 2009;25(1):15–20.
40. Van Mieghem T, Al-Ibrahim A, Deprest J, et al. Minimally invasive therapy for fetal sacrococcygeal teratoma: case series and systematic review of the literature. Ultrasound Obstet Gynecol 2014;43(6):611–9.
41. Adzick NS, Crombleholme TM, Morgan MA, et al. A rapidly growing fetal teratoma. Lancet 1997;349(9051):538.
42. Lin EE, Moldenhauer JS, Tran KM, et al. Anesthetic management of 65 cases of ex utero intrapartum therapy: a 13-year single-center experience. Anesth Analg 2016;123(2):411–7.
43. Roybal JL, Moldenhauer JS, Khalek N, et al. Early delivery as an alternative management strategy for selected high-risk fetal sacrococcygeal teratomas. J Pediatr Surg 2011;46(7):1325–32.
44. Baumgarten HD, Gebb JS, Khalek N, et al. Preemptive delivery and immediate resection for fetuses with high-risk sacrococcygeal teratomas. Fetal Diagn Ther 2019;45(3):137–44.
45. Hoagland MA, Chatterjee D. Anesthesia for fetal surgery. Paediatr Anaesth 2017;27(4):346–57.
46. Graves CE, Harrison MR, Padilla BE. Minimally invasive fetal surgery. Clin Perinatol 2017;44(4):729–51.

47. Nassr AA, Erfani H, Fisher JE, et al. Fetal interventional procedures and surgeries: a practical approach. J Perinat Med 2018;46(7):701–15.

48. Marwan A, Crombleholme TM. The EXIT procedure: principles, pitfalls, and progress. Semin Pediatr Surg 2006;15(2):107–15.

49. Liechty KW. Ex-utero intrapartum therapy. Semin Fetal Neonatal Med 2010; 15(1):34–9.

50. Moldenhauer JS. Ex utero intrapartum therapy. Semin Pediatr Surg 2013; 22(1):44–9.

51. Walz PC, Schroeder JW. Prenatal diagnosis of obstructive head and neck masses and perinatal airway management: the ex utero intrapartum treatment procedure. Otolaryngol Clin North Am 2015;48(1):191–207.

52. Mohammad S, Olutoye O. Airway management for neonates requiring ex utero intrapartum treatment (EXIT). Paediatr Anaesth 2020. https://doi.org/10.1111/pan.13818.

53. Ferschl MB, Feiner J, Vu L, et al. A comparison of spinal anesthesia versus monitored anesthesia care with local anesthesia in minimally invasive fetal surgery. Anesth Analg 2020;130(2):409–15.

54. Robinson MB, Crombleholme TM, Kurth CD. Maternal pulmonary edema during fetoscopic surgery. Anesth Analg. 2008;107(6):1978–80.

55. Van de Velde M, Van Schoubroeck D, Lewi LE, et al. Remifentanil for fetal immobilization and maternal sedation during fetoscopic surgery: a randomized, double-blind comparison with diazepam. Anesth Analg 2005;101(1):251–8.

56. Al-Refai A, Ryan G, Van Mieghem T. Maternal risks of fetal therapy. Curr Opin Obstet Gynecol 2017;29(2):80–4.

57. Sacco A, Van der Veeken L, Bagshaw E, et al. Maternal complications following open and fetoscopic fetal surgery: A systematic review and meta-analysis. Prenat Diagn 2019;39(4):251–68.

58. Gregoir C, Engels AC, Gomez O, et al. Fertility, pregnancy and gynecological outcomes after fetoscopic surgery for congenital diaphragmatic hernia. Hum Reprod 2016;31(9):2024–30.

59. Ferschl M, Ball R, Lee H, et al. Anesthesia for in utero repair of myelomeningocele. Anesthesiology 2013;118(5):1211–23.

60. Rychik J, Cohen D, Tran KM, et al. The role of echocardiography in the intraoperative management of the fetus undergoing myelomeningocele repair. Fetal Diagn Ther 2015;37(3):172–8.

61. Boat A, Mahmoud M, Michelfelder EC, et al. Supplementing desflurane with intravenous anesthesia reduces fetal cardiac dysfunction during open fetal surgery. Paediatr Anaesth 2010;20(8):748–56.

62. Donepudi R, Huynh M, Moise KJ, et al. Early administration of magnesium sulfate during open fetal myelomeningocele repair reduces the dose of inhalational anesthesia. Fetal Diagn Ther 2019;45(3):192–6.

63. Howley L, Wood C, Patel SS, et al. Flow patterns in the ductus arteriosus during open fetal myelomeningocele repair. Prenat Diagn 2015;35(6):564–70.

64. Johnson MP, Bennett KA, Rand L, et al. MOMS: obstetrical outcomes and risk factors for obstetrical complications following prenatal surgery. Am J Obstet Gynecol 2016;215(6):778.e1-9.

65. Garcia PJ, Olutoye OO, Ivey RT, et al. Case scenario: anesthesia for maternal-fetal surgery: the Ex Utero Intrapartum Therapy (EXIT) procedure. Anesthesiology 2011;114(6):1446–52.

66. Fink RJ, Allen TK, Habib AS. Remifentanil for fetal immobilization and analgesia during the ex utero intrapartum treatment procedure under combined spinal-epidural anaesthesia. Br J Anaesth 2011;106(6):851–5.
67. George RB, Melnick AH, Rose EC, et al. Case series: Combined spinal epidural anesthesia for Cesarean delivery and ex utero intrapartum treatment procedure. Can J Anaesth 2007;54(3):218–22.

Anesthetic Implications of Common Congenital Anomalies

Ji Yeon Jemma Kang, MD

KEYWORDS

- Down syndrome • Cleft lip • Cleft palate • Pharyngoplasty • Neural tube defect
- Myelomeningocele • Spina bifida

KEY POINTS

- The most common congenital anomalies are congenital heart defects, cleft lip and palate, Down syndrome, and neural tube defects.
- Anesthetic considerations for Down syndrome involve evaluation for the presence of congenital heart defects, cervical spine instability, upper airway obstruction, and behavioral considerations for induction and emergence.
- Congenital anomalies should be investigated in patients with cleft lip and palate prior to proceeding with an anesthetic.
- The most common complications after a cleft palate repair and pharyngoplasty are vomiting, pain, airway obstruction, and bleeding.
- Fetal surgery for myelomeningocele has been shown to reduce the need for ventriculoperitoneal shunting and improve motor outcomes, but it increases the risk of preterm delivery and uterine dehiscence at delivery.

INTRODUCTION

The World Health Organization defines congenital anomalies as structural or functional defects (eg, metabolic disorders) that occur during intrauterine life. They can be identified prenatally, at birth, or later in life. Anomalies can be caused by single gene defects, chromosomal disorders, multifactorial inheritance, environmental teratogens, and micronutrient deficiencies.[1]

Because congenital anomalies may be the result of 1 or more genetic, infectious, nutritional, and environmental factors, it often is difficult to identify the exact cause. Worldwide, approximately 303,000 newborns die within 4 weeks of birth every year due to congenital anomalies.[2] These anomalies can contribute to long-term disability, which also may have a significant impact on individuals, families, health care systems, and societies.

Department of Anesthesia, University of Cincinnati College of Medicine, Cincinnati Children's Hospital Medical Center, 3333 Burnet Avenue, MLC 2001, Cincinnati, OH 45229, USA
E-mail address: Jiyeon.kang@cchmc.org

Anesthesiology Clin 38 (2020) 621–642
https://doi.org/10.1016/j.anclin.2020.06.002
1932-2275/20/© 2020 Elsevier Inc. All rights reserved.
anesthesiology.theclinics.com

The most common congenital anomalies are congenital heart defects, cleft lip and palate, Down syndrome (DS), and neural tube defects.[3] This article discusses anesthetic implications associated with DS, cleft lip and palate, and neural tube defects. Congenital heart disease (CHD) is covered in Adam C. Adler and Aruna T. Nathan's article, "Perioperative Considerations for the Fontan Patient Requiring Non-cardiac Surgery," in this issue. Congenital defects repaired in utero are covered in Kha M. Tran and Debnath Chatterjee's article, "New Trends in Fetal Anesthesia," in this issue.

DOWN SYNDROME
Introduction

DS, otherwise known as trisomy 21, is the most common chromosomal condition in the United States,[3] occurring in 1 in 700 infants, or approximately 5400 of nearly 4 million infants born yearly.[4] It is caused by the inheritance of an additional chromosome 21.

Several important conditions are associated with DS, including CHD and gastrointestinal malformations, such as duodenal atresia, annular pancreas, and Hirschsprung disease. Other conditions associated with DS include polydactyly, cleft palate, and cataracts.[4] Due to major and minor malformations related to DS, patients with DS frequently present for diagnostic and/or surgical procedures that require anesthesia. Anesthetic considerations unique to DS are reviewed by organ system. **Fig. 1** demonstrates associated defects in DS.

Cervical Instability

Although DS patients are known to have the potential for cervical spine instability, predicting the likelihood of instability is difficult and the incidence is diverse. The American Academy of Pediatrics previously recommended 1 set of lateral cervical spine radiographs for children between 3 years and 5 years of age, but current guidelines no longer recommend routine cervical spine radiographs for asymptomatic children with DS. It is estimated that although only 1% to 2% actually show significant symptoms of cervical spine instability, the frequency of separation of the odontoid process from the body of the axis, which could contribute to instability, may be as high as 6%.[4]

All children with DS should be treated as having the potential for an acute dislocation and should receive a basic neurologic examination to assure equal motion and strength. Repeat assessment postoperatively also is important. Special consideration should be given to positioning during intubation and surgery. It may be prudent to forego the shoulder roll and make sure the intubation occurs with in-line cervical stabilization. Instead of turning the neck to access the side of the head or ear, the operating room table can be airplaned to the appropriate position. There also is an increased incidence and severity of degenerative changes at higher spinal levels with increasing age.[5] This is an important concern in adult DS patients.

Cardiac Considerations

Congenital heart disease

DS is the most frequent genetic syndrome among children born with CHD.[6] Congenital cardiac lesions are present in 40% to 50% of affected children. The most common cardiac lesions are atrioventricular septal defects (AVSDs) (50%–60%), followed by ventricular septal defects (VSDs) (15.5%), atrial septal defects (ASDs) (9.6%), and tetralogy of Fallot (7.3%).[6]

All infants with known or suspected DS should have a cardiac evaluation, including echocardiography, within the first few days to weeks of life. Prior to proceeding with a

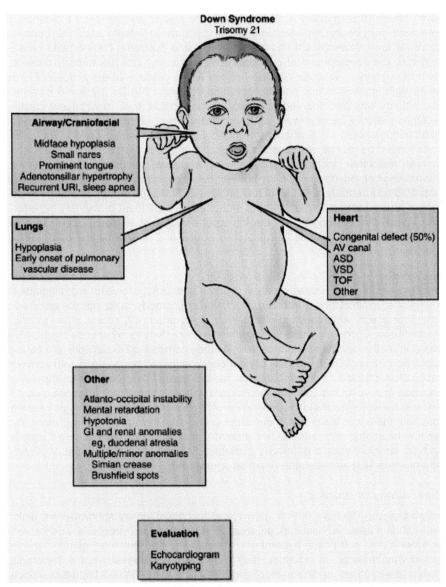

Fig. 1. Associated defects of DS. ASD, atrial septal defect; AV, Atrioventricular; TOF, tetralogy of Fallot; URI, upper respiratory infection; VSD, ventricular septal defect. (*From* Landis BJ, Lisi MT. Syndromes, Genetics and Heritable Heart Disease. In: Critical Heart Disease in Infants and Children, 3rd edition. Philadelphia: Elsevier; 2019. p. 893-894; with permission.)

procedure that necessitates an anesthetic, the most recent cardiac evaluation and studies should be reviewed if a child has CHD.

DS patients are at higher risk for developing pulmonary vascular disease even in the absence of predisposing CHD. This risk is high particularly in those children with a complete AVSD or large VSD, resulting in additional pulmonary blood flow. Chronic upper airway obstruction and hypoventilation can contribute to the development of pulmonary hypertension. There also is an increased incidence of persistent pulmonary hypertension of the neonate in infants with DS because abnormal lung development has both prenatal and postnatal components predisposing to the development of pulmonary hypertension.[4] The risk of early development of pulmonary vascular disease has led to the practice of early repair of large left-to-right interventricular shunts, including complete AVSDs, by age 6 months.[7] For patients with documented pulmonary hypertension, their most recent cardiac evaluation should be reviewed, and administration of all pulmonary hypertensive medications should be continued throughout the perioperative period. The anesthetic must be managed carefully, avoiding triggers that increase pulmonary vascular resistance, including hypoxemia, hypercapnia, acidosis, and hypothermia. Maintaining hemodynamic stability is essential; a balanced anesthetic often is best for providing adequate anesthesia and analgesia for this patient population. For patients with unrepaired cardiac defects or those with significant pulmonary hypertension, invasive monitoring and/or the intraoperative use of inotropic agents may be required depending on the surgical procedure and the patient's preoperative condition.

Bradycardia

Sevoflurane induction is used widely in children because it allows for rapid induction/emergence, minimal airway irritation, and favorable hemodynamic stability compared with other agents while allowing placement of intravenous (IV) access after induction of anesthesia. Children with DS are significantly more likely to experience bradycardia during and after sevoflurane induction. In a study comparing DS patients to a control population, 28% of DS versus 9% of controls experienced bradycardia with administration of sevoflurane.[4] For most patients, the bradycardia resolved with an immediate decrease in sevoflurane concentration or airway instrumentation.[8] There were no differences between groups in the prevalence of hypotension or pharmacologic interventions, but there was a significant decrease in end-tidal sevoflurane immediately after the low heart rate with subsequent increase in heart rate. Anticholinergic agents, such as atropine, should be readily available; if a patient does not have IV access, intramuscular (IM) administration may be considered.

Upper Airway Obstruction

Individuals with DS have both anatomic and functional airway abnormalities, which can include a flattened nasal bridge, macroglossia, midface hypoplasia, adenotonsillar hypertrophy, soft palate hyperplasia, tracheal and congenital subglottic stenosis, and airway malacia. In addition, they may have pharyngeal muscle hypotonia, increased secretions, and frequent respiratory infections.[4] All these factors contribute to upper airway obstruction and, as a result, patients with DS tend to have multiple sites of airway obstruction. Unfortunately, this means that even after surgical procedures to address upper airway obstruction, they may continue to have residual obstruction that can contribute to the development of pulmonary hypertension or complications during emergence from anesthesia. Obesity, more common in this population, can also involve soft tissues of the upper airway, which affects ventilation and oxygenation during and after anesthesia. One study found that by age 5, 79% of DS patients either had current symptoms of airway obstruction or had undergone an adenotonsillectomy. The prevalence of obstructive sleep apnea on polysomnogram in this population was 57%.[9]

Although most patients with DS have some degree of subglottic stenosis, a study found that only around 6% are symptomatic.[9] Subglottic stenosis may be from previous intubations or may be congenital. Because these patients are at risk for post-extubation stridor, it may be prudent to use a smaller endotracheal tube than predicted. A laryngeal mask airway (LMA) should be considered for shorter procedures.

Hematologic/Immunologic Disturbances

DS is associated with a large spectrum of hematologic findings and typically these vary over time. During the second trimester, there is dysmegakaryopoiesis and dyserythropoiesis, with an increase of megakaryocyte-erythrocyte progenitors in the liver. This can lead to abnormalities, such as neutrophilia (80%), thrombocytopenia (66%), and polycythemia (33%), in neonates. This typically regresses within a week.[10] A complete blood cell count, which should be drawn prior to surgery, identifies these issues.

Approximately 3% to 10% of neonates have a transient myeloproliferative disorder (TMD), also known as transient megakaryoblastic leukemia. Clinical presentation can vary from being asymptomatic to hepatosplenomegaly to bleeding/petechias and effusions (hydrops fetalis, ascites, and pleural and pericardial effusions). It usually resolves in the first 3 months, although death is reported in 15% to 20% of cases. One institution has proposed a peripheral blood smear at approximately 2 months of life or if the infant displays symptoms of TMD or leukemia.[10] Significant cytopenias or peripheral blasts may require a bone marrow examination prior to any elective surgery.[4] Severely increased white blood cell count can increase the risk of thrombosis and stroke. Plasmapheresis may be utilized if the white blood cell count is over 125,000/μL. Decreased blood counts can produce anemia and/or thrombocytopenia and may require red blood cell and/or platelet transfusion.[4]

DS patients are at a 10-times to 20-times increased risk of developing acute lymphoblastic leukemia compared with non-DS patients. There is a 150-times increased risk of myeloid leukemia for patients below 5 years old compared with non-DS patients.[10] These patients may have procedures such as line placements or chemotherapy treatments under anesthesia.

DS patients also have a higher frequency of infections, usually in the upper respiratory tract, characterized by increased severity and prolonged disease course, which are partially attributed to immune system defects.[11] This decrease in immunity is associated with mild to moderate T-cell and B-cell lymphopenia, marked decrease of naïve lymphocytes, impaired mitogen-induced T-cell proliferation, reduced specific antibody responses to immunizations, and defects of neutrophil chemotaxis. Nonimmune factors, such as abnormal airway and ear anatomy and the inability to clear secretions, also may be contributing factors to the high frequency of upper respiratory tract infections.[11]

Endocrinological Issues

Autoimmune conditions are prevalent in DS patients. Autoimmune thyroiditis is the most frequent disorder, affecting approximately 39% of adult patients with DS.[5] Abnormalities in clinical and subclinical thyroid function are frequent and increase with age. Although hypothyroidism occurs in the highest frequency, hyperthyroidism also is possible, emphasizing the need for yearly thyroid surveillance. Because thyroid hormone abnormalities can have an impact on cardiac function, thyroid screening also should be performed as part of the preoperative evaluation if not already done. Abnormalities should receive adequate treatment and the patient should be euthyroid at the time of any nonemergent procedure.

Other autoimmune conditions that may affect DS patients include hemolytic anemia and celiac-like enteropathy.[4]

Behavioral/Psychological Considerations

Currently, the average life expectancy of a DS patient is approximately 60 years old. In 1947, the life expectancy was 12 years old.[12] With this longer life expectancy comes an increasing number of adult DS patients presenting for procedures under anesthesia. They have not only developmental delay but also higher rates of dementia, autism, attention-deficit/hyperactivity disorder, and depression compared to the rest of the population.[13] With these potential behavioral issues comes the concern of inducing anesthesia for these patients as safely as possible (for both patient and medical personnel), while also decreasing the patient's anxiety. Parental presence has not been shown to improve preoperative anxiety[14] but, in this case, may improve a patient's compliance on induction. Various pharmacologic interventions, such as midazolam (oral or intranasal), dexmedetomidine (intranasal), and ketamine (oral or IM), have been used. Some pharmacologic agents, such as midazolam, may worsen airway obstruction and should be used judiciously, especially if a patient has obstructive sleep apnea or adeno-tonsillar hypertrophy. Options, such as midazolam and dexmedetomidine, may allow a patient to undergo an inhalation induction more easily. Sevoflurane, however, can cause bradycardia and airway obstruction, and inhalational induction of anesthesia is prolonged in larger patients. Therefore, an IV induction of anesthesia may be preferable. IM injection of ketamine may induce a faster and more profound response, allowing IV access to be obtained. The patient may recall the IM administration, however, and then have increased anxiety for future medical visits. For larger patients who may have a more aggressive personality, the use of either a ketamine IM injection or inhalational induction without previous premedication may be dangerous for the staff involved. There is no single clear best approach; each case must be individually considered according to the patient size, cardiac and/or airway pathophysiology, and psychological condition. The anesthetic approach to individual patients also should utilize their known support systems, along with the knowledge of what has worked for them in the past. Studies to better understand passive and interactive distraction to improve induction for these patients are ongoing.

CLEFT LIP AND CLEFT PALATE
Introduction

1 to 2 in 1000 children in the United States are born with cleft lip and cleft palate.[3] The incidence is estimated to be 1 per 500 to 700 births worldwide, with the ratio varying considerably across geographic areas or ethnic grouping.[15] It can be unilateral or bilateral and affects boys more than girls. Causes are multifactorial, with both environmental and genetic causes contributing.

Cleft lip and palate are associated with many syndromes. Some of the associated syndromes are illustrated in **Tables 1** and **2**.[16,17] Identification of syndromes prior to delivering anesthesia is important because many of these associated syndromes are associated with difficult tracheal intubation.

Patients with cleft lip and/or palate likely need multiple procedures and anesthetics throughout their lives. **Table 3**[18] gives a summary of these possible procedures. Major procedures include cleft lip repair, palatoplasty, and pharyngoplasty for velopharyngeal dysfunction. This article focuses on the anesthetic implications for these procedures.

Preoperative Considerations

Prior to proceeding with the following procedures, several common anesthetic considerations should be considered. First, as discussed previously, syndromes can affect

Table 1
Multiple malformation syndromes associated with cleft lip with or without cleft palate and features with possible anesthetic implications

Genetic Disorders	Possible Features with Anesthetic Implications
Down syndrome	See DS section of this article.
Smith-Lemli-Opitz syndrome	• Micrognathia and dysmorphic facial features—possible difficult intubation • Renal abnormalities—renal hypoplasia, renal cysts/duplication hydronephrosis, ureteropelvic junction obstruction • Vomiting and gastroesophageal reflux • CLD from recurrent aspiration and pneumonia • CHD—TOF and VSD
Aarskog syndrome	• Vertebral laxity and odontoid abnormalities—avoid excessive neck manipulation
Coffin-Siris syndrome	• Facial dysmorphism—microcephaly, short neck, macroglossia, cleft palate—possible difficult intubation • Upper and lower respiratory tract infections • Choanal atresia • Joint hypermobility • Renal abnormalities • CHD–PDA, ASD, VSD, TOF
Van der Woude syndrome	• Dental abnormalities with missing incisors, canines, and bicuspids • Oral synechiae—limited mouth opening, difficult intubation • Oral syngnathia—possible nasal intubation required
Waardenburg syndrome	• Hearing loss • Scoliosis
Ectodermal dysplasia syndromes (ectrodactyly-ectodermal dysplasia-clefting, Hay-Wells and Rapp-Hodgkin syndromes)	• Hearing loss • Hypoplasia of sweat glands and abnormal temperature regulation • Ectodermal dysplasia affecting teeth • Lacrimal duct hypoplasia—decreased tear production • Fragile skin • Choanal atresia • Renal abnormalities—renal dysplasia, hydronephrosis, vesicoureteral reflux
Distal arthrogryposis type 2	• Micrognathia, microstomia, neck shortening, cephalad positioning of larynx—possible difficult intubation • Pharyngeal airway obstruction from pharyngeal muscle myopathy • Recurrent aspiration pneumonia—CLD • Scoliosis, extremity contractures, deformities of hands and feet
Fryns syndrome	• Congenital diaphragmatic hernia, lung hypoplasia • Microretrognathia—possible difficult intubation • Delayed gastric emptying • Hydrocephalus • CHD: VSD, aortic arch anomalies • Renal disease—renal dysplasia, ureteral dilation

(continued on next page)

Table 1 (continued)	
Genetic Disorders	**Possible Features with Anesthetic Implications**
Popliteal pterygium syndrome	• Intraoral webbing may severely limit mouth opening and access to larynx—possible difficult intubation • Possible posterior displacement of tongue • Careful positioning of lower extremities due to sciatic and popliteal artery contained within popliteal webs
22q deletion syndromes (DiGeorge syndrome, Shprintzen syndrome)	• Hypocalcemia • Micrognathia/retrognathia—possible difficult intubation • Choanal atresia • T-cell defects—may need irradiated blood to prevent graft-versus-host disease • Hypothyroidism • CHD, such as TOF • May have right aortic arch, vascular ring, displacement of carotid arteries, aberrant subclavian arteries
Wolf-Hirschhorn syndrome	• Micrognathia—possible difficult intubation • Recurrent aspiration • CHD: ASD, VSD, pulmonary stenosis • Scoliosis and congenital hip dislocation
Basal cell nevus syndrome	• Dental abnormalities and caries predisposing to loss during laryngoscopy • Scoliosis and cervical vertebral abnormalities • Hydrocephalus
Kallmann syndrome	• Hypertelorism, sensorineural hearing loss • High arched palate • Choanal atresia • Hypogonadism
Nail patella syndrome	• Renal insufficiency • Proteinuria—leading to hypoalbuminemia • Weakened teeth • Glaucoma • Limited joint mobility and tendency to join dislocation

Abbreviations: CLD, chronic lung disease; TOF, tetralogy of Fallot; PDA, patent ductus arteriosus.
Adapted from Arosarena OA. Cleft lip and palate. *Otolaryngol Clin North Am.* 2007;40(1):27-60, vi. *and* Baum VC, O'Flaherty JE. Anesthesia for Genetic, Metabolic, & Dysmorphic Syndromes of Childhood, 3rd edition. Philadelphia: Walters Kluwer; 2015; with permission.

several organ systems that may need to be investigated. If a patient has any form of CHD, the most recent cardiac evaluations and studies should be reviewed. Second, these patients also may have potential airway problems that need careful assessment and management. An example is mandibular hypoplasia in patients with Pierre Robin sequence. The frequency of difficult tracheal intubation in children with cleft lip and palate varies from 4.7% to 8.4%.[19] Third, if a patient has an upper respiratory tract infection on the day of the procedure, the risks and benefits of the procedure need to be discussed with the surgeon due to the increased risk of respiratory complications, such as bronchospasm and laryngospasm. These risks take on particular significance in children with coexisting CHD or a known difficult airway. **Table 2** [16,17] summarizes common anesthetic risks of genetic disorders associated with cleft palate.

Table 2
Multiple malformation syndromes associated with cleft palate and features with possible anesthetic implications

Genetic Disorders	Possible Features with Anesthetic Implications
Down syndrome	See DS section of this article.
Prader-Willi syndrome	• Morbid obesity and risk of OSA • Rumination—high-risk gastric aspiration • Insatiable hunger and hypoglycemia at approximately 1 y of age • Non-insulin dependent diabetes mellitus as adolescent/ adult
Campomelic dysplasia	• Micrognathia, short neck—possible difficult intubation • May require smaller than expected endotracheal tube • Cervical vertebral anomalies and unstable cervical spine • Possible respiratory insufficiency and risk of perioperative apnea • Possible hydronephrosis and renal dysfunction • Tracheobronchomalacia and airway obstruction
Stickler syndrome	• Micrognathia—possible difficult intubation • Joint laxity and arthritis—careful positioning • Glaucoma—avoid anticholinergic medications
Holoprosencephaly sequence	• Oral/midline facial defects—nasal defects, absence of philtrum/labial frenulum, cleft lip and palate—possible difficult mask ventilation and intubation • Seizures • Perioperative temperature instability • Hypernatremia—subclinical diabetes insipidus
Cornelia de Lange syndrome	• Severe mental and motor delay—possible autistic, self-destructive behavior • Micrognathia, high-arched palate, short neck—possible difficult intubation • Possible choanal atresia • High risk for pulmonary aspiration—high incidence of gastroesophageal reflux • Risk of apnea in infancy • CHD—VSD, valvular pulmonary stenosis • Micromelia—possible difficult vascular access • Flexion contractures—careful positioning
Spondyloepiphyseal dysplasia congenita	• Short neck and limited flexion—possible difficult intubation • Cervical spine instability • Small stature—possible smaller than expected endotracheal tube • Restrictive lung disease • Limited joint mobility—careful positioning
Treacher Collins syndrome	• Severe mandibular hypoplasia, small mouth, narrow airway—difficult intubation • Laryngoscopy often becomes more difficult with aging. • OSA
22q deletion syndromes (DiGeorge syndrome, Shprintzen syndrome, and CHARGE association)	Refer to **Table 1**.

(continued on next page)

Table 2
(continued)

Genetic Disorders	Possible Features with Anesthetic Implications
Diastrophic dysplasia	• Laryngotracheobronchomalacia or laryngotracheal stenosis—airway obstruction • May require smaller endotracheal tube • Micrognathia—possible difficult intubation • Restrictive lung disease • Risk for subluxation at C2-3 and baseline cord compression—avoid hyperextension • Limited joint mobility—careful positioning
Orofaciodigital syndrome type I	• Dental abnormalities • Choanal atresia • Small mandible—possible difficult intubation
Otopalatodigital syndrome type I	• Dental abnormalities • Small mouth, micrognathia—possible difficult intubation
Nager syndrome	• Small mouth, micrognathia, hypoplasia of the larynx–difficult intubation • Choanal atresia • Limb abnormalities—difficult arterial/IV access
Smith-Lemli-Opitz syndrome	• Dysmorphic facial features and micrognathia—possible difficult intubation • Increased risk for perioperative aspiration (reflux and vomiting) • CLD • Behavior problems, including autism • TOF and VSD
Apert syndrome	• Small nasopharynx, choanal atresia/stenosis, tracheal stenosis, abnormal cartilage—possible difficult intubation • Cervical anomalies, including fusion • OSA • Eye protection for proptosis • Possible elevated intracranial pressure • CHD—pulmonary stenosis, overriding aorta, VSD • Possible genitourinary anomalies—polycystic kidneys, hydronephrosis, bicornuate uterus, vaginal atresia, cryptorchidism
Marfan syndrome	• Aortic or pulmonary artery dilatation, aortic dissection, aortic insufficiency, mitral prolapse • Risk for aortic dissection—avoid hypertension • Development of medial necrosis in coronary arteries • Pulmonary blebs with risk of pneumothoraces • OSA from pharyngeal laxity • Joint laxity—careful positioning • Dural ectasia—inadequate spread of spinal anesthesia • Glaucoma
Turner syndrome	• Short webbed neck—possible difficult intubation and short tracheal lengths • Hypothyroidism • Coarctation of aorta and bicuspid aortic valve • At risk for aortic dissection • Hypertension

(continued on next page)

Table 2 (continued)	
Genetic Disorders	**Possible Features with Anesthetic Implications**
Cleidocranial dysostosis	• Hypoplasia/aplasia of clavicles—alters subclavian artery/vein/plexus landmarks • Vertebral abnormalities—difficult neuraxial techniques • Narrow thoracic cage—decreased perioperative respiratory reserve • Dental abnormalities—predisposition to loss • Joint laxity and fragile bones—careful positioning

Abbreviations: CLD, chronic lung disease; OSA, obstructive sleep apnea; TOF, tetralogy of Fallot.
Adapted from Arosarena OA. Cleft lip and palate. *Otolaryngol Clin North Am.* 2007;40(1):27-60, vi. *and* Baum VC, O'Flaherty JE. Anesthesia for Genetic, Metabolic, & Dysmorphic Syndromes of Childhood, 3rd edition. Philadelphia: Walters Kluwer; 2015; with permission.

Cleft Lip Repair

Cleft lip repairs usually are performed at around 3 months to 4 months of age but sometimes may be done earlier. Traditionally, the recommendations for repair were referred to as the rule of 10. In a study done in 1966, it was shown that if the infant was less than 10 lb, had a hemoglobin less than 10 g/dL, and had a white blood cell count of less than 10×10^9/L, there was an increased risk of complications.[20] This thinking has been challenged due to increased prenatal screening technology. Not only may early lip repair improve the appearance of scarring but weight gain from improved feeding also has the potential to improve the capacity for correction of the nasal deformity. These improvements are due to the increased malleability of neonatal cartilage in the first 6 weeks of life.[21]

Table 3 Basic cleft care		
Age	**Medical Treatments**	**Surgery**
Prenatal to birth	• Genetic counseling • SLP consultation for feeding	—
0–5 mo	• SLP for feeding and growth • Monitor hearing • Nasoalveolar molding (if indicated)	• CL repair • Ear tubes (if COM)
9–12 mo	—	• Palatoplasty • Ear tubes (if COM)
1–4 y	• Introduction to pediatric dentist • Assess language development	—
4–6 y	• Assess for velopharyngeal dysfunction	• Corrective speech surgery • Lip revision if needed • Minor nasal surgery if needed
6–12 y	• Orthodontics • Assess school/psychosocial adjustment	• Alveolar bone grafting
12–21 y	• Orthodontics	• Orthognathic surgery • Definitive rhinoplasty

Abbreviations: COM, chronic otitis media; SLP, speech-language pathology.
From Worley ML, Patel KG, Kilpatrick LA. Cleft Lip and Palate. *Clin Perinatol* 2018;45(4):661–678; with permission.

Preoperative considerations
Similar to patients presenting with cleft palate, a complete review of systems should be performed prior to proceeding with anesthesia, including identifying the presence of possible syndromes, the possibility of a difficult airway, and the presence of concurrent respiratory illness. In addition, infants at this age typically are at the nadir for their hemoglobin, with a hemoglobin of 9 g/dL to 11 g/dL; lower hemoglobin levels may imply an underlying issue. A type and screen usually are sufficient for infants with a hematocrit less than 30%.[22]

Intraoperative considerations
For most infants, an inhalational induction can be performed without issue. For those who already have IV access, an IV induction may be performed. Difficult mask ventilation and intubation are recognized issues in certain patients with craniofacial abnormalities and micro/retrognathia. Continuous positive airway pressure and an oropharyngeal airway can be utilized to assist ventilation when necessary. Known risk factors for difficult laryngoscopy include infants with congenital anomalies, especially micrognathia, age less than 6 months, combined cleft lip and palate, left cleft lip and alveolus deformity, and combined bilateral cleft lip and palate.[19] For infants with cleft palate, further details are discussed later.

Local anesthesia with epinephrine often is infiltrated by surgeons for analgesia and to reduce surgical bleeding. An infraorbital nerve block is an effective block for this type of surgery. The use of IV or a preoperatively placed acetaminophen suppository also may be considered to augment analgesia and decrease opioid requirements in these patients.

Postoperative considerations
A smooth emergence limits the risk of damage of delicately sutured repairs. Analgesia with an infraorbital block assists in a smooth emergence. Little, if any, opioid is needed, and pain control usually is adequate with acetaminophen. Dexmedetomidine also can be used, but its use must be balanced with the risk of prolonged emergence or excessive sedation.

Cleft Palate Repair and Pharyngoplasty

Cleft palate repairs are performed to obtain velopharyngeal competence and normal speech. This repair typically is performed at around 9 months to 12 months of age. Surgery involves hard palate repair, repair of the nasal lining flaps, velar repair, and mobilization of the soft palate tissue to the midline.[13] The raw areas are expected to heal by granulation during the first few postoperative days with serosanguineous drainage during the postoperative period.

A pharyngoplasty is performed to reduce velopharyngeal incompetence and improve speech for patients who previously have undergone a cleft palate repair. This can be done by a pharyngeal flap, sphincter pharyngoplasty, and palatal lengthening. A posterior pharyngeal flap is a flap of tissue raised off the posterior pharyngeal wall and sewn to the middle of the velum, creating velopharyngeal ports on either side. The velopharyngeal ports function essentially as nasal airways and connect the posterior nasal cavity and the pharynx. Pharyngoplasties alter the anatomy of the velopharyngeal port and the posterior pharynx and carry the lifetime risk of overcorrection, hyponasality, and, more importantly, obstructive sleep apnea.[23]

Preoperative considerations
As discussed previously, a complete review of systems should be performed, screening for the presence of possible syndromes, the possibility of a difficult airway,

and any concurrent respiratory illness. By this point, the patient likely already has undergone several anesthetics. Therefore, review of these records, if available, should be done, with a particular focus on the details of previous airway management.

Intraoperative considerations
Most patients can be induced with a standard inhalational induction without difficulty. Due to the possibility of difficult ventilation and/or intubation, however, those with craniofacial abnormalities and retrognathia should be kept spontaneously breathing if possible until the trachea is secured. Patients with both cleft lip and palate, bilateral cleft lip and palate, and micrognathia are at special risk for difficult laryngoscopy.[19] Intubation through an LMA with the aid of a fiberoptic scope has also been described. Another technique described for intubation of patients with cleft palates is the use of a straight blade via the paraglossal approach. This technique involves inserting a laryngoscope with a Miller blade from the left corner of the mouth along the groove between the tonsil and tongue. The blade then is advanced, and the epiglottis lifted to expose the glottis, taking care to avoid inserting the blade into the cleft.[24]

An oral Ring-Adair-Elwyn (RAE) tube is used most commonly for endotracheal intubation for palate surgery. This tube, placed centrally, allows the Dingman mouth retractor to be placed in a convenient location. Due to the preformed nature of the RAE tube, it may need to be pulled back to prevent endobronchial intubation in small infants. Neck flexion may advance the tube and extension may result in inadvertent extubation. A reinforced tube is a suitable alternative for patients requiring a smaller than expected oral RAE because it does not kink like a standard endotracheal tube.

Blood loss in a palatoplasty typically is insignificant in patients without coagulopathy. In patients with underlying coagulopathy, however, soft tissue dissection may result in significant bleeding. As such, a type and screen should be obtained, and blood loss should be monitored closely.

During surgery, the pharyngeal space is reduced dramatically. Hence, extubation must occur when airway reflexes have returned, and the child is fully awake. Nasopharyngeal airways often are placed at the end of the procedure, typically by a surgeon, to ensure airway patency. Swelling of the tongue due to use of the mouth retractor (**Fig. 2**A) may cause airway obstruction. These children also are at risk for acute upper airway obstruction as a result of airway narrowing, edema, blood, and residual anesthetic effects.[25] A tongue suture (**Fig. 2**B) may be placed to exert traction and facilitate immediate postoperative control of the airway in the recovery area. The surgeon also may intermittently release the retractor throughout the procedure to reduce the risk of tongue edema.

The use of both inhalational and total IV anesthesia for anesthetic maintenance has been described. A balanced anesthetic with an inhalational agent, an opioid, and a muscle relaxant generally is considered safe. Opioids should be used judiciously due to the possibility of airway obstruction at the end of the case. Blocks (as discussed later) also should be considered. Dexmedetomidine has been shown to decrease emergence delirium and may assist in achieving a smooth emergence to help maintain the delicate sutures from the repair; a recent study assessing the impact of dexmedetomidine on emergence agitation found a 90% incidence of emergence agitation in the placebo group versus 15% in the dexmedetomidine group.[26] In this study, the respiratory recovery and extubation times were similar between the 2 groups and there was no significant difference in time of discharge from the postanesthetic care unit.

At the conclusion of a pharyngoplasty, nasal/oral airways become narrowed due to edema, the nasopharynx becomes obstructed by the flap, and the oropharynx becomes smaller due to flap construction. The resultant tissue edema after repair as

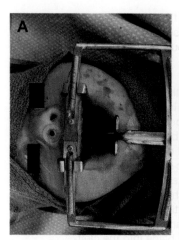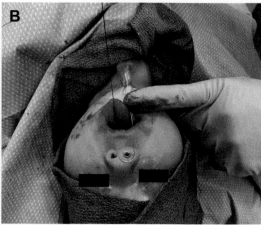

Fig. 2. (*A*) Picture of repaired palate with retractor in place. (*B*) Completion of palate surgery with nasopharyngeal airway and tongue stitch. (*Courtesy of* Ji Yeon Jemma Kang MD, Department of Anesthesia, Cincinnati Children's Hospital Medical Center, University of Cincinnati, College of Medicine.)

well as the residual effect of anesthetic drugs causing reduced respiratory drive may severely impair airway patency in the early postoperative period.[27] The surgeon may place nasopharyngeal airways or small endotracheal tubes in the bilateral nares for the first 4 hours to 6 hours to maintain airway patency. **Figs. 3**A and **3**B illustrate how a 3.5 mm and 4.0 mm cut endotracheal tracheal tube can be placed in the velopharyngeal ports. **Fig. 3**B shows the tubes positioned in the posterior pharynx demonstrating patency.

Postoperative considerations

When considering the postoperative management of these patients, the goals are to minimize airway obstruction, provide analgesia, and minimize postoperative nausea, vomiting, respiratory depression, and suture disruption. Arm restraints are used in some centers to prevent suture disruption and removal of the airways. These patients are monitored for upper airway obstruction for 48 hours. In 1 study, the incidence of airway obstruction after a palatoplasty was 57% in the operating room, 21% during the first 24 hours, and 21% during the 24 hours to 48 hours post-repair.[25] These findings emphasize the need for close monitoring of these patients.

Postoperative pain can be managed with a combination of acetaminophen and opioids. Palatal nerve block (nasopalatine or greater and lesser palatine) or a bilateral suprazygomatic maxillary nerve block can reduce postoperative pain[28] and favor early feedings.[29]

For those experiencing worsening respiratory distress in the recovery area, reintubation and mechanical ventilation need to be considered because it may take several days for tissue edema to resolve.[25] The presence of other congenital anomalies has been associated with a significantly increased risk of airway obstruction. In 1 study, 5.7% of patient had airway issues after a palatoplasty, and 13 of the 14 affected patients had an underlying congenital anomaly.[25]

In a 23-year retrospective chart review, the complications described most commonly for pharyngoplasties were vomiting (16%), pain (14%), airway obstruction (5%), and bleeding (4%); 2% of surgeries were revised due to severe cases of

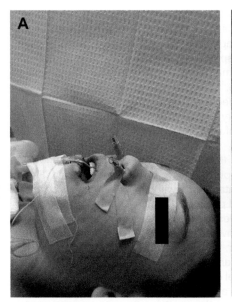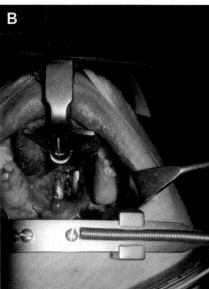

Fig. 3. (A) Patient with 4.0 mm endotracheal tubes positioned in the nasal passages to maintain patency after a pharyngeal flap construction. (B) View of the posterior pharynx with 4.0 mm endotracheal tubes positioned in the velopharyngeal ports to maintain airway patency. (*Courtesy of* Ji Yeon Jemma Kang MD, Department of Anesthesia, Cincinnati Children's Hospital Medical Center, University of Cincinnati, College of Medicine.)

bleeding, airway obstruction, or both.[27] Fewer complications were seen if sevoflurane and propofol were used as the main inhalational or IV anesthetic, respectively. Other potential airway complications include hyponasality, nasal obstruction, nasal apnea, and sleep apnea.[27] Obstructive sleep apnea is more common in patients with craniofacial anomalies.[30] Chronic airway obstruction may persist after surgery and may lead to obstructive sleep apnea and contribute to the development of pulmonary hypertension.

Another factor influencing airway obstruction is the number of other airway procedures performed at the time of pharyngeal flap palatoplasty. Patients who undergo concomitant palatoplasty and pharyngeal flap surgery are at significantly higher risk of airway obstruction.[30] When pharyngeal flap surgery is combined with tonsillectomy, there may be increased bleeding complications and the potential for adherent scars to form in the areas of the tonsillar pillars, palate, and pharyngeal wall with resultant increased risk of airway obstruction.

Finally, any subsequent procedures involving a nasal intubation should be done with caution to preserve the integrity of the cleft palate and pharyngeal flap repair. A nasal fiberoptic intubation may be helpful. Care also should be taken prior to placing an LMA in a patient with a history of cleft palate repair because disruption of previous cleft palate repair during LMA placement has been described.[31]

NEURAL TUBE DEFECTS
Introduction

Neural tube defects arise from the failure of the neural tube to fuse in the fetus. As the neural plate develops, the bone and muscle form a protective barrier over the spinal cord. Defects occur from abnormal neurulation in which a portion of the neural plate fails to join; as a result, bone and muscle are unable to grow over this open section of the developing spinal column. This dysraphism may occur anywhere along the neural axis, from the head (encephalocele) or spine (spina bifida). The defect may be relatively minor, affecting only superficial and membranous structures, or it may include a large segment of malformed neural tissue.[32] The severity of the symptoms is determined by the level of the defect and the degree of damage and/or maldevelopment. Although the degree of motor and sensory disability is associated with the level of the vertebral defect, the functional level of neurologic deficit frequently is 1 or more levels higher than the anatomic defect.[33]

Encephaloceles are neural tube defects that are protrusions of the brain and cerebrospinal fluid (CSF) arising from the occiput to the frontal area of the brain (**Fig. 4**). When there is a defect in the spine that contains CSF without spinal tissue and the spinal cord and spinal root are in their normal position, it is called a meningocele. Spinal cord and root abnormalities can be seen despite their normal location. If neural tissue is present in the defect, it is defined as a myelomeningocele. The incidence of myelomeningoceles is 5 to 10 pregnancies per 10,000 in the United States and 3.4 per 10,000 live births.[33] Myelomeningoceles are more common than meningocele and cause neurologic deficits inferior to the level of the protruding sac. They are most common in the lumbar region but can occur anywhere along the spinal cord. Severity ranges from minor types to spina bifida occulta (malformation of vertebrae only) to myelomeningoceles. It is estimated that 1 in every 10,500 babies is born with an encephalocele in the United States.[34]

Neural tube defects are associated with hydrocephalus, which can occur in 80% of infants with myelomeningocele or encephaloceles.[35] An Arnold-Chiari malformation is an abnormality in the posterior fossa and upper cervical spine. There are several different types depending on the severity. Type II is when there is caudal displacement of the cerebellar vermis, fourth ventricle, and lower brainstem below the foramen

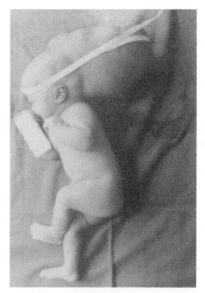

Fig. 4. Photograph showing neonate with giant occipital encephalocele. (*From* Walia B, Bhargava P, Sandhu K. Giant Occipital Encephalocele: Case Report. Medical Journal Armed Forces India 2005;61(3):293–4; with permission.)

magnum and is the most commonly encountered in patients with myelomeningoceles.[32] Encephaloceles constitute 8% to 19% of craniospinal dysraphisms, and 15.6% are larger than the size of the patient's head.[36]

Initial repair of a myelomeningocele is completed during the first few days of life to prevent rupture and infection of the defect. Many encephaloceles in otherwise healthy individuals can be carried out electively based on the general condition of the child. In cases of giant swellings (as big as the head), however, excision and repair should be planned as early as possible to prevent rupture and minimize further herniation. Specific anesthetic conditions for the initial repair are discussed.

Other spinal anomalies (lipomeningoceles, lipomyelomeningoceles, diastematomyelias, and dermoid tracts) may manifest themselves as tethered cords. Children who have had a myelomeningocele repaired after birth also may develop an ascending neurologic deficit from tethered spinal cord as growth occurs.[37] Persistence of the anatomic anomaly can lead to cord or nerve root distortion and impaired perfusion of the spinal cord, resulting in progressive neurologic deficit and chronic pain. This ultimately can lead to fecal urinary incontinence and exacerbation of lower extremity neurologic dysfunction. Early detection is more common with use of magnetic resonance imaging. Untethering of the cord is an option and neuromonitoring using electromyography may be utilized to identify the functional nerve roots. Injury during surgical dissection is a risk as identification of the functional nerve roots may be difficult.

Preoperative Considerations

A majority of studies support delivery of neonates with myelomeningoceles by planned cesarean section, thus allowing more careful delivery of the baby to protect the spinal cord from injury and prevent possible rupture of the meningeal sac.[38]

Most myelomeningoceles present for primary closure within the first 24 hours to 48 hours of life to minimize infection.[38] Some neurosurgeons insert a ventriculoperitoneal (VP) shunt at the time of initial surgery, whereas others may wait a few days or defer it all together if there is no evidence of hydrocephalus at birth.

Symptoms of Arnold-Chiari malformation usually come from 1 of 3 areas of the central nervous system: the cerebellum, the lower brain stem, and/or the spinal cord. Lower brainstem symptoms present most often in newborns and young infants and include difficulty swallowing, inspiratory stridor, weak/poor cry, and sustained arching of the head.[38] When severe, these symptoms may lead to respiratory insufficiency. The initial step is to relieve intracranial pressure using a VP shunt. It is important to identify any respiratory symptoms in the preoperative evaluation when considering analgesia and possible postoperative ventilation.

Spina bifida occurs more often than expected in both trisomy 13 and 18. Additionally, it is associated with many genetic syndromes, including acrocallosal syndrome, cerebrocostomandibular syndrome, congenital hemidysplasia with ichthyosiform erythroderma and limb defects (CHILD syndrome), Fraser syndrome, Jarcho-Levin syndrome, Meckel-Gruber syndrome, and Waardenburg syndrome types I and II.[38] The possibility of syndromes should be considered in the preoperative evaluation.

Intraoperative Considerations

One of the major anesthetic considerations involves positioning of the neonate for induction. It is of utmost importance to prevent rupture of the defect prior to surgical intervention. For most cases of myelomeningoceles, the defect can be placed in a donut pillow typically used for the head. The uninvolved portions of the infant can be placed on sheets or blankets. Occasionally, the infant may need to be placed in the lateral position for induction and intubation.

Airway management, mask ventilation, and intubation may be difficult for infants with massive hydrocephalus or very large defects. The difficult airway cart should be readily available. For a frontoethmoidal encephalocele, mask ventilation may need to occur below the lesion while compressing the nasal alae.[39] For the more common occipital lesions, neck extension may be limited. A second assistant may need to support the neck with the infant's body on sheets for the baby to be intubated in the supine position.[40] Intubation in the lateral decubitus position is another possibility. Inhalation induction is favorable because spontaneous ventilation can be maintained and volatile agents can be discontinued and rapidly eliminated should a difficult airway ensue. Once mask ventilation has been established, muscle relaxant can be given. In a series of 29 giant encephalocele cases, intubation was attempted in the lateral position in 82.8%. Difficult intubation was experienced in 15.3%; these patients were subsequently placed supine with the head off the end of the table. In 10.3% of patients, the encephalocele was decompressed with a needle under sterile conditions to facilitate proper positioning of the head. This aspiration of CSF allowed for more extension of the neck and an improved view of the glottis.[36]

Sudden decompression of the ventricles from CSF aspiration may cause traction on the brainstem leading to bradycardia and cardiac arrest. Hemodynamic instability and electrolyte imbalance may also occur.[36] Therefore, resuscitation medications including atropine and epinephrine should be readily available.

Arnold-Chiari malformation may also cause brainstem compression during excessive flexion or extension of the head, which should be taken into consideration during laryngoscopy.[36] Fiberoptic bronchoscopy intubation or intubation via an LMA also is a consideration.

Blood loss may be considerable for both conditions, particularly when large amounts of skin need to be undermined to cover the defect. Blood loss can be considerable, especially for patients undergoing encephalocele repair. This can happen during the dissection of the large encephalocele sac, while cutting through vascular suboccipital bone, and if venous sinuses are damaged.[36] It is important to keep track of blood loss because soaked sponges and blood on drapes may rapidly equate to a large percentage of blood volume in a neonate or small child. Adequate IV access, generally 2 peripheral IVs, should be obtained and blood products should be available. Fluid and blood loss should be replaced as appropriate. It is important not to get behind with resuscitation.

Due to the patient's prone positioning and the small size of the patient, it may be difficult to maintain an appropriate body temperature. Forced air blankets should be used and the temperature of the operating room should be raised to maintain appropriate warmth.

Postoperative Considerations

When a Chiari malformation coexists, ventilatory responses to hypoxia can be diminished or absent.[41] Careful titration of narcotics and possible postoperative ventilation in the intensive care unit should be considered.

In patients with encephaloceles, attempts are made to keep the neural tissue present in the sac inside the cranial cavity; this may lead to raised intracranial pressure, which occasionally can lead to respiratory arrest.[42]

Patients with myelomeningocele suffer from multisystem disease that results from severe injury of the developing central nervous system during gestation. Commonly involved systems include the musculoskeletal system, genitourinary system, and immune system. Common orthopedic problems in spina bifida patients include club-foot, hip dysplasia, and spinal deformities, including scoliosis and kyphosis.[38] These abnormalities may require multiple procedures (surgical and nonsurgical) that frequently involve anesthesia. VP shunts may need multiple revisions and bear an ongoing risk of infection. It is important to consider the implications of multiple anesthetics on development. The impact of anesthetics on the developing brain is discussed in Sulpicio G. Soriano and Mary Ellen McCann's article, "Is Anesthesia Bad for the Brain? Current Knowledge on the Impact of Anesthetics on the Developing Brain," in this issue.

Myelodysplasia patients are at high risk of developing allergic reactions to latex,[43] most likely as a result of repeated exposures to latex products encountered during surgery. These patients should be treated with a latex alert and anaphylaxis must be considered when appropriate. Those who develop latex allergy can exhibit cross-reactivity with some antibiotics and foods, especially tropical fruits, such as avocados, kiwis, and bananas. Many institutions have replaced most of their latex-containing supplies with nonlatex alternatives; this has resulted in complete elimination of latex anaphylactic reactions during anesthesia in some institutions.[44]

Fetal Procedures

A 2-hit theory of nerve damage has been postulated regarding central and peripheral nerve damage for myelomeningocele. The first is the failure of the neural tube formation and the second is the nerve damage caused by exposure to the uterine environment. The option for in utero repair was developed because it has the potential to decrease neurologic deficits and associated comorbidities by reducing intrauterine exposure, improving the function and quality of life in these children.[33] Technical advances in ultrasonography and improved prenatal diagnosis of anomalies have also paved the way for fetal surgery. The Management of Myelomeningocele Study was stopped because it showed a reduced need for VP shunting and improved motor outcomes. There was, however, an increased risk of preterm delivery and uterine dehiscence at delivery.[45] More detail about fetal surgery can be found in Kha M. Tran and Debnath Chatterjee's article, "New Trends in Fetal Anesthesia," in this issue.

SUMMARY

The most common congenital anomalies are CHD, DS, cleft lip/palate, and neural tube defects. This article has illustrated the perioperative anesthetic considerations for DS, cleft lip/palate and neural tube defects. Anesthetic considerations for DS include cervical spine instability; history of CHD; risk of bradycardia; and hematologic, endocrine, and behavioral considerations. Patients with cleft lip and palate can have associated syndromes and the potential for underlying abnormalities should be investigated prior to their anesthetic. The most common anesthetic complications for cleft palate and pharyngoplasties are vomiting, pain, airway obstruction, and bleeding. Neural tube defects can occur anywhere along the neuroaxis, from encephaloceles to spina bifida. Spina bifida includes meningoceles and myelomeningoceles. A major anesthetic consideration for neural tube defect surgery is positioning for intubation. Fetal surgery for myelomeningocele has been shown to reduce the need for VP shunting and improved motor outcomes. Finally, although each condition has general anesthetic considerations, it is important to tailor the anesthetic to the individual patient. Previous anesthetic records are especially helpful.

> **Clinics Care Points**
>
> - Down syndrome patients should be evaluated for the presence of congenital heart defect, cervical spine instability and upper airway obstruction. Other important considerations involve hematologic, endocrinological and behavioral concerns.
>
> - Congenital anomalies should be investigated in patients with cleft lip and palate prior to proceeding with an anesthetic.
>
> - Two major anesthetic considerations for neural tube defect surgery are optimal positioning for intubation and appropriate rescuscitation.

ACKNOWLEDGMENTS

Laura Berenstain, MD, Professor, University of Cincinnati College of Medicine, Department of Anesthesia, Cincinnati Children's Hospital Medical Center.

Brian S. Pan MD, FACS, FAAP, Associate Professor, Division of Pediatric Plastic Surgery, Cincinnati Children's Hospital Medical Center, University of Cincinnati College of Medicine.

J. Paul Willging, MD, Professor, University of Cincinnati College of Medicine, Department of Otolaryngology, Cincinnati Children's Hospital Medical Center.

DISCLOSURE

The author has nothing to disclose.

REFERENCES

1. World Health Organization. Health Topics: Congenital anomalies. 1. 2020. Available at: https://www.who.int/topics/congenital_anomalies/en/. Accessed December 7, 2020.
2. World Health Organization. Congenital Anomalies: Key facts. 2016. Available at: https://www.who.int/en/news-room/fact-sheets/detail/congenital-anomalies. Accessed December 2, 2019.
3. March of Dimes. Rare Birth defects. 2013. Available at: https://www.marchofdimes.org/baby/rare-birth-defects.aspx. Accessed December 10, 2019.
4. Lewanda AF, Matisoff A, Revenis M, et al. Preoperative evaluation and comprehensive risk assessment for children with Down syndrome. Paediatr Anaesth 2016;26(4):356–62.
5. Santamaria LB, Di Paola C, Mafrica F, et al. Preanesthetic evaluation and assessment of children with Down's syndrome. ScientificWorldJournal 2007;7:242–51.
6. Ferencz C, Neill CA, Boughman JA, et al. Congenital cardiovascular malformations associated with chromosome abnormalities: an epidemiologic study. J Pediatr 1989;114(1):79–86.
7. Landis BJ, Lisi MT. Syndromes, Genetics, and Heritable Heart Disease. In: Ungerleider RM, Meliones JN, McMillon KN, et al, editors. Critical heart disease in infants and children E-Book. 3rd edition. Philadelphia: Elsevier Health Sciences; 2019. p. 893–4.
8. Bai W, Voepel-Lewis T, Malviya S. Hemodynamic changes in children with Down syndrome during and following inhalation induction of anesthesia with sevoflurane. J Clin Anesth 2010;22(8):592–7.
9. Hamilton J, Yaneza MM, Clement WA, et al. The prevalence of airway problems in children with Down's syndrome. Int J Pediatr Otorhinolaryngol 2016;81:1–4.

10. Bruwier A, Chantrain CF. Hematological disorders and leukemia in children with Down syndrome. Eur J Pediatr 2012;171(9):1301–7.

11. Ram G, Chinen J. Infections and immunodeficiency in Down syndrome. Clin Exp Immunol 2011;164(1):9–16.

12. Esbensen AJ. Health conditions associated with aging and end of life of adults with Down syndrome. Int Rev Res Ment Retard 2010;39(C):107–26.

13. Startin CM, D'Souza H, Ball G, et al. Health comorbidities and cognitive abilities across the lifespan in Down syndrome. J Neurodev Disord 2020;12(1):4.

14. Manyande A, Cyna AM, Yip P, et al. Non-pharmacological interventions for assisting the induction of anaesthesia in children. Cochrane Database Syst Rev 2015;7: CD006447.

15. World Health Organization. Human genomics in global heath: International Collaborative Research on Craniofacial Anomalies 2020. Available at: https://www.who.int/genomics/anomalies/en/. Accessed March 1, 2020.

16. Arosarena OA. Cleft lip and palate. Otolaryngol Clin North Am 2007;40(1): 27–60, vi.

17. Baum VC, O'Flaherty JE. Anesthesia for Genetic, Metabolic, & Dysmorphic Syndromes of Childhood. 3rd edition. Philadelphia: Walters Kluwer; 2015.

18. Worley ML, Patel KG, Kilpatrick LA. Cleft lip and palate. Clin Perinatol 2018;45(4): 661–78.

19. Xue FS, Zhang GH, Li P, et al. The clinical observation of difficult laryngoscopy and difficult intubation in infants with cleft lip and palate. Paediatr Anaesth 2006;16(3):283–9.

20. Millard, Ralph D. Cleft craft. The evolution of its surgery: The unilateral deformity. 1st edition. Boston; 1976. p. 69–74.

21. Hammoudeh JA, Imahiyerobo TA, Liang F, et al. Early cleft lip repair revisited: a safe and effective approach utilizing a multidisciplinary protocol. Plast Reconstr Surg Glob Open 2017;5(6):e1340.

22. Adeyemo WL, Adeyemo TA, Ogunlewe MO, et al. Blood transfusion requirements in cleft lip surgery. Int J Pediatr Otorhinolaryngol 2011;75(5):691–4.

23. Cladis FP, Grunwaldt L, Losee J. Anesthesia for Pediatric Plastic Surgery. In: Davis PJ, Cladis FP, editors. Smith's Anesthesia for Infants and Children e-book. 9th edition. Philadelphia: Elsevier; 2017.

24. Sen I, Kumar S, Bhardwaj N, et al. A left paraglossal approach for oral intubation in children scheduled for bilateral orofacial cleft reconstruction surgery–a prospective observational study. Paediatr Anaesth 2009;19(2):159–63.

25. Antony AK, Sloan GM. Airway obstruction following palatoplasty: analysis of 247 consecutive operations. Cleft Palate Craniofac J 2002;39(2):145–8.

26. Peng W, Zhang T. Dexmedetomidine decreases the emergence agitation in infant patients undergoing cleft palate repair surgery after general anesthesia. BMC Anesthesiol 2015;15:145.

27. Schwerdtfeger CM, Almeida AM, Trindade IE, et al. Influence of anesthetics on pharyngeal flap surgery: a 23-year study. Int J Oral Maxillofac Surg 2009;38(3): 224–7.

28. Jonnavithula N, Durga P, Madduri V, et al. Efficacy of palatal block for analgesia following palatoplasty in children with cleft palate. Paediatr Anaesth 2010;20(8): 727–33.

29. Mesnil M, Dadure C, Captier G, et al. A new approach for peri-operative analgesia of cleft palate repair in infants: the bilateral suprazygomatic maxillary nerve block. Paediatr Anaesth 2010;20(4):343–9.

30. Pena M, Choi S, Boyajian M, et al. Perioperative airway complications following pharyngeal flap palatoplasty. Ann Otol Rhinol Laryngol 2000;109(9):808–11.
31. Somerville NS, Fenlon S, Boorman J, et al. Disruption of cleft palate repair following the use of the laryngeal mask airway. Anaesthesia 2004;59(4):401–3.
32. Mcclain CD, Soriano SG, Rockoff M A. Pediatric Neurosurgical Anesthesia. In: Coté CJ, Lerman J, Anderson BJ, editors. A Practice of Anesthesia for Infants and Children e-book. 5th edition. Philadelphia: Elsevier; 2013.
33. Ferschl M, Ball R, Lee H, et al. Anesthesia for in utero repair of myelomeningocele. Anesthesiology 2013;118(5):1211–23.
34. Mai CT, Isenburg JL, Canfield MA, et al. National population-based estimates for major birth defects, 2010-2014. Birth Defects Res 2019;111(18):1420–35.
35. Lerman J, Coté CJ, Steward DJ. Neurosurgery and Invasive Neuroradiology. In: Lerman J, Coté CJ, Steward DJ, editors. Manual of pediatric anesthesia. 7th edition. Switzerland: Springer; 2016.
36. Mahajan C, Rath GP, Bithal PK, et al. Perioperative Management of Children With Giant Encephalocele: A Clinical Report of 29 Cases. J Neurosurg Anesthesiol 2017;29(3):322–9.
37. Vavilala MS, Soriano SG, Krane EJ. Anesthesia for Neurosurgery. In: Davis PJ, Cladis FP, editors. Smith's Anesthesia for Infants and Children e-book. 9th edition. Philadelphia: Elsevier; 2017.
38. Northrup H, Volcik KA. Spina bifida and other neural tube defects. Curr Probl Pediatr 2000;30(10):313–32.
39. Geddam LM, Mahmoud MA, Pan BS, et al. Frontoethmoidal encephalocele: a pediatric airway challenge. Can J Anaesth 2018;65(2):208–9.
40. Pahuja HD, Deshmukh SR, Lande S, et al. Anaesthetic management of neonate with giant occipital meningoencephalocele: Case report. Egypt J Anaesth 2015; 31(4):331–4.
41. Patel DM, Rocque BG, Hopson B, et al. Sleep-disordered breathing in patients with myelomeningocele. J Neurosurg Pediatr 2015;16(1):30–5.
42. Mahapatra AK. Giant encephalocele: a study of 14 patients. Pediatr Neurosurg 2011;47(6):406–11.
43. Holzman RS. Clinical management of latex-allergic children. Anesth Analg 1997; 85(3):529–33.
44. De Queiroz M, Combet S, Berard J, et al. Latex allergy in children: modalities and prevention. Paediatr Anaesth 2009;19(4):313–9.
45. Adzick NS, Thom EA, Spong CY, et al. A randomized trial of prenatal versus postnatal repair of myelomeningocele. N Engl J Med 2011;364(11):993–1004.

Managing the Adult Patient with Congenital Heart Disease

Meagan King, MD[a,b,*], Kumar Belani, MD[b]

KEYWORDS

- Adult congenital heart disease • Congenital heart disease • CHD
- Noncardiac surgery • Single ventricle

KEY POINTS

- Patients with congenital heart disease are increasingly surviving to adulthood and may present for noncardiac surgery.
- Congenital heart disease is exceedingly heterogeneous, and repairs and perioperative concerns depend on individual anatomy and the resultant physiology.
- Anesthesia for adult congenital heart patients should be individualized to the patient's specific lesion, physiology, and operation.

Congenital heart disease (CHD) is the most common birth defect, present in almost 1% of live births comprising approximately 40,000 births in the United States and 1.35 million births worldwide per year.[1,2] The incidence has climbed from 0.6% in the 1930s to current rates, with ventricular septal defect (VSD), atrial septal defect (ASD), and patent ductus arteriosus being the most common.[1] Although some increase can likely be attributed to incidental findings of subclinical lesions often found incidentally owing to increased and improved screening techniques, there is undoubtedly a large public health concern regardless of cause of CHD.[1] Interestingly, geographic factors appear to influence both prevalence and type of CHD, with Asia having the highest incidence overall and predominantly right ventricular outflow tract obstructive lesions.[3] European and North American children have a higher incidence of left ventricular obstructive lesions.[4] African populations showed the lowest overall prevalence of CHD, suggesting a strong genetic component for all lesions.[5] Because the United States is home to people of all populations, providers can expect to encounter all types of CHD during their practice.

[a] Department of Anesthesiology, Cincinnati Children's Hospital Medical Center, 3333 Burnet Avenue, Cincinnati, OH 45229, USA; [b] Department of Anesthesiology, University of Minnesota, B515 Mayo, 420 Delaware Street Southeast, Minneapolis, MN 55455, USA
* Corresponding author. Department of Anesthesiology, University of Minnesota, B515 Mayo, 420 Delaware Street Southeast, Minneapolis, MN 55455.
E-mail address: king1449@umn.edu

Anesthesiology Clin 38 (2020) 643–662
https://doi.org/10.1016/j.anclin.2020.05.008
1932-2275/20/© 2020 Elsevier Inc. All rights reserved.
anesthesiology.theclinics.com

Patients with CHD are increasingly surviving long term, with between 85% and greater than 90% expected to reach adulthood,[6,7] and providers should expect to see adults with congenital heart disease (ACHD) patients in the operating room for noncardiac surgeries. When undergoing anesthesia for a procedure, patients with CHD had a higher instance of morbidity and mortality than the general population.[8–10] Given the heterogeneity of cardiac disease, consideration of not only the patient's operation but also the individual lesion is critical for the provider. Long-term sequelae from ACHD, including repaired versus unrepaired lesions, right and left heart function, arrhythmias, conduction defects, hypertension, aneurysms, previous vascular access including possible extracorporeal membrane oxygenation, residual intracardiac shunts, valvular lesions, and need for endocarditis prophylaxis are all factors influencing clinical decision making.[9] Independent risk factors for mortality in ACHD patients admitted to the hospital are related to their existing comorbidities, including respiratory dysfunction, the use of a ventricular assist device, sepsis, acute myocardial infarction, and acute renal failure.[6,11]

ATRIAL SEPTAL DEFECT
Prevalence

ASDs (**Fig. 1**) comprise 6% to 10% of all CHD, affect women and girls more than men and boys. More than 75% of all ASDs are ostium secundum types, arising from enlargement of the foramen ovale, reabsorption of the septum primum, or inadequate growth of the septum resulting in a secundum type.[10]

Overview and Anesthetic Implications

Left-to-right shunts in patients with ASD cause increased right heart (RH) circulation and possible RH dilation leading in some to arrhythmias (atrial fibrillation in up to 23% of adults) and placing the patient at risk of atrially originating embolism.[2] Volume overload of the RH can eventually cause right ventricular dilation.[12] Increased pulmonary blood flow may eventually lead to pulmonary congestion and pulmonary hypertension. Noxious stimuli, hypothermia, acidosis, hypoxia, and hypercarbia associated with surgery can worsen pulmonary hypertension and right-to-left shunting.

Although most solo ASDs will have a predominantly left-to-right shunt, it is possible for patients to have right-to-left shunt when pulmonary vascular resistance (PVR) increases above systemic vascular resistance (SVR), causing a risk of paradoxic embolus. It is therefore vital to remove all air bubbles from intravenous lines in order to prevent stroke. The effects of anesthesia on SVR increase the likelihood of a right-to-left (hypoxic) shunt.[12]

Concerns:
Right heart over circulation
Arrhythmias
Pulmonary hypertension
Hypoxic shunt
Paradoxic embolus

VENTRICULAR SEPTAL DEFECTS
Prevalence

VSDs are the most common lesion, found in approximately 30% of patients with CHD.[2,11] VSDs (**Fig. 2**) are often diagnosed after discovery of a pansystolic murmur. Small VSDs are rarely clinically significant. Upwards of 40% resolve spontaneously

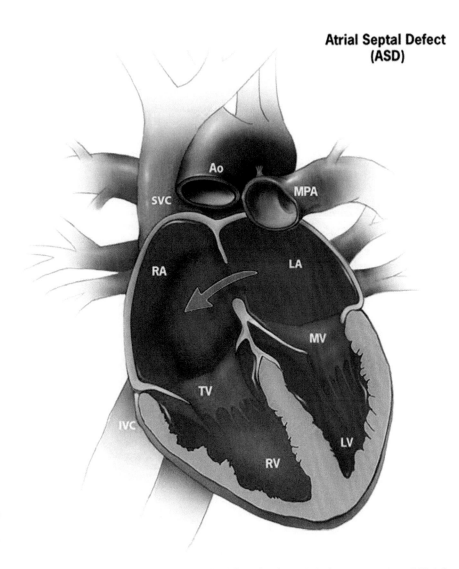

**Atrial Septal Defect
(ASD)**

Fig. 1. ASD. A communication between the left and right atria is shown. Ao, aorta; IVC, inferior vena cava; LA, left atrium; LV, left ventricle; MPA, main pulmonary artery; MV, mitral valve; RA, right atrium; RV, right ventricle; SVC, superior vena cava; TV, tricuspid valve. (*Courtesy of* the Centers for Disease Control and Prevention, Bethesda, MD; https://www. cdc.gov/ncbddd/heartdefects/AtrialSeptalDefect-graphic2.html.)

during childhood, specifically muscular VSDs.[2,11] Larger VSDs, which produce significant shunting, may require repair as early as infancy or may not be discovered until they become clinically significant later in life.[11]

Overview and Anesthetic Implications

Patients with VSD often have a volume-overloaded left heart, leading to left atrial and ventricular dilation.[2] Up to 5% of patients with VSDs has a conduction defect,

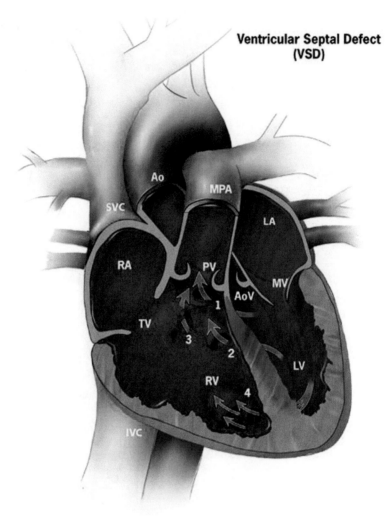

Ventricular Septal Defect (VSD)

1. Conoventricular, malaligned
2. perimembranous
3. inlet
4. muscular

Fig. 2. VSD. Examples of conoventricular, perimembranous, inlet, and muscular ventricular defects creating a communication between the left and right ventricles are shown. AoV, aortic valve; PV, pulmonary valve. (*Courtesy of* the Centers for Disease Control and Prevention, Bethesda, MD; https://www.cdc.gov/ncbddd/heartdefects/images/vsd_simple-lg.jpg.)

sometimes requiring a pacemaker.[13] Many VSDs that require closure are now occluded with devices in the catheterization laboratory.[2] However, larger or more complex VSDs require surgical intervention.[2] Most adult patients with clinically significant VSDs will have had either device closure or surgical repair before adulthood. Because of significant shunting with larger VSDs, patients who have been repaired may already have developed pulmonary overcirculation resulting in a residual pulmonary hypertension and right ventricular hypertrophy, or Eisenmenger syndrome.[11] This state of higher right-sided cardiac pressures puts the patient at risk for paradoxic embolus.[13] Patients who remain unrepaired may present with biventricular hypertrophy as compensation for dramatic over circulation.[11]

Along with SVR decreases owing to anesthesia, noxious stimuli, hypoxia, and hypercarbia may lead patients with pulmonary hypertension to have a decrease in Qp:Qs and therefore subsequent oxygen desaturation secondary to right-to-left shunting. Conversely, in patients with large, unrestricted VSDs who have an increased SVR, hyperoxia and hypocarbia may result in pulmonary overcirculation under anesthesia and subsequent hypotension and pulmonary edema.[13] However, most adults with unrepaired VSDs do not have lesions large enough to cause significant hemodynamic instability.[11] It should be noted that all patients with unrepaired VSDs are at risk for endocarditis before repair.[11]

Concerns:
    Left heart overcirculation and dilation
    Right heart overcirculation
    Arrhythmias
    Eisenmenger syndrome
    Pulmonary hypertension
    Hypoxic shunt
    Paradoxic embolus
    Endocarditis

VALVE ABNORMALITIES
Prevalence

Of all valvular CHD lesions, bicuspid aortic valve is by far the most common, encompassing almost 2% of the general population and accounting for more than half of patients requiring aortic valve replacement before age 70.[14]

Overview and Anesthetic Implications

The 2 main subcategories of congenital valvular heart disease are obstructive and stenotic, although both may be present. For example, patients born with bicuspid aortic valve will often develop both aortic valve stenosis and regurgitation in adulthood.[10] Often there is no need for operation in childhood, but eventually many valvular diseases require surgical intervention.

Obstructive lesions, such as aortic stenosis or pulmonary atresia (**Fig. 3**), place the patient at increased risk of perioperative morbidity and mortality. Severity of the lesion and symptoms including but not limited to congestive heart failure determine the timing of need for surgical repair.[10] As the obstructive lesion worsens, the ventricle hypertrophies, leading to increased dependence on atrial contraction for contribution to left ventricular end diastolic volume.[14] Therefore, sinus rhythm and preload are both vital to maintaining cardiac output, and adequate SVR is required for coronary perfusion to avoid myocardial ischemia.[14,15] Regurgitant valve lesions require that the patient be maintained in a normal to high heart rate in order to maintain cardiac output and forward flow, and bradycardia should be avoided.[15] In addition, a normal or mildly reduced SVR is needed for adequate end-organ perfusion, and providers should prevent hypertension.[15]

Although both types of valvular lesions present unique anesthetic implications, often the patients have already had surgical repair and will therefore have another additional set of perioperative risks for the consideration by the anesthesia provider. For patients who have undergone valve repair, risks for noncardiac surgery include inadequate

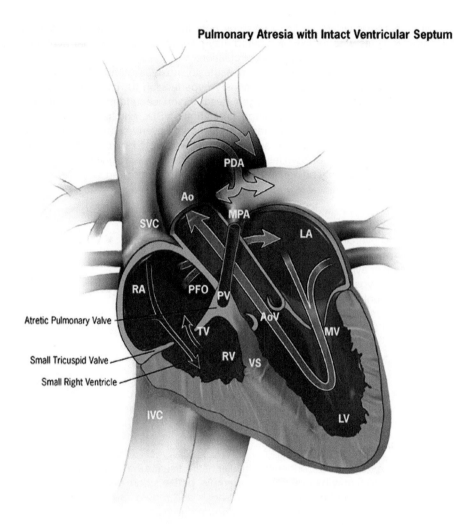

Pulmonary Atresia with Intact Ventricular Septum

Fig. 3. Pulmonary atresia with intact ventricular septum. An atretic pulmonary valve with intact ventricular septum leading to a small right ventricle is shown. PDA, patent ductus arteriosis; PFO, patent foramen pvale; VS, ventricular septum. (*Courtesy of* the Centers for Disease Control and Prevention, Bethesda, MD; https://www.cdc.gov/ncbddd/heartdefects/images/PulmonaryAtresia-intact-600px.jpg.)

repair with a residual lesion, leaflet perforation, perivalvular pseudoaneurysm, annular dilation leading to regurgitation, hematoma, and endocarditis.[16] Patients who have valve replacement in lieu of repair will have an entirely different set of implications for the perioperative period. Regardless of autograft, homograft, or mechanical valve replacement, complications include valve dysfunction and endocarditis.[17] Furthermore, mechanical valves have additional risks, such as thromboembolism and need for anticoagulation, leading to bleeding.[17] Other rarer cardiac valve lesions include Ebstein anomaly, which is characterized by a downwardly displaced, often dysplastic tricuspid valve, and atrialization of a portion of the right ventricle.[2] These lesions often need surgical repair as well as lifelong follow-up with cardiology owing to risk of arrhythmias, including Wolff-Parkinson-White syndrome and sudden cardiac death in adulthood.[2]

Concerns:
  Obstructive lesions:
    Maintenance of sinus rhythm
    Ventricular hypertrophy
    Maintenance of SVR for coronary perfusion
  Regurgitant lesions:
    Maintenance of normal/fast heart rate
    Reduction of SVR to maintain normal flow
  After valve surgery
    Inadequate repair
    Postrepair complications: hematoma, aneurysm
    Endocarditis
  After valve replacement
    Thromboembolism
    Bleeding secondary to anticoagulation
    Endocarditis

COARCTATION OF THE AORTA
Prevalence

Coarctation of the aorta (**Fig. 4**) is a common defect seen in 6% to 8% of patients with CHD[15] and in 0.06% to 0.08% of the general population; it is more common in men and boys than in women and girls. It may be isolated but often occurs with other cardiac and vascular lesions, including VSD, bicuspid aortic valve, mitral valve stenosis, and circle of Willis aneurysms.[15,16] The most common genetic cause of coarctation of the aorta is Turner syndrome, characterized by XO sex chromosomes and often associated with left-sided heart defects.[15] First-degree relatives of patients with coarctation of the aorta have a 10-fold increase in risk of having an obstructive left-sided lesion.[17]

Overview and Anesthetic Implications

Aortic coarctation is characterized by a discrete narrowing of the aorta, usually adjacent to the location of the ductus arteriosus. Symptoms include precoarctation hypertension found in the upper extremities, hypotension in the lower extremities, and left ventricular hypertrophy on electrocardiogram.[15] Long-term survival without repair is significantly reduced, because without surgical intervention, mortality is 75% by age 50. Untreated coarctation of the aorta can be associated with premature coronary artery disease, left ventricular dysfunction, aortic aneurysm/dissection, and cerebral vascular disease, despite development of significant collateral blood flow.[15]

Although there is increased morbidity and mortality without intervention, surgical repair has its own set of associated complications, including most commonly restenosis, which is seen in up to 10% of patients.[16] Other issues include aortic root aneurysm, aortic dissection, collateral vessel aneurysm, and less commonly, lower-extremity paralysis or other perfusion-related spinal cord injuries from aortic cross-clamp time during the procedure.[16] Furthermore, age of the patient at time of repair also has implications for long-term outcomes and associated issues. Thus, 90% of patients repaired in childhood has no hypertension, but 50% of those repaired after age 40 has persistent hypertension.[16]

Coarctation of the Aorta

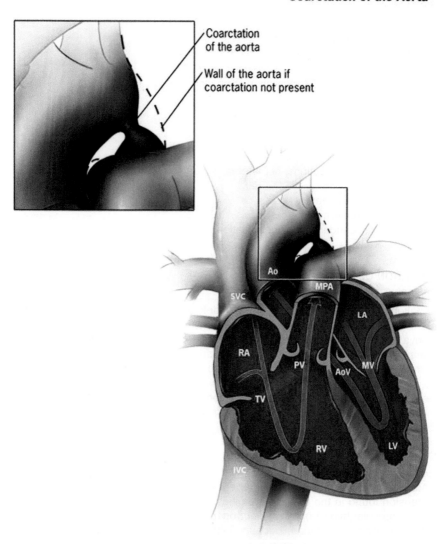

Coarctation
of the aorta

Wall of the aorta if
coarctation not present

Fig. 4. Coarctation of the aorta. A coarct, or abrupt narrowing, of the aorta is shown. (*Courtesy of* the Centers for Disease Control and Prevention, Bethesda, MD; https://www.cdc.gov/ncbddd/heartdefects/images/coarctationlayoutv2-575px.jpg.)

Several considerations are needed when caring for patients with coarctation of the aorta during noncardiac surgery, starting with if the patient has had surgical repair. Issues such as hypertension, left ventricular hypertrophy, aortic root aneurysm, spinal cord hypoperfusion injuries, and other associated issues can influence the surgical plan and must be thoroughly investigated before noncardiac surgery.[15,16] The timing of the operation or intervention also heavily influences the types of likely sequelae, with later–in-life operations having more long-term issues, including coronary artery disease and long-standing hypertension.[16] The type of repair also affects the possible long-term effects, with end-to-end anastomotic repair more frequently (3%) causing restenosis, but patch repair more commonly causing aortic root aneurysm.[16,18] Regardless of treatment, patients born with coarctation of the aorta have a lifelong increase in the risk of cerebral artery aneurysm.[15] Therefore, all patients with coarctation should be followed long term by a congenital cardiologist.[15]

Concerns:
  Associated cardiac defects and genetic syndromes
  Management of hypertension
  Coronary artery disease
  Cerebral vascular disease
  Restenosis
  Aortic root aneurysm
  Aortic root dissection
  Collateral blood vessels
  Paraplegia
  Spinal cord hypoperfusion injuries from repair
  Age of patient at time of repair

SINGLE-VENTRICLE PATIENTS
Prevalence

The 10- and 20-year survival of patients receiving a Fontan shunt is greater than 90% and 84%, respectively.[15] Because palliative surgery can be between 18 months and 2 years of age, but on average childhood to early teen years, patients will present as adults with palliated single-ventricle (Fontan) physiology for noncardiac surgery.[15] The number of adults with univentricular physiology is increasing.[19]

Overview and Anesthetic Implications

Congenital cardiac lesions that are not amenable to biventricular repair are palliated with Fontan physiology, resulting in total cavopulmonary connection (TCPC).[16] In TCPC, the superior vena cava and inferior vena cava are directly connected to the pulmonary arteries (Glenn and Fontan anastomoses, respectively),[16] which takes the circulation of patients with single-ventricle physiology from parallel to series. Several lesions may require Fontan palliation, including hypoplastic left heart syndrome (HLHS) (**Fig. 5**), tricuspid atresia (**Fig. 6**), double-outlet right ventricle, right ventricle hypoplasia, severe Ebstein anomaly, double-inlet right ventricle, and unbalanced atrioventricular canal (AVC).[15] Regardless of the original lesion, the resulting physiology causes total dependence of cardiac output on passive pulmonary blood return. The 1 exception seen to this complete dependence occurs in patients with a fenestrated Fontan conduit. The fenestration allows augmentation of cardiac output by directly supplying additional volume to an underfilled ventricle.[16]

Although long-term survival has greatly improved, most patients over 30 years of age with Fontan physiology are New York Heart Association (NYHA) class III.[16] Patients with a palliated single ventricle have a progressive systolic dysfunction that often leads to systemic valvular regurgitation, causing a dilated cardiomyopathy.[16] There is no current tool for assessment of risk stratification for patients with Fontan physiology.[16] Therefore, preoperative evaluation and optimization is critical for palliated single-ventricle patients and may necessitate delay of nonemergent surgery.[16]

A thorough history should include current functional status, any recent changes in exercise capacity, overall health, and hospital admissions. Physical examination should also be performed with a focus on signs of poor end-organ perfusion, such

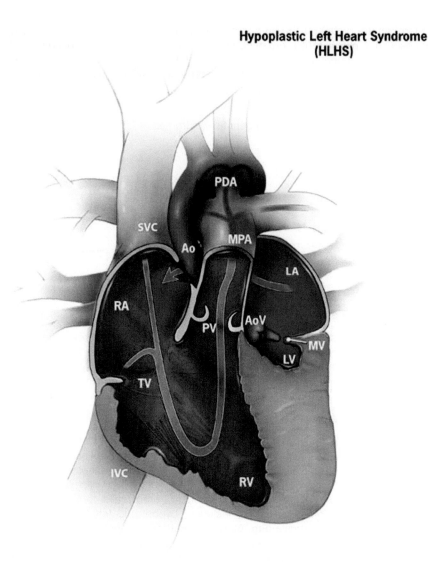

Fig. 5. Hypoplastic left heart syndrome. A hypoplastic left ventricle, aortic valve, and ascending aorta along with ASD comprise an example of HLHS. (*Courtesy of* the Centers for Disease Control and Prevention, Bethesda, MD; https://www.cdc.gov/ncbddd/heartdefects/images/hlhs-web.jpg.)

as digital clubbing, cyanosis, and arterial oxygen saturations less than 90% as well as indications of increased pulmonary pressures, such as hepatomegaly and ascites. Following comprehensive history and physical examination, a chest radiograph, recent echocardiogram, electrocardiogram, liver function tests, electrolytes, blood chemistry, and baseline coagulation profile should be obtained. Interrogation of a pacemaker (if present) is also important.[15,16] The provider should identify signs of a failing Fontan, including cardiomegaly, pleural effusions, arrhythmias (seen in more than 50% of patients at 20-year follow-up), atrioventricular valve (AVV) disease, diastolic and systolic heart failure, cyanosis, cerebrovascular accidents, renal

Tricuspid Atresia

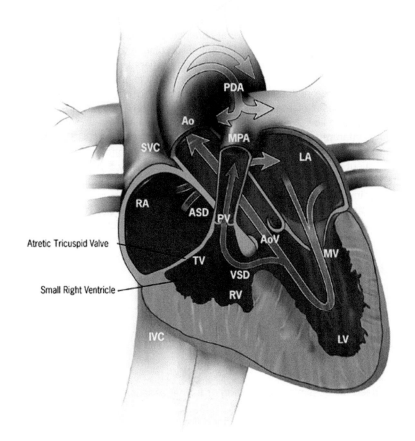

Fig. 6. Tricuspid atresia. A hypoplastic right ventricle, pulmonary valve, and main pulmonary artery along with a VSD comprise an example of tricuspid atresia and its sequelae. ASD, atrial septal defect; VSD, ventricular atrial septal defect. (*Courtesy of* the Centers for Disease Control and Prevention, Bethesda, MD; https://www.cdc.gov/ncbddd/heartdefects/images/tricuspid_atresia.jpg.)

failure, cirrhosis, protein-losing enteropathy, vascular occlusions, collateral circulation, and coagulopathies.[15,16] If patients show signs of failure, further workup, such as cardiac catheterization, is necessary to assess for need for optimization and possible intervention before noncardiac surgery.[16] Optimization may include antiarrhythmic medications, interventional cardiac procedures, pulmonary vasodilators, and inotropes.[17]

Patients with Fontan palliation present unique challenges in the perioperative period, particularly with the frequent increase in venous capacitance caused by several anesthetics. Venous dilation resulting from general anesthesia can dramatically decrease cardiac output by reducing return of blood to the heart, which is entirely based on the combination of PVR and venous capacitance.[16] Therefore, avoidance of prolonged nothing by mouth times and underresuscitation should be avoided.[16]

Furthermore, avoidance of pulmonary hypertension is essential in patients with Fontan physiology. Noxious stimuli, hypercarbia, acidosis, and hypoxia are all to be avoided in order to avoid increased pulmonary vascular resistance.

The goal of anesthetic maintenance for patients with a Fontan includes minimization of intrathoracic pressure, avoidance of positive pressure ventilation if possible (optimizing transpulmonary gradient), maintaining adequate preload and sinus rhythm, avoiding hypotension, and underresuscitation to allow for optimal cardiac output.[15,16] Strategies for optimizing and augmenting cardiac output in a Fontan patient include ventilating with 100% oxygen, using the lowest-peak airway pressure possible, maintaining low partial pressures of carbon dioxide, maintaining an appropriate depth of anesthesia, maintaining preload with intravenous fluids, maintaining normothermia, and appropriate use of pulmonary vasodilators and lusitropic/inotropic agents, such as milrinone.[16,18]

Patients with Fontan physiology should be adequately monitored based on current severity of disease and operation performed. In general, the standard guidelines for intraoperative patient monitoring set forth by the American Society of Anesthesiologists are adequate for most cases. The exceptions would be, based on the case performed, possible need for invasive blood pressure and central venous pressure monitoring.[16] It should be noted that upper-extremity blood monitoring should be performed on the contralateral side as the patient's former subclavian artery to pulmonary artery anastomosis, or Blalock-Taussig shunt (BTS), in order to avoid falsely low readings.[16] Other considerations include need for perioperative endocarditis prophylaxis, and providers should follow current guidelines set forth by the American Heart Association.[11,20]

Concerns:
    Preoperative evaluation
        Thorough history and physical examination
        Echocardiogram
        Chest radiograph
        Electrocardiogram
        Baseline laboratory tests
        Assess need for possible optimization or further assessment
    Intraoperative
        Maintenance of passive pulmonary blood flow
            Optimize preload
            Avoid long nothing by mouth times and hypotension (new nothing by mouth guidelines will help)
            Avoid hypoxia, hypercarbia, noxious stimuli
            Optimize transpulmonary gradient: avoid positive pressure ventilation if possible
            Avoid laparoscopic procedures if able (consider open approach)
        Arrhythmias; external pacing pads
        Systolic function
            Avoidance of myocardial depressants
            Need for possible inotropes
        Avoidance of blood pressure measurements on side of previous BTS

ATRIOVENTRICULAR CANAL AND TETRALOGY OF FALLOT
Prevalence

Tetralogy of Fallot (TOF; **Fig. 7**) is the most common of all cyanotic CHDs, encompassing upwards of 10% of all lesions and occurring in 3 of every 10,000 live births.[21,22] It is associated with chromosomal abnormalities, including trisomy 21, 18, and 13 as well as

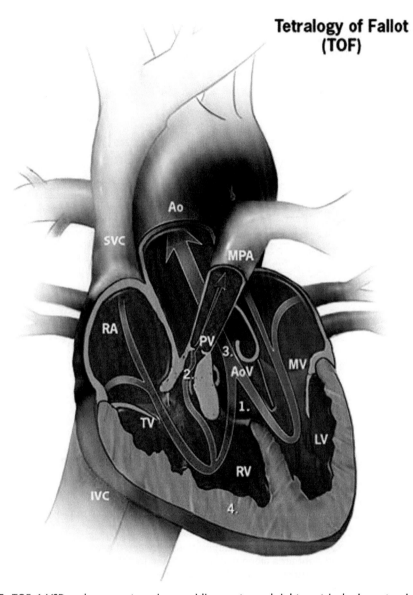

Tetralogy of Fallot (TOF)

Fig. 7. TOF. A VSD, pulmonary stenosis, overriding aorta, and right ventricular hypertrophy comprisingTOF are shown. (*Courtesy of* the Centers for Disease Control and Prevention, Bethesda, MD; https://www.cdc.gov/ncbddd/heartdefects/images/Teralogy_web.jpg.)

microdeletions of chromosome 22.[22] The 30-year survival rate is 85%.[22] TOF can occur as the sole lesion, but often occurs with other congenital heart defects, most often AVC, also known as atrioventricular septal defect (AVSD).[22] Other commonly coexisting lesions are pulmonary atresia, double-outlet right ventricle, and anomalous coronary artery.[22] Complete atrioventricular canal (CAVC) accounts for approximately 3% of congenital cardiac lesions and has a strong association with trisomy 21.[23] Unrepaired, more than half of patients with CAVC (**Fig. 8**) will die in infancy owing to heart failure.[23]

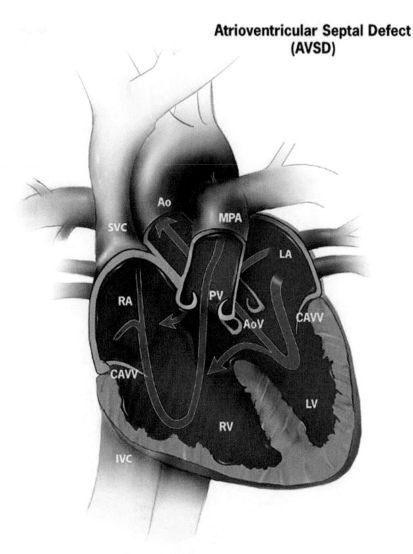

Atrioventricular Septal Defect (AVSD)

Fig. 8. AVSD or CAVC, comprising communications between the left and right ventricle as well as the left and right atria along with tricuspid and mitral valve involvement is shown. CAVV, common atrioventricular valve. (*Courtesy of* the Centers for Disease Control and Prevention, Bethesda, MD; https://www.cdc.gov/ncbddd/heartdefects/images/avsd-575px.jpg.)

Overview and Anesthetic Implications

The 4 components comprising the TOF are VSD, right ventricular outflow tract obstruction, right ventricular hypertrophy, and overriding aorta.[21] The type of surgical repair depends on the severity of pulmonary outflow obstruction and coexisting lesions, such as AVC or pulmonary atresia. Common long-term sequelae after surgical repair are pulmonary regurgitation, residual pulmonary stenosis, and arrhythmias, including complete heart block and ventricular tachycardia, which can lead to sudden cardiac death.[22] Although most patients undergo surgical correction in infancy or early childhood, some do not have palliation until adulthood.[24] These patients have an increased risk of atrial arrhythmias, low-cardiac output syndrome, junctional ectopic tachycardia, and complete heart block.[24]

AVCs are characterized by a common AVV, an ostium primum ASD, and a VSD.[23] Surgical repair is generally before 6 months of age in order to prevent development of pulmonary hypertension.[23] The type of repair is dependent on the patient's individual anatomy, but often includes an atrial patch, ventricular patch, and valvuloplasty to make the atrioventricular valve into 2 ventricular valves.[23] One exception to biventricular repair is in patients with concurrent moderate to severe hypoplasia of either ventricle who may be unable to undergo biventricular repair. Instead, in these patients, a single-ventricle route is followed, and patients are palliated in the same way as other single-ventricle lesions.[25–32] The most common postsurgical sequelae in patients undergoing full intracardiac repair is left AVV regurgitation, subaortic stenosis, complete heart block, and residual VSD.[25]

When encountering patient with TOF, AVC, or both concurrently for noncardiac surgery, it is important to consider the individual's anatomy and previous repairs or palliation. Lifetime cardiology follow-up is required despite good long-term outcomes for both lesions after surgical intervention.[2] It is important to consider all of the patient's current sequelae as well as anticipate known possible complications. Therefore, in addition to the conduct of a thorough history and physical examination other evaluations, including possible stress test and electrocardiogram or Holter monitor study may be necessary before surgery.[2] Intraoperative care should be based on the most current data available and type of surgery being performed.

Concerns:
  TOF
    Pulmonary regurgitation
    Arrhythmias
    Complete heart block
    Sudden cardiac death
  AVC
    Left AVV regurgitation
    Complete heart block
    Residual VSD
    Subaortic stenosis
    Single-ventricle palliation with cavopulmonary anastomosis

TRANSPOSITION OF THE GREAT ARTERIES
Prevalence

More than 1 in 3500 to 5000 infants each year in the United States are born with transposition of the great arteries (TGA).[33] More than 1200 of those TGA are categorized as D-type with isolated ventriculoarterial discordance,[34] which is in contrast to the rarer L-type transposition (also known as congenitally corrected TGA), in which the patient has both atrioventricular and ventriculoarterial discordance.[34] Frequently TGA is associated with other cardiac lesions, such as VSD and left ventricular outflow obstruction.[33]

Both conditions result in the morphologic right ventricle being the systemic ventricle. However, L-type TGA results in the morphologic right ventricle pumping oxygenated blood systemically, whereas the D-type TGA results in the right ventricle pumping deoxygenated blood to the systemic circulation. Both present their own unique problems and perioperative considerations.

Overview and Anesthetic Implications

D-type TGA (**Fig. 9**) patients have parallel pulmonary and systemic circulations, which, without additional shunting to allow for oxygenated and deoxygenated blood to mix, are not compatible with life. Upwards of 90% mortality is seen in patients who are not surgically corrected in infancy.[34,35] It is important to know not only the type of transposition that the patient had but also the type of surgical repair because surgical

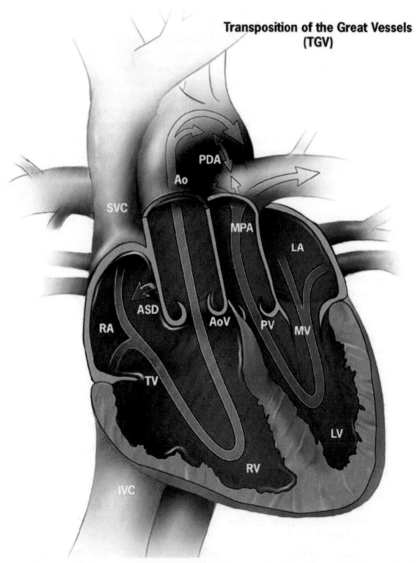

Fig. 9. TGA. A D-TGA or transposition of the great vessels, where the aorta arises from the right ventricle and the pulmonary artery arises from the left ventricle, is shown. (*Courtesy of* the Centers for Disease Control and Prevention, Bethesda, MD; https://www.cdc.gov/ncbddd/heartdefects/images/d-tga-575px.jpg.)

corrections have changed drastically since the first repairs were performed in the 1950s.[34]

Although current surgical technique involves arterial switch, there are an estimated 9000 patients in the United States who have had atrial switches for palliation, also known as Mustard (autologous pericardium repair) and Senning (synthetic material repair) procedures for baffle creation.[34] With an 80% survival at almost 30 years after operation, it is likely for these patients to eventually present for noncardiac surgery.[19,34] Because these patients are repaired in a way that maintains the morphologic right ventricle as the systemic ventricle, the most common concern is right ventricular dysfunction, which is seen in 18% of patients[19] and which is assessed by NYHA functionality, echocardiography, and presence of tricuspid regurgitation and pulmonary venous congestion.[19,36] Given the atriotomy and extensive atrial sewing required during repair, the other major consideration in patients with atrial switch palliation is arrhythmia, which is the most common cause of sudden death.[19] Another concern in up to 7% of patients is development of pulmonary hypertension.[37,38]

As opposed to the Mustard and Senning atrial switches, improved long-term survival of more than 97% over 20 years in patients receiving the arterial switch makes it the current preferred method of repair for dextro-TGA. The arterial switch includes switching the pulmonary and aortic roots, and reimplanting the coronary arteries to the aorta.[33,36] Several variations exist, including the Rastelli procedure, which uses a conduit to connect the right ventricle to the pulmonary arteries for patients with concurrent pulmonary stenosis.[37] Common long-term concerns in this population include aortic root dilation, possibly leading to aortic valve regurgitation and need for further surgical intervention, atrial arrhythmias, and conduit stenosis.[37]

Patients with the rare L-type TGA may or may not need surgical repair depending on the presence of other cardiac defects, such as a large VSD (70% of patients), which could lead to congestive heart failure without closure.[37] Pulmonary stenosis occurs in up to 40% of patients and is most commonly valvular.[37] Because of the transposition, patients with L- Transposition of the Great Arteries have abnormal positioning and course of their conduction system, leading to progressive fibrosis of the conduction system and risk of complete atrioventricular nodal block, the risk of which increases with need for tricuspid valve repair and VSD closure.[37]

Concerns:
  Type of defect
    D-type: ventriculoarterial discordance
    L-Type: atrioventricular discordance
  Type of repair
  Atrial switch
    Right ventricular dysfunction
    Arrhythmias
  Arterial switch
    Aortic root dilation
    Aortic valve regurgitation
    Right ventricle to pulmonary artery conduit stenosis
    Arrhythmias
  L-type TGA
    Concurrent congenital cardiac defects
    Pulmonary stenosis
    Arrhythmias including complete heart block

SUMMARY

The authors have provided information for the common lesions that will be encountered during the perioperative care of adult patients with CHD presenting for noncardiac surgery. Before surgery, all patients will need a preanesthetic evaluation to determine the type and status of the uncorrected, corrected, or palliatively repaired CHD. The adult patient's physical status and comorbidities should be determined based on bedside evaluation, echocardiographic, and other diagnostic information when available.[39] When planning for the anesthetic care, one needs to give full consideration to the anatomic lesion and physiologic status of the patient.[40,41] When indicated, the physiologic status should be optimized before the anesthetic and perioperative period. As for children with CHD, one should pay attention to prevent air in the intravenous tubing to minimize the risk of air embolism, ensure a proper preload, and ensure a proper hematocrit when indicated to minimize the risk of thrombosis, hypotension, and hypoxia. Furthermore, it is imperative for the caregiver to remain up-to-date on current recommendations for endocarditis prophylaxis based on the surgical procedure and patient's specific repair or remaining lesion. Although many providers may safely care for adult patients with CHD for noncardiac surgery, it is always advisable to seek collaborative assistance with colleagues trained in CHD should questions arise.

Clinics Care Points

- A complete and thorough preoperative evaluation is vital for congenital heart disease patients.
- A patient's specific lesions, repairs, and current physiology will significantly change the intraoperative management and hemodynamic goals during surgery.
- Induction of anesthesia and operations can greatly change the hemodynamics of patients with intracardiac shunts.
- A patient's previous surgical repairs and history of intravascular catheters can compromise future venous access and arterial monitoring capability.
- Even small air bubbles in vascular access lines can lead to coronary air embolism or stroke in patients with intracardiac shunts, regardless of pre-anesthetic shunt direction.

REFERENCES

1. Denise van der Linde E, Konings EEM, Slager MA, et al. Birth prevalence of congenital heart disease worldwide: a systemic review and meta-analysis. J Am Coll Cardiol 2011;58(21):2241–7.
2. Moodie D. Adult congenital heart disease. Oschner 2002;4(4):221–6.
3. Jacobs EG, Leung MP, Karlberg J. Distribution of symptomatic congenital heart disease in Hong Kong. Pediatr Cardiol 2000;21:148–57.
4. Ferencz C, Rubin JD, McCarter RJ, et al. Congenital heart disease: prevalence at live birth. Am J Epidemiol 1985;121:31–6.
5. Correa-Villaseñor A, McCarter R, Downing J, et al. White-black differences in cardiovascular malformations in infancy and socioeconomic factors: the Baltimore-Washington Infant Study Group. Am J Epidemiol 1991;134:393–402.
6. Moodie D. Adult congenital heart disease. Tex Heart Inst J 2011;38(6):705–6.
7. Ramamoorthy C, Haberkern CM, Bhananker SM, et al. Anesthesia-related cardiac arrest in children with heart disease: data from the Pediatric Perioperative Cardiac Arrest (POCA) registry. Anesth Analg 2010;110:1376–82.

8. Brown M, DiNardo JA, Odegard KC. Patients with single ventricle physiology undergoing noncardiac surgery are at high risk for adverse events. Paediatr Anaesth 2015;8:846–51.

9. Cannesson M, Earing MG, Collange V, et al. Anesthesia for noncardiac surgery in adults with congenital heart disease. Anesthesiology 2009;111(2):432–40.

10. Hoffman JL, Kaplan S. The incidence of congenital heart disease. J Am Coll Cardiol 2002;39:1890–900.

11. Ashley EA, Niebauer J. Adult congenital heart disease," in cardiology explained. London: Remedica; 2004.

12. Menghraj SJ. Anaesthetic considerations in children with congenital heart disease undergoing non-cardiac surgery. Indian J Anaesth 2012;56(5):491–5.

13. Phillip Yen D. ASD and VSD flow dynamics and anesthetic management. Anesth Prog 2015;62(3):125–30.

14. Brown J, Morgan-Hughes NJ. Aortic stenosis and non-cardiac surgery. Continuing Education in Anaesthesia Critical Care & Pain 2005;5(1):1–4.

15. M. e. a. Edmund Just, "Anesthesia for adults with congenital heart disease undergoing noncardiac surgery, 12. 2019. Available at: www.UptoDate.com. Accessed January 16, 2020.

16. Van Dyck M, Glineur D, de Kerchove L, et al. Complications after aortic valve repair and valve-sparing procedures. Ann Cardiothorac Surg 2013;2(1):130–9.

17. Misawa Y. Valve-related complications after mechanical heart valve implantation. Surg Today 2015;45(10):1205–9.

18. Law MA, Tivakaran VS. Coarctation of the aorta. StatPearls Publishing; 2019.

19. Warnes C. "Single ventricle physiology," in adult congenital heart disease. American Heart Association; 2011. p. 170–84.

20. Serfontein SJ, Kron IL. Complications of coarctation repair. Semin Thorac Cardiovasc Surg Pediatr Card Surg Annu 2002;5:206–11.

21. Wilson W, Taubert KA, Gewitz M, et al. Prevention of infective endocarditis. Circulation 2007;116(15):1736–54.

22. Lovell A. Anaesthetic implications of grown-up congenital heart disease. Br J Anaesth 2004;93(1):129–39.

23. Frederique Bailliard RA. Tetralogy of Fallot. Orphanet J Rare Dis 2009;4:2.

24. Rafaele Calabro GL. Complete atrioventricular canal. Orphanet J Rare Dis 2006; 1:8.

25. Khan I, Tufail Z, Afridi S, et al. Surgery for tetralogy of Fallot in adults: early outcomes. Braz J Cardiovasc Surg 2016;31(4):300–3.

26. Craig B. Atrioventricular septal defect: from fetus to adult. Heart 2006;92(12): 1879–85.

27. Paula Martins EC. Transposition of the great arteries. Orphanet J Rare Dis 2008; 3:27.

28. Baskaran J, March KS, Thenappan T. Late-onset pulmonary arterial hypertension in repaired D-transposition of great arteries: an uncommon complication. Pulm Circ 2017;7(2):547–50.

29. Barbanti M, Webb JG, Hahn RT, et al. Impact of preoperative moderate/severe mitral regurgitation on 2-year outcome after transcatheter and surgical aortic valve replacement: insight from the placement of aortic transcatheter valve (PARTNER) trail cohort A. Circulation 2013;128(25):2776–84.

30. Wilson NJ, Clarkson PM, Barratt-Boyes BG, et al. Long-term outcome after the mustard repair for simple transposition of the great arteries. J Am Coll Cardiol 1998;32(3):758–65.

31. Kiener A, Kelleman M, McCracken C, et al. Long-term survival after arterial versus atrial switch in D-transposition of the great arteries. Ann Thorac Surg 2018;106: 1827–33.
32. Warnes C. Transposition of the great arteries. Circulation 2006;114:24.
33. Yetman AT, Starr L, Sanmann J, et al. Clinical and echocardiographic prevalence and detection of congenital and acquired cardiac abnormalities in girls and women with the Turner syndrome. Am J Cardiol 2018;122(2):327–30.
34. Beckmann E, Jassar S. Coarctation repair—redo challenges in the adults: what to do? J Vis Surg 2018;4:76.
35. Windsor J, Townsley MM, Briston D, et al. Fontan palliation for single-ventricle physiology: perioperative management for noncardiac surgery and analysis of outcomes. J Cardiothorac Vasc Anesth 2017;31(6):2296–303.
36. Eagle SS, Daves SM. The adult with Fontan physiology: systematic approach to perioperative management for noncardiac surgery. J Cardiothorac Vasc Anesth 2011;25(2):320–44.
37. Ghanayem NS, Berger S, Tweddell JS. Medical management of the failing Fontan. Pediatr Cardiol 2007;28:465–71.
38. Bailey PD Jr, Jobes DR. The Fontan patient. Anesthesiol Clin 2009;27:285–300.
39. Brida MG, Gatzoulis MA. Adult congenital heart disease: past, present and future. Acta Paediatr 2019;108(10):1757–64.
40. Neidenbach RC, Lummert E, Vigl M, et al. Non-cardiac comorbidities in adults with inherited and congenital heart disease: report from a single center experience of more than 800 consecutive patients. Cardiovasc Diagn Ther 2018;8(4): 423–31.
41. Maxwell BG, Wong JK, Kin C, et al. Perioperative outcomes of major noncardiac surgery in adults with congenital heart disease. Anesthesiology 2013;119(4): 762–9.

Trends in Pediatric Pain
Thinking Beyond Opioids

Charlotte M. Walter, MD*, Niekoo Abbasian, MD,
Vanessa A. Olbrecht, MD, MBA

KEYWORDS

- Pediatric pain management • Regional anesthesia • ERAS protocol • Virtual reality

KEY POINTS

- Newly described regional anesthetic techniques provide novel ways to control postoperative pain in the pediatric population.
- Several different adjuvants can be added safely to pediatric peripheral nerve blocks to prolong and improve postoperative pain control.
- Several nonopioid medications can be used in a multimodal analgesia technique to control pain in the pediatric population.
- Incorporation of enhanced recovery after surgery (ERAS) protocols, which utilize opioid-sparing multimodal analgesia and regional/neuraxial techniques to aid in decreased length of stay and improved early ambulation, is becoming more common in the pediatric population.
- Virtual reality is a new and innovative way to help reduce pain in the pediatric population.

INTRODUCTION

Changing landscapes have made pediatric pain management providers think beyond traditional opioid management to help alleviate pediatric pain. Newly described blocks are being utilized more, whether to avoid the risks of neuraxial anesthesia or to facilitate earlier ambulation or to minimize other side effects from regional techniques. Various adjuvants are also added to pediatric nerve blocks to prolong their effects. Medications besides opioids frequently are used to provide a multimodal analgesia model to control pediatric pain. Often, these techniques are blended together in enhanced recovery after surgery (ERAS) protocols to facilitate shorter length of stays and earlier ambulation. Finally, advances in technology are allowing virtual reality (VR) to become a useful tool in alleviating pediatric pain.

Cincinnati Children's Hospital Medical Center, 3333 Burnet Avenue, MLC 2001, Cincinnati, OH 45229-3026, USA
* Corresponding author.
E-mail address: charlotte.walter@cchmc.org

Anesthesiology Clin 38 (2020) 663–678
https://doi.org/10.1016/j.anclin.2020.04.002   **anesthesiology.theclinics.com**
1932-2275/20/© 2020 Elsevier Inc. All rights reserved.

DISCUSSION
Emerging Regional Techniques

Several newly described regional techniques are utilized in the pediatric population.

Quadratus lumborum block

The quadratus lumborum (QL) is a deep abdominal muscle and the quadratus lumborum block (QLB) is an ultrasound-guided block that finds its key to success in the thoracolumbar fascia (TLF). The TLF is a connective structure that links the anterolateral abdominal wall with the lumbar paravertebral space.[1] The block is possibly effective from local anesthetic bathing the nerves lying within the fascia or from local anesthetic diffusing from the TLF into the paravertebral space.[1] There are 4 different types of QLBs.

In the QLB 1, the lateral side of the QL muscle that is in contact with the transversalis fascia is targeted.[1] The patient is placed in the supine position with a pillow under the spine; a transversely placed probe near the iliac crest is used to identify all 3 layers of the abdominal wall and followed until they taper off into an aponeurosis with the QL posterior to this[1] (**Fig. 1**). Local anesthetic is deposited into this space.[1]

In the QLB 2 (QLB 2), the area targeted is the posterior QL between the QL and the latissimus dorsi and paraspinal muscles; injecting into this space, local anesthetic spreads to the paravertebral space and bathes sympathetic fibers and mechanoreceptors found in the fascia.[2] To achieve this block, the patient is placed in the supine position and the posterior aspect of the QL is identified; the needle tip is then placed in the TLF and local is injected.[2]

In the QLB 3 (QLB 3), the front of the QL at its attachment to the L4 transverse process is targeted; this block sometimes is referred to as the transmuscular QLB .[3] The

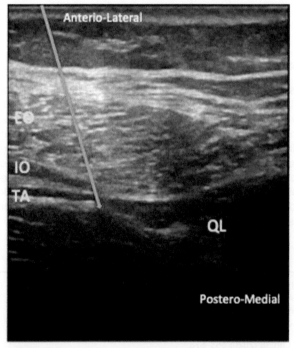

Fig. 1. QL 1 block. Arrow, projected needle path; EO, external oblique; IO, internal oblique; TA, transversus abdominus.

patient is placed in the lateral position and the probe is placed transversely over L4. A needle is inserted transmuscularly through the QL in the anterolateral position with the needle tip positioned between the QL and psoas major.[2,3] The local anesthetic has been shown to spread cephalad with this technique and enter the thoracic paraverte- bral space.[3] The correct ultrasound image for this block has been described as the shamrock sign, with the transverse process of L4 as the center of the shamrock and the QL, psoas muscle, and erector spinae muscles forming the 3 leaves of the shamrock[3] **(Fig. 2)**.

In the QLB 4, the local anesthetic is deposited into the muscle itself.[1] The patient is placed in the supine position and the QL is identified on ultrasound; a needle then is placed within the muscle body of the QL and local anesthetic is injected.[1]

The QLB has been found to offer more local anesthetic spread and better pain con- trol than a transverse abdominis plane (TAP) block.[4] In adults, it has been successfully utilized for a myriad of surgical procedures, including abdominal, transplant, and renal surgeries.[4] In pediatrics, it has also been shown useful in many abdominal procedures, including lower abdominal procedures.[5] It too has been shown to be more effective for postoperative analgesia than the TAP block in children.[5] Complications of the QLB include local anesthetic toxicity; damage to the underlying organs, in particular the kidney; and unwanted/inadvertent femoral nerve (FN) block with the QL 3.[1,4]

Erector spinae plane block

The erector spinae plane (ESP) block is a regional technique where local anesthetic is injected into a plane deep to the erector spinae muscle and is utilized to provide analgesia to the thoracic and abdominal walls.[6] It has been described as techni- cally simpler than the paravertebral and thoracic epidural injections and has an additional layer of safety because it is more remote from the pleura and neuraxial structures.[6,7]

To perform an ESP block, an ultrasound is used to scan both longitudinally and transversely up and down the thoracic spine to confirm positioning of the transverse process at the appropriate level to be anesthetized.[7] The probe then is placed longi- tudinally over the transverse process and the needle inserted in plane until the tip of

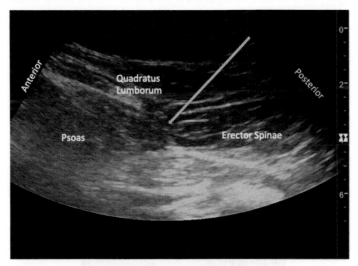

Fig. 2. QL 3 block: shamrock view—3 leaves of the shamrock depicted by 3 muscles shown (erector spinae, QL, and psoas muscles). Arrow, projected needle path.

the needle touches bone; this is directly under the erector spinae muscle and is where local anesthetic is injected[7] **(Fig. 3)**. The block can be performed in the sitting, lateral, or prone position. In pediatrics, some clinicians have found that the ESP block technically is more difficult than in adults, secondary to thinner layers of muscle and sliding fascial planes, and finer needle manipulation is required.[8]

Indications for the ESP block are vast. In adults, it has been used for treatment of acute, postoperative, and chronic pain.[6] In pediatrics, it also has been shown to effective in a multitude of operations in the thoracic and abdominal cavities.[8,9] Complications are rare; the ESP block is further removed from the pleura compared with the paravertebral block but the risk of pneumothorax still remains.[6]

Suprainguinal fascia iliaca block

The suprainguinal fascia iliaca (FI) block is a newer approach of the FI block, which first was described infrainguinally, to better cover pain after hip and knee surgery. The lateral femoral cutaneous nerve (LFCN), FN, and obturator nerve (ON) all provide sensation to the hip joint; the LFCN leaves the FI at the inguinal ligament whereas the branches of the FN that innervate the hip leave proximal to the inguinal ligament.[10] The ON, FN, and LFCN, however, all are found in the suprainguinal FI.[10]

To perform the suprainguinal FI block under ultrasound guidance, an ultrasound transducer is placed longitudinally medial to the anterior superior iliac spine and rotated 30° toward the umblilicus.[11] The iliacus muscle lies between the oblique muscle and the ilium, and the local anesthetic is deposited below the fascia but above the muscle cephalad[11] **(Fig. 4)**.

The suprainguinal FI block has been shown effective in adults after total hip arthroplasty as demonstrated by decreasing opioid consumption.[12] It also has been shown to treat perioperative pain in children after arthroscopic surgery, with a low complication rate.[11] Overall, the suprainguinal FI block results in more reliable spread of local anesthetic to the LFCN, FN, and ON and more completely provides a sensory block of the medial, anterior, and lateral thigh compared with the infrainguinal approach.[13]

Knee sensory blocks

A desire to provide a sensory block of the knee with little to no motor deficit allowing for early ambulation after knee surgery has led to the development of two blocks. The first, the adductor canal block, provides analgesia to the anterior knee. The second,

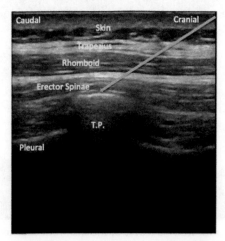

Fig. 3. Erector spinae nerve block. Arrow, projected needle path; T.P., transverse process.

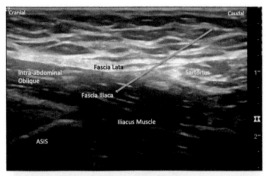

Fig. 4. Suprainguinal FI block: bowtie made by boundary of fascia lata, FI, sartorius muscle, and intra-abdominal oblique muscles. Arrow, projected needle path; ASIS, anterior superior iliac spine.

the interspace between the popliteal artery and posterior knee (IPACK) block, provides analgesia to the posterior knee.[14,15]

Adductor canal block The adductor canal is a tunnel extending from the start of the femoral triangle to the adductor hiatus on the thigh; it is bound medially by the adductor magnus, laterally by the vastus medialis, and superiorly by the sartorius.[14] Its contents include the superficial femoral vessels, the saphenous nerve, and the nerve to the vastus medialis. The nerve to the vastus medialis is the only motor nerve in the canal; therefore, blocking in the adductor canal is associated with minimal muscle weakness and an ability to ambulate safely faster compared with the traditional FN block.[14]

The block is performed at the midthigh level, halfway to two-thirds down from a line between the anterior superior iliac spine and the patella.[14] A transducer is placed longitudinally at this level and the superficial femoral artery is identified in the canal; the saphenous nerve, a hyperechoic structure, should be seen anteriolateral to the artery (more distally toward the patella, the saphenous nerve will appear medial to the artery)[14] (**Fig. 5**). The canal is filled with local anesthetic with needle infiltration.[14]

The primary indication for the adductor canal block is postoperative analgesia to the anterior knee. Compared with continuous FN blocks, continuous adductor canal blocks demonstrate equivalent analgesia and opioid requirements in adult patients undergoing total knee arthroplasty (TKA).[14] A large comparative analysis demonstrated that opioid consumption was comparable between FN block and adductor canal block but that the adductor canal block was associated with better quadriceps power, longer ambulation distance, and shorter hospital length of stay in adults undergoing TKA.[16] In pediatrics, there is a single case series report following patients who received an adductor canal block for their patellar dislocation surgery.[17] All subjects demonstrated acceptable numerical rating scale scores for postoperative pain control and there were no adverse effects during the 48 hours after surgery.[17] An adductor canal block has a low risk of long-term neurologic injury; one other adverse effect is that even though the block seems to be quadriceps sparing, the quadriceps function is not completely normal, so fall precautions are needed.[14]

Interspace between the popliteal artery and posterior knee block IPACK block is a motor-sparing block to provide posterior knee analgesia to facilitate early ambulation while sparing the tibial and common peroneal nerves, thereby maintaining strength and sensation to the leg.[15,18] Anatomically, this block targets the articular branches

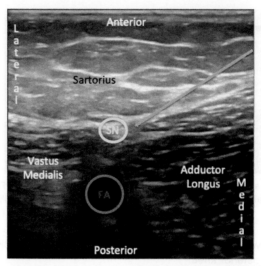

Fig. 5. Adductor canal nerve block. Arrow, projected needle path; FA, femoral artery; SN, saphenous nerve.

of the tibial nerve and obturator nerve that travel through the space between the popliteal artery and posterior knee.[15,18]

To perform the block, the ultrasound probe is placed to view the adductor canal in the lower third of the medial thigh and then slid distally to visualize the popliteal artery diving into the popliteal fossa. The probe then is moved to visualize the space between the popliteal artery and shaft of the femur just above the femoral condyles, approximately 1 fingerbreadth above the patella[18] (**Fig. 6**). The needle then is inserted in plane to 2 cm beyond the artery; local anesthetic is given in divided doses as the needle is withdrawn.[18]

Indications for the IPACK block include posterior knee pain after TKA and major ligament repair.[18] One recent study has shown that in addition to adductor canal block, addition of the IPACK block allowed for better pain control, range of motion, and ambulation distance in TKA patients compared with adductor canal block alone.[19] In pediatrics, a single case series has looked at IPACK blocks for anterior cruciate ligament repairs; they found that patients who received the IPACK block had minimal opioid needs in the postanesthesia care unit with no sciatic motor weakness.[20] Adverse effects are thought to be low. Cadaver studies have shown the potential for local anesthetic spread to unintended locations, such as the tibial nerve and common peroneal nerve.[15] Intra-articular injection is also possible.[15]

Block Adjuvants

Block adjuvants are medications that can be used in addition to local anesthetics in regional anesthesia techniques to prolong the length of the block and/or increase the analgesic effect of the block. Some investigators argue that block adjuvants should always be used in pediatric regional anesthesia.[21]

α_2-Agonists

Clonidine Clonidine is an α_2-agonist that prolongs local anesthetic blockade in 2 ways: indirectly, by vasoconstrictor properties, and directly, by interfering with hyperpolarization.[22] The interference with the hyperpolarization-activated cation channel, however, likely contributes more effect.[21] A large meta-analysis demonstrated

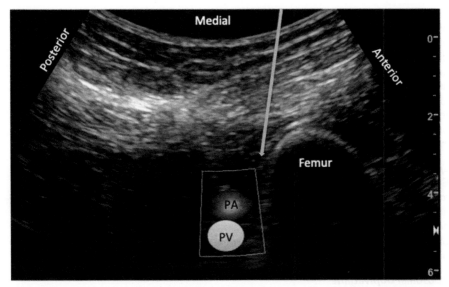

Fig. 6. IPACK block. Arrow, projected needle path; PA, popliteal artery; PV, popliteal vein.

evidence-based support of clonidine use in pediatrics.[23] Clonidine use in pediatrics has been shown to prolong the block by 20% to 50%, depending on the type of block performed.[24] In addition to block prolongation, clonidine may be beneficial in case of inadvertent interneural injection, where it has been shown to have a protective effect at the site of nerve injury.[25] Adding clonidine to blocks can be associated with side effects, such as bradycardia and hypotension, especially at higher doses; the recommended dose is no higher than 0.5 μg/kg.[25]

Dexmedetomidine Like clonidine, dexmedetomidine is a potent α_2-agonist. It has been shown to prolong peripheral nerve blockade, similar to clonidine.[26] Most literature supports that dexmedetomidine can prolong blocks by approximately 200 minutes, at doses of approximately 1 μg/kg.[26] Side effects are the same as with clonidine and include bradycardia and hypotension.[27] A large meta-analysis also supports the use dexmedetomidine in pediatric regional blocks.[28]

Dexamethasone
Dexamethasone has also been used to prolong blocks. It has an unknown mechanism of action and both perineural and systemic administration seem to prolong the block.[22] It is hypothesized that it may prolong a block by attenuation of the C-fiber response, anti-inflammatory action, and/or immunosuppressive actions.[28] A meta-analysis has demonstrated, however, that perineural dexamethasone prolongs analgesia more than dexamethasone given intravenously (IV).[29] A Cochrane review found that the use of dexamethasone in upper limb surgeries prolongs peripheral nerve blocks, reduces opioid consumption, and reduces pain scores.[30] The review could not find enough evidence, however, to support its use for lower limb surgery and found no evidence supporting its use in pediatric populations.[30] More studies are needed to assess whether dexamethasone given perineurally prolongs blocks in pediatric patients.

Opioids
Various opioids have been added to peripheral nerve blocks with varying success. Morphine use has been studied the most extensively but the routine use of morphine

in peripheral nerve blocks cannot be recommended because the benefits of its use do not surpass IV morphine and the side effects are increased.[22] Buprenorphine, a partial opioid receptor agonist with local anesthetic-like capacity to block voltage-gated sodium channels, has been shown to prolong blocks but also has been shown to increase nausea.[31] As such, its use is recommended only with coadministration of antiemetics.[22] Numerous studies have shown that it can significantly prolong blocks in adults and provides better analgesia and longer duration of action compared with the addition of morphine.[28] Tramadol has also been studied. It has analgesic effects on the mu-opioid and other nonopioid receptors; however, there have been only inconsistent results in adults with the addition of tramadol to blocks.[28]

Epinephrine
Epinephrine has been used to prolong the effect of peripheral nerve blocks. It has 2 main effects on peripheral nerves blocks: it allows for an increased amount of local anesthetic that can be given and it prolongs the duration of the block.[28] Epinephrine, however, can compromise neural blood flow and has shown only mixed efficacy for block prolongation.[27] Therefore, it is not recommended for routine use of block prolongation.[22]

Liposomal bupivacaine
Liposomal bupivacaine is a recent addition to peripheral nerve blocks. Liposomes act as a medication depot; as they slowly break down in the body, they slowly release the medication in their matrix.[32] Therefore, liposomal bupivacaine allows for the extended release of bupivacaine.[32] It initially was approved for local infiltration by the US Food and Drug Administration (FDA); it recently has gained approval for use in interscalene blocks in adults. It has been shown more effective than bupivacaine alone in TAP blocks; it has also been shown more effective than bupivacaine alone in lower extremity blocks but that is an off-label use.[32] A Cochrane review demonstrated that liposomal bupivacaine infiltration at the surgical site reduced pain compared with placebo but was not superior to regular bupivacaine infiltration.[33] It is not FDA approved for use in pediatric patients. There are studies in pediatrics that demonstrate a benefit in wound infiltration but no studies to date have looked at the use of liposomal bupivacaine in peripheral nerve blocks in children.[34]

Medication Management

A variety of medications are used to treat both acute and chronic pain in children. For some of the medications, the data supporting its use are poor or extrapolated from the adult literature. Continued studies on effective pharmacologic management for pediatric pain are needed.

Opioids
Opioids remain a mainstay of managing pediatric pain. Some opioids have mixed antagonist and agonist actions or act on other nonopioid receptors. These medications are used in the hope of providing pain relief while minimizing unwanted side effects. Buprenorphine is a partial mu agonist, partial or complete opioid receptor like-1 agonist, and kappa and delta opioid antagonist.[35] It has many benefits compared with pure opioid agonists. In addition, it causes internalization of opioid receptors, which decreases the risk of tolerance or dependence.[36] Adding to its safety profile, it has a ceiling effect on respiratory depression.[35] There are few studies, however, demonstrating its efficacy in pediatrics and its use is considered off-label in children.[35] Nalbuphine is a kappa receptor agonist and mu receptor antagonist.[37] Nalbuphine and morphine are considered equianalgesic but nalbuphine carries a lower risk of

respiratory depression, itching, and euphoria.[37] A Cochrane review, however, was unable to definitively show superiority of nalbuphine over placebo; the review could also not comment on the side effects of nalbuphine and recommends more studies to further assess its use in children.[37] Lastly, tramadol is a weak mu opioid receptor agonist that also inhibits the reuptake of norepinephrine and serotonin.[38] In studies, tramadol has shown to provide adequate analgesia for postsurgical pain compared with placebo but not compared with morphine.[38] Pediatric patients who have overactive CYP2D6, however, have an increase in the active metabolites of tramadol, which can lead to an increase in side effects, including respiratory depression, oversedation, and death.[39] The FDA has recently issued a recommendation against the use of tramadol in patients under 12 years of age.[39]

Nonsteroidal anti-inflammatory drugs

Nonsteroidal anti-inflammatory drugs (NSAIDs) are often used for pediatric pain. Perioperative NSAIDs have been shown to decrease pain and opioid consumption in some pediatric surgical populations.[40] A meta-analysis also demonstrated that perioperative NSAID use was associated with less postoperative nausea and vomiting in pediatric patients.[36] In a trial comparing ibuprofen to morphine to control post-tonsillectomy pain, there was no difference in analgesic effectiveness or tonsillar bleeding in the 2 groups.[41] The number of respiratory adverse events, however, was higher in the morphine group.[41] Unfortunately, a Cochrane review could not be certain of the efficacy or safety of ketorolac in treating postoperative pain in children.[42]

Few studies have looked at NSAID use in the treatment of pediatric noncancer chronic pain.[43] A Cochrane review concluded that the amount and quality of evidence for the use of NSAIDs to treat pediatric noncancer chronic pain is very low and that NSAID use in children for this indication is supported only by inference from adult guidelines.[43] In comparison with acetaminophen, however, NSAIDs have shown superior at standard doses for the treatment of both acute and chronic pain.[44]

Acetaminophen

The mechanism of action for acetaminophen is still not completely understood. Acetaminophen inhibits cyclooxygenase (COX) activities in the brain. It does not appear to be a direct COX inhibitor but rather seems to reduce the overall levels of COX.[45] Studies have shown that compared with placebo, acetaminophen is superior for the treatment of postsurgical pain.[46] This same review found that acetaminophen has equal safety compared with placebo.[46] Other systemic reviews have shown that acetaminophen can decrease pain and opioid use when used perioperatively in the pediatric surgical patient.[40] Since the arrival of IV acetaminophen, studies also have shown efficacy in the use of IV acetaminophen to treat acute pain in children.[47] When comparing oral to IV formulations, the oral formulation offers a significant cost savings over the IV formulation.[45] The IV formulation, however, has superior cerebrospinal bioavailability of the drug.[45] A meta-analysis in adult literature showed no difference in pain control and opioid consumption between IV and oral acetaminophen.[45] The benefit of IV versus oral acetaminophen has not been clearly established.

Ketamine

Ketamine is an N-methyl-D-aspartate (NMDA) antagonist that has been used for its anesthetic, analgesic, and antidepressant properties.[48] The American Society of Regional Anesthesia and Pain Medicine consensus guidelines recommend ketamine in the perioperative setting both as a stand-alone treatment of pain and as an opioid adjunct.[49] Studies have shown safety and efficacy in using low-dose ketamine (less than 0.3 mg/kg/h) in the non–critical care setting for acute pain.[50] Although side effects frequently are reported with the use of ketamine infusions, these side effects tend to be minimal or mild and often do not result in discontinuation of the infusion.[50] In pediatric populations, perioperative ketamine has been shown to reduce postoperative pain and opioid use.[40]

Antiepileptics

Gabapentin and pregabalin are 2 antiepileptics that are now also used as pain medications. They are both potent inhibitors of the mechanisms that play a role in neuropathic pain models.[51] They are well-tolerated medications with few side effects, which can include dizziness, fatigue, and worsening depression.[51] In pediatric populations undergoing the Ravitch procedure, patients who received perioperative gabapentin had lower anxiety and needed fewer rescue antiemetics compared with patients who did not receive gabapentin.[52] In pediatric patients presenting for amputation, perioperative gabapentin started 4 days before surgery and continued for 30 days after surgery was associated with less development of phantom limb pain and less acute postoperative pain.[53] In the neonatal intensive care units, gabapentin also has been trialed and shown effective in reducing overall opioid consumption.[54]

There are, however, some caveats with gabapentin use. A Cochrane systemic review found no evidence to support or refute the use of gabapentin or pregabalin to treat chronic noncancer pain in children and adolescents.[55] In the adult literature, a recent review could not recommend gabapentinoids for use in postoperative pain.[56]

Antidepressants

Antidepressant medications are often used to help treat adult, chronic noncancer pain. A recent review of the literature revealed few studies related to treating chronic noncancer pain in children with antidepressants.[57] Adult trials show that some antidepressants, such as amitriptyline, can provide pain relief in noncancer pain.[57] For pediatric functional abdominal pain, however, a recent review of the literature came to the conclusion that there is no evidence to support the routine use of antidepressants.[58] More research on the efficacy of antidepressants and pediatric pain is needed.

Enhanced Recovery After Surgery Protocols

ERAS protocol development describes a comprehensive process of perioperative management aimed at improving outcomes and shortening in-hospital length of stay while minimizing complications and resource wasting in the adult population. The main principal of ERAS is to reduce the body's stress response to surgery with a significant role of multimodal analgesia, which includes nonopioid pharmacologic agents and regional analgesia.[59] Common ERAS elements include minimization of preoperative fasting with encouraged use of clear carbohydrate drink 2 hours before surgery, judicious fluid administration with avoidance of volume overload, early enteral nutrition in the postoperative period, and daily postoperative mobilization. Selection of the surgical technique is also stressed, with emphasis on minimally invasive surgeries and reduction in surgical drains and tubes.[60] Studies of comprehensive protocols in adults are abundant for the past 2 decades beginning with colorectal surgery and now expanded to many different intra-abdominal and orthopedic surgeries.

The majority of enhanced recovery protocol (ERP) research in the pediatric population is limited to the inclusion of 6 or fewer components of the 20 published ERAS Society adult recommendations.[61] One such example of an adjusted pediatric ERAS protocol for urologic surgery at an academic pediatric tertiary medical center is demonstrated in **Table 1**. Although many of the pediatric studies cited in the literature

Table 1
Common elements of enhanced recovery after surgery protocols

Avoid preoperative bowel preparation	Normothermia (36°C–38°C esophageal)
Preoperative clear liquid carbohydrate load (10 mL/kg up to 350 mL max)	DVT prophylaxis
Antibiotic prophylaxis (within 60 min prior to incision)	Minimally invasive (laparoscopy assisted)
Intraoperative euvolemia (3–7 mL/kg/h)	No postoperative NG tube
Minimize intraoperative opioids (<0.3 mg/kg morphine equivalents for case)	Early enteral feeding (POD 0 clear liquids; POD 1 regular)
Minimize postoperative opioids (<0.15 mg/ kg/d morphine equivalents)	Use of nonopioid analgesics (acetaminophen, ketorolac)
Regional anesthesia (wound soakers, nerve catheters, etc.)	Early mobilization (POD 1)

Abbreviations: DVT, deep vein thrombosis; max, maximum; NG, nasogatric; POD, postoperative day.

evaluate individual aspects of ERPs like preoperative counseling, a standardized anesthetic protocol, antimicrobial prophylaxis, modification of surgical access, nonroutine nasogastric intubation, minimized perioperative fasting, and early mobilization, relatively few address multiple components in a systematic approach. Nevertheless, these studies suggest that ERPs, when applied to appropriate pediatric surgical populations, may be associated with decreased length of stay and decreased narcotic use with no detectable increase in complications.[62] More pediatric studies are critical to investigate further ERAS component efficacy in order to alter the disparity in ERAS literature between adult and pediatric populations.

Virtual Reality

Although many nonopioid options exist to help manage pain in pediatric patients, the management of pain must look beyond pharmacologic treatment. There are a growing number of nonpharmacologic options to help manage pain, including the use of VR. VR has been shown to be an innovative way to help decrease pain in a wide variety of situations in both children and adults. Distraction-based VR reduces pain by redirecting attention.[62–69] In particular, VR has been effective in helping to manage pain in children during acutely painful procedures. In 2006, Gold and colleagues[62] published a report on the use of VR to help decrease pain and anxiety during venipuncture in a group of 20 children undergoing IV placement for magnetic resonance imaging/ computed tomography scan. The investigators found that the use of VR was effective as a pain distraction tool during IV placement and that the use of VR was rated favorably by parents, children, and nurses.[62] As such, the investigators suggest that this type of therapy holds promise for pain and anxiety management during acutely painful procedures. In 2018, these investigators published a follow-up randomized controlled trial evaluating the use of VR to reduce pain and anxiety in a cohort of children between the ages of 10 years and 21 years.[66] This study supported their previous findings. The use of VR, however, may go beyond its use of managing pain for acutely painful procedures. In a recent study published in 2019, Spiegel and colleagues assessed the use of VR to help treat pain in hospitalized patients via a prospective, randomized, comparative effectiveness trial.[70] In the 120 patients included, VR was able to reduce pain more significantly compared with a control condition; furthermore, these investigators found that VR was more successful at pain reduction in patients with higher levels of baseline pain (≥7/10 on the numerical rating scale). Similar findings were reported by Tashjian and colleagues in 2017.[68] VR offers patients an innovative, nonpharmacologic modality to help manage pain.

SUMMARY

In treating pediatric pain, thinking beyond opioids is possible. Regional techniques, including newly described methods, are being increasingly used to treat acute post-operative pain, with successes noted in the pediatric populations. The analgesic benefits of regional techniques can be maximized by addition of various block adjuvants to the local anesthetic. When it comes to treating pediatric acute and chronic pain medically, many various nonopioid medications have been used in the pediatric populations. Frequently, opioid-sparing techniques for pain control are being incorporated into ERAS protocols to allow for shorter length of stays and early ambulation. Finally, thinking past pharmacologic management, advances in VR show increasing promise as useful tools to help pediatric pain.

Clinics Care Points

- Newly described regional techniques have been used in pediatric populations to alleviate postoperative pain.

- Several adjuvants can be safely added to pediatric peripheral nerve blocks to prolong and improve postoperative pain control.

- Many nonopioid pain medications have been used successfully to treat acute and chronic pediatric pain.

- Although ERAS research and integration in pediatrics are lagging behind the adult literature, the limited research available indicates improved outcomes, including decreased length of hospital stay and reduced opioid use.

- VR offers a novel way to help manage acute pain in children, including acute procedural pain; the use of VR not only can be associated with decreased pain but also with high patient satisfaction.

DISCLOSURE

The authors have nothing to disclose.

REFERENCES

1. Akermarn M, Pejcic N, Velickovic I. A review of quadratus lumborum block and ERAS. Front Med 2018;5:44.
2. Ueshima H, Otake H, Lin JA. Ultrasound guided quadratus lumborum block: an updated review of anatomy and technique. Biomed Res Int 2017;2017:2752976.
3. Dam M, Moriggl B, Hansen CK, et al. The pathway of injectate spread with the transmuscular quadratus lumborum block; a cadaver study. Anesth Analg 2017;125(1):3030–312.
4. Urits I, Ostling PS, Novitch MB, et al. Truncal regional nerve blocks in clinical anesthesia practice. Best Pract Res Clin Anaesthesiol 2019;33(4):559–71.
5. Oksuz G, Bilal B, Gurkan Y, et al. Quadratus lumborum block versus trasversus abdominis place block in children undergoing low abdominal surgery: a randomized controlled trial. Reg Anesth Pain Med 2017;42(5):674–9.

6. Urits I, Charipova K, Gress K, et al. Expanding role of the erector spinae plane block for the postoperative and chronic pain management. Curr Pain Headache Rep 2019;23(10):71.
7. Ivanusic J, Konishi Y, Barrington MJ. A cadaveric study investigating the mechanism of action of erector spinae blockade. Reg Anesth Pain Med 2018;43(6): 567–71.
8. Aksu C, Gurkan Y. Ultrasound guided erector spinae block for postoperative analgesia in pediatric nephrectomy surgeries. J Clin Anesth 2018;45:35–6.
9. Munoz F, Cubillos J, Bonilla AJ, et al. Erector spinae plane block for posteroperative analgesia in pediatric oncological thoracic surgery. Can J Anesth 2017;64: 880–2.
10. Hebbard P, Ivanusic J, Sha S. Ultrasound-guided supra-inguinal fascia iliaca block: a cadaveric evaluation of a novel approach. Aneaesthesia 2011;66(4): 300–5.
11. Eastburn E Hernandez MA, Boretsky K. Technical success of the ultrasound-guided supra-inguinal fascia iliaca compartment block in older children and adolescents for hip arthroscopy. Paediatr Anaesth 2017;27(11):1120–4.
12. Desmet M, Vermeylen K, Van Herreweghe I, et al. A longitudinal supra-inguinal fascia iliaca compartment block reduces morphine consumption after total hip arthroplasty. Reg Anesth Pain Med 2017;43(3):327–33.
13. Vermeylen K, Desmet M, Leunen I, et al. Supra-inguinal injection for fascia iliaca compartment block results in more consistent spread towards the lumbar plexus than a infra-inguinal injection: a volunteer study. Reg Anesth Pain Med 2019;100092 [Epub ahead of print].
14. Vora MA, Nicholas TA, Kassel CA, et al. Adductor canal block for knee procedures: review article. J Clin Anesth 2016;35:295–303.
15. Nissen AD, Harris DJ, Johnson CS, et al. Interspace between popliteal artery and posterior capsule of the knee (IPACK) injectate spread a cadaver study. J Ultrasound Med 2019;38:741–5.
16. Karkhur Y, Mahajan R, Kakralia A, et al. A comparative analysis of femoral nerve block with adductor canal block following total knee arthroplasty: A systemic literature review. J Anaesthesiol Clin Pharmacol 2018;34(4):433–8.
17. Chen JY, Li N, Xu YQ. Single shot adductor canal block for postoperative analgesia of pediatric patellar dislocation surgery: a case-series report. Medicine (Baltimore) 2015;94(48):e2217.
18. Sinha S. How do I do it: infilatration between popliteal artery and capsule of the knee (iPACK). ASRA News 2019. Available at: www.asra.com.
19. Sankinieani SR, Reddy ARC, Eachempati KK, et al. Comparison of adductor canal block and IPACK block (interspace between the popliteal artery and capsule of the posterior knee) and adductor canal block alone after total knee arthroplasty: a prospective control trial on pain and knee function in immediate postoperative period. Eur J Orthop Surg Traumatol 2018;28:1391–5.
20. Nguyen KT, Marcelino R, Jagannathan N. Infiltration between popliteal artery and capsule of the knee to augment continuous femoral nerve catheter for adolescent anterior cruciate ligament reconstruction: a case series. A A Pract 2020; 14(2):37–9.
21. Lonnqvist PA. Adjuncts should always be used in a pediatric regional anesthesia. Paediatr Anesth 2015;25:100–6.
22. Kirksey MA, Haskins SC, Cheng J, et al. Local anesthetic peripheral nerve block adjuvants for prolongation of analgesia: a systematic qualitative review. PLoS One 2015;10(9):e0137312.

23. Lundblad M, Trifa M, Kaabachi O, et al. Alpha-2 adrenoceptor agonists as adjuncts to peripheral nerve blocks in children: a meta-analysis. Paediatr Anaesth 2016;26(3):232–8.
24. Cucchiaro G, Ganesh A. The effects of clonidine on postoperative analgesia after peripheral nerve blockade in children. Anesth Analg 2007;104:532–7.
25. McCartney CJ, Duggan E, Apatu E. Should we add clonidine to local anesthetics for peripheral nerve blockade? A qualitative systemic review of the literature. Reg Anesth Pain Med 2007;32(4):330–8.
26. Agarwal S, Aggarwal R, Gupta P. Dexmedetomidine prolongs the effect of bupivacaine In supraclavicular brachial plexus blocks. J Anaesthesiol Clin Pharmacol 2014;30(1):36–40.
27. Al-Zaben KR, Qudaisat IY, Alja'bari AN, et al. The effects of caudal or intravenous dexmedetomidine on postoperative analgesia produced by caudal bupivacaine in children: a randomized controlled double blinded study. J Clin Anesth 2016;33: 386–94.
28. Koyyalamudi V, Sen S, Patil S, et al. Adjuvant agents in regional anesthesia in the ambulatory setting. Curr Pain Headache Rep 2017;21:6.
29. Chong MA, Berbenetz NM, Lin C, et al. Perineural versus intravenous dexamethasone as an adjuvant to peripheral nerve blocks: a systemic review and meta-analysis. Reg Anesth Pain Med 2017;42(3):319–26.
30. Phenoa C, Pearson AM, Kaushal A, et al. Dexamethasone as an adjuvant to peripheral nerve block. Cochrane Database Syst Rev 2017;(11):CD011770.
31. Leffler A, Frank G, Kistner K, et al. Local anesthetic -like inhibition of voltage-gated Na(+) channels by the partial mu-opioid receptor agonist buprenorphine. Anesthesiology 2012;116(6):1335–46.
32. Ilfeld B. Continuous peripheral nerve blocks; an update of the published evidence and comparison with novel, alternative analgesic modalities. Anesth Analg 2017;124(1):308–35.
33. Hamilton TW, Athanassoglou V, Mellon S, et al. Liposomal bupivacaine infiltration at the surgical site for the management of postoperative pain. Cochrane Database Syst Rev 2017;(2):CD0011419.
34. Cloyd C, Moffett BS, Bernhardt MB, et al. Efficacy of liposomal bupivacaine in pediatric patients undergoing spine surgery. Paediatr Anesth 2018;28:982–6.
35. Vicencio-Rosas E, Perez-Guille MG, Flores-Perez C. Buprenorphine and pain management in pediatric patients: a update. J Pain Res 2018;11:549–59.
36. Michelet D, Andreu-Gallien J, Bensalah T, et al. A meta-analysis of the use of nonsteroidal anti-inflammatory drugs for pediatric postoperative pain. Anesth Analg 2012;114(2):393–406.
37. Schnabel A, Reichl SU, Zahn PK. Nalbuphine for postoperative pain treatment in children. Cochrane Database Syst Rev 2014;(7):CD009583.
38. Schnabel A, Reichl SU, Meyer-Friedbem C, et al. Tramadol for the postoperative pain treatment in children. Cochrane Database Syst Rev 2015;(3):CD009574.
39. Fortenberry M, Crowder J, So TY. Tramadol in the pediatric population – What is the verdict now? J Pediatr Health Care 2019;33(1):117–23.
40. Zhu A, Benzon HA, Anderson TA. Evidence for the efficacy of systemic opioid-sparing analgesics in pediatric surgical populations: a systemic review. Anesth Analg 2017;125(5):1569–87.
41. Kelly LD, Sommer DD, Ramakrishna J, et al. Morphine or ibuprofen for post-tonsillectomy analgesia: a randomized trial. Pediatrics 2015;135(2):307–13.
42. McNicol ED, Rowe E, Cooper TE. Ketorolac for postoperative pain in children. Cochrane Database Syst Rev 2018;(7):CD012294.

43. Eccleston C, Cooper TE, Fisher E, et al. Non-steroidal anti-inflammatory drugs (NSAIDS) for chronic non-cancer pain in children and adolescents. Cochrane Database Syst Rev 2017;(8):CD012537.

44. Moore RA, Derry S, Wiffen PJ, et al. Overview review: comparative efficacy of oral ibuprofen and paracetamol (acetaminophen) across acute and chronic pain conditions. Eur J Pain 2015;19(9):1213–23.

45. Sun L, Zhu X, Zou J, et al. Comparison of intravenous and oral acetaminophen for pain control for total knee and hip arthroplasty: a systemic review and meta-analysis. Medicine (Baltimore) 2018;97(6):e9751.

46. Boric K, Dosenovic S, Kadic AJ. Interventions for postoperative pain in children: an overview of systemic review. Paediatr Anaesth 2017;27(9):893–904.

47. Baichoo P, Asuncion A, El-Chaar G. Intravenous acetaminophen for the management of pain during vaso-occlusive crises in pediatric patients. P T 2019; 44(1):5–8.

48. Abdallah CG, Adams TG, Kelmendi B, et al. Ketamine's mechanism of action: a path to rapid-acting antidepressants. Depress Anxiety 2016;33(8):689–97.

49. Schwenk ES, Viscusi ER, Buvanendran A, et al. Consensusu guidelines on the use of intravenous ketamine infusions for acute apin management from the American Society of Regional Pain Medicine, and the American Society of Anesthesiologists. Reg Anesth Pain Med 2018;43(5):456–66.

50. Masaracchia MM, Sites BD, Lee J, et al. Subanesthetic ketamine infusions for the management of pediatric pain in non-critical care settings: An observational analysis. Acta Anaesthesiol Scand 2019;63:1225–30.

51. Rose MA, Kam PCA. Gabaepentin: pharmacology and its use in pain management. Anaesth 2002;57:451–62.

52. Tomaszek L, Fenikoswski D, Maciejewski P, et al. Perioperative gabapentin in pediatric thoracic surgery patients – randomized, placebo-controlled, phase 4 study. Pain Med 2017;pnz207.

53. Wang X, Yi Y, Tang D, et al. Gabapentin as a adjuvant therapy for prevention of acute phantom-limb pain in pediatric patients undergoing amputation for malignant bone tumors: a prospective double-blind randomized controlled trial. J Pain Symptom Manage 2018;55(3):721–7.

54. Squillaro A, Mahdi EM, Tran N, et al. Managing procedural pain in the neonate using an opioid sparing approach. Clin Ther 2019;41:1701–37.

55. Cooper TE, Wiffen PJ, Heathcote LC. Antiepileptic drugs for chronic non-cancer pain in children and adolescents. Cochrane Database Syst Rev 2017;(8):CD012536.

56. Fabritius ML, Strom C, Koyuncu S, et al. Benefit and harm of pregabalin in acute pain treatment: a systemic review with meta-analyses and trial sequential analyses. Br J Anaesth 2017;119(4):775–91.

57. Cooper TE, Heathcote LC, Clinch J, et al. Antidepressants for chronic non-cancer pain in children and adolescents. Cochrane Datatbase Syst Rev 2017;(8):CD012535.

58. Korterink JJ, Rutten JM, Venmans L, et al. Pharmacologic treatment in pediatric functional abdominal pain disorders: a systemic review. J Pediatri 2015;166(2): 424–31.

59. Beverly A, Kaye AD, Ljungovist O, et al. Essential elements of multimodal analgesia in Enhanced Recovery After Surgery (ERAS) guidelines. Anesthesiol Clin 2017;35:e115–43.

60. Rove KO, Edney JC, Brockel MA. Enhanced recovery after surgery in children: promising, evidence-based multidisciplinary care. Paediatr Anesth 2018;28: 482–92.
61. Shinnick JA, Short HL, Heiss KF, et al. Enhancing recovery in pediatric surgery: a review of the literature. J Surg Res 2017;202:165–76.
62. Gold JI, Kim SH, Kant AJ, et al. Effectiveness of virtual reality for pediatric pain distraction during i.v. placement. Cyberpsychol Behav 2006;9:207–12.
63. Malloy KM, Milling LS. The effectiveness of virtual reality distraction for pain reduction: a systematic review. Clin Psychol Rev 2010;30:1011–8.
64. Li A, Montano Z, Chen VJ, et al. Virtual reality and pain management: current trends and future directions. Pain Manag 2011;1:147–57.
65. Dascal J, Reid M, IsHak WW, et al. Virtual reality and medical inpatients: a systematic review of randomized, controlled trials. Innov Clin Neurosci 2017;14: 14–21.
66. Gold JI, Mahrer NE. Is virtual reality ready for prime time in the medical space? A randomized control trial of pediatric virtual reality for acute procedural pain management. J Pediatr Psychol 2018;43:266–75.
67. van Twillert B, Bremer M, Faber AW. Computer-generated virtual reality to control pain and anxiety in pediatric and adult burn patients during wound dressing changes. J Burn Care Res 2007;28:694–702.
68. Tashjian VC, Mosadeghi S, Howard AR, et al. Virtual reality for management of pain in hospitalized patients: results of a controlled trial. JMIR Ment Health 2017;4:e9.
69. Indovina P, Barone D, Gallo L, et al. Virtual reality as a distraction intervention to relieve pain and distress during medical procedures: a comprehensive literature review. Clin J Pain 2018;34:858–77.
70. Spiegel B, Fuller G, Lopez M, et al. Virtual reality for management of pain in hospitalized patients: a randomized comparative effectiveness trial. PLoS One 2019; 14:e0219115.

Sustainability in the Operating Room

Reducing Our Impact on the Planet

Diane Gordon, MD

KEYWORDS

• Sustainability • Environmental impact • Climate change • Greenhouse gas • Waste

KEY POINTS

- Anesthesia providers have the ability to choose an anesthetic plan that minimizes environmental impact without affecting patient care.
- Volatile anesthetic agents are greenhouse gases with significant environmental impacts that can be reduced by choosing to avoid desflurane and nitrous oxide and to use low fresh gas flows.
- Wasted medications and single-use devices, particularly disposable laryngoscopes, contaminate the environment and are a source of considerable cost.
- Anesthesia sustainability initiatives save money and decrease the carbon footprint of the operating room, which is appealing not only to clinicians' individual sense of responsibility and stewardship but also to the collective duty of physicians to improve global health.

INTRODUCTION

Climate change will be the defining health crisis of the twenty-first century and represents the greatest threat to global health.[1] Although severe acute respiratory syndrome coronavirus 2 (SARS-CoV-2) has captured attention and will be at the forefront of public health measures for the foreseeable future, the effects of climate change on public health are further reaching, longer lasting, and more difficult to mitigate than even this very contagious virus. The scope of the problems arising from climate change is immense, including a rise in sea levels, increases in extreme weather events, increases in atmospheric carbon dioxide (CO_2) to unprecedented levels, the spread of infectious diseases, the loss of biodiversity, and the declining health status of the population as a whole. Efforts are underway in many countries to curb CO_2 emissions and thus slow and, it is hoped, eventually reverse the current trends. Ironically, in striving to improve population and individual health, the health care system contributes significantly to climate change, which ultimately negatively affects human

Department of Anesthesiology, University of Colorado School of Medicine, 13123 East 16th Avenue B 090, Aurora, CO 80045, USA
E-mail address: diane.gordon@childrenscolorado.org

Anesthesiology Clin 38 (2020) 679–692
https://doi.org/10.1016/j.anclin.2020.06.006
1932-2275/20/© 2020 Elsevier Inc. All rights reserved.

anesthesiology.theclinics.com

well-being. Many analyses have verified the contribution of developed countries' national health care systems to their countries' greenhouse gas (GHG) emissions to be between 3% and 10%. The UK National Health Service was estimated to contribute 4.6% of national GHGs in 2015,[2,3] whereas an analysis of 36 generally first-world countries as well as India and China found that the health care sector was responsible for an average of 5.5% of each nation's overall emissions in 2014.[4] The United States is the second-largest emitter of GHGs globally[5] and the US health care sector is responsible for 10% of US GHG emissions.[6] If the US health care sector were a country, it would rank 13th in the world for GHG emissions, ahead of the entire United Kingdom (**Box 1**).[6] Thus, a decrease in US health care GHG emissions would result in a significant decrease in overall US GHG emissions.

In 2012, the Institute of Medicine suggested that the health sector should lead by example by greening itself and reducing its ecological footprint to improve global health and the health of the planet. Anesthesia providers have considerable freedom in making the care plans for patients and it is important to make choices that minimize the environmental impact of anesthetics without affecting the quality of patient care.

The environmental impact of volatile anesthetics, nitrous oxide (N_2O), intravenous medication waste, single-use devices, and the energy consumption of the heating, ventilation, and air conditioning (HVAC) systems are discussed here, along with practical suggestions to reduce environmental impact.

VOLATILE ANESTHETIC AGENTS

In response to the growing hole in the ozone layer above Antarctica that formed as a result of atmospheric GHGs, the Montreal protocol of 1987 aimed to phase out global chlorofluorocarbon use, with hydrofluorocarbons subsequently targeted through the 2016 Kigali amendment.[7] Anesthetic gases are chlorofluorocarbons (isoflurane) and hydrofluorocarbons (desflurane, sevoflurane), but volatile anesthetic use was not restricted by either protocol because of medical necessity. In 2014, the release of hydrofluorocarbon and chlorofluorocarbon anesthetic gases was equivalent to 3 million tons of CO_2, with 80% of the emissions from desflurane alone. GHGs differ in their abilities to trap heat. The effect of this heat trapping over a 100-year period is described using a scale called the global warming potential over 100 years (GWP_{100}), as shown in **Table 1**. Although other GHGs, such as methane, are emitted in much larger quantities, the environmental impact of volatile anesthetics is significant because volatile anesthetics have much higher GWP_{100} values. For example, despite small quantities, anesthetic gases represented 2% of the United Kingdom's acute National Health Service organizations' carbon footprint in 2012.[8] Desflurane has far higher GWP_{100} values than the other commonly used agents sevoflurane and isoflurane. The use of desflurane results in nearly 20 times the global warming impact of using sevoflurane. Thus, the choice of volatile agent has the most impact in determining the carbon footprint of an anesthetic (**Box 2**). To put it in more practical terms, the environmental impact of volatile anesthetics can be expressed in equivalent miles driven in a car per MAC-hour of anesthesia, as shown in **Table 2**.

Box 1
If the US health care sector alone were a country, it would rank 13th in the world for GHG emissions.

Table 1
Atmospheric lifetime and global warming potential of volatile anesthetics compared with other known greenhouse gases

	Atmospheric Lifetime (y)	GWP_{100}
CO_2	5–200[a]	1
Methane (CH_4)	10	30
Sevoflurane	1.1	130
Isoflurane	3.2	510
Desflurane	14	2540

[a] No single lifetime can be defined for CO_2 because of the different rates of uptake by different removal processes.[40]

Data from U.S. Environmental Protection Agency,[39] Sulbaek Andersen MP et al,[16] Intergovernmental Panel on Climate Change (IPCC).[40]

Low Flow

After the choice of volatile anesthetic agent, the fresh gas flow (FGF) rate is the next most important determinant of the carbon footprint of a typical anesthetic (**Box 3**). Any FGF that exceeds the patient's needs and the system requirements will be delivered directly out the roof of the hospital via the anesthesia machine's scavenging system. Thus, the importance of low (<2 L/min) flow cannot be overemphasized. Low flow is most easily accomplished during the maintenance phase of anesthesia. There are several considerations when using low-flow delivery that should be addressed, including the production of compound A and carbon monoxide (CO) and ensuring adequate inspired fraction of oxygen.

Compound A is formed by the degradation of sevoflurane by CO_2 absorbents, most notably those containing the strong bases sodium hydroxide and potassium hydroxide (NaOH and KOH) in desiccated conditions.[9] Early studies with sevoflurane found a theoretical risk of nephrotoxicity in humans from compound A. However, the literature does not support the evidence of renal injury caused by compound A in humans undergoing anesthesia. Nevertheless, the US Food and Drug Administration (FDA) has included a warning in the package insert for sevoflurane that states: "sevoflurane exposure should not exceed 2 MAC·hours at flow rates of 1 to <2 L/min. Fresh gas flow rates of <1 L/min are not recommended."[10] Although KOH-based CO_2 absorbents are no longer available, NaOH-based CO_2 absorbents are still in use. More modern CO_2 absorbents are calcium hydroxide [$Ca(OH)_2$]–based or lithium hydroxide (LiOH)–based, which interact minimally with sevoflurane but can still produce compound A when dessicated.[11] Overall, the ability to use CO_2 absorbents that do not interact with sevoflurane and the absence of compelling human data that compound A is injurious seem to allow for reasonable doubt regarding FGF limitations with

Box 2

The GHG emissions generated by a 2-hour anesthetic with desflurane (1 L/min fresh gas flow [FGF]) are equivalent to driving a car 608 km (378 miles), roughly the distance from New York City to Akron, Ohio, or from Los Angeles, California, to Phoenix, Arizona. The same anesthetic with sevoflurane (2 L/min FGF) is equivalent to driving 26 km (16 miles).

Table 2	
Equivalent miles driven per minimum alveolar concentration hour of each volatile anesthetic	
	Equivalent Miles Driven per MAC-Hour
Sevoflurane	8 (FGF 2 L/min)
Isoflurane	7 (FGF 1 L/min)
Desflurane	189 (FGF 1 L/min)

Abbreviations: FGF, fresh gas flow; MAC, minimum alveolar concentration.
Data from Sherman JS, Feldman J, Berry JM. Reducing Inhaled Anesthetic Waste and Pollution. Anesthesiology News April 13, 2017. Available at https://www.anesthesiologynews.com/Commentary/Article/04-17/Reducing-Inhaled-Anesthetic-Waste-and-Pollution/40910 Accessed 2/1/2020.

sevoflurane. However, the FDA recommendation mentioned earlier currently still stands and warrants compliance.[12]

CO can be formed by the degradation of any of the volatile agents by desiccated CO_2 absorbents that contain the strong bases NaOH and KOH in large quantities, such as Baralyme and soda lime.[9] Low FGF maintains moisture in the circuit and in the CO_2 absorbent, thus decreasing the risk of CO production with these absorbents. More modern absorbents [$Ca(OH)_2$ based or LiOH based] do not produce CO when they interact with volatile agents.[11]

Fraction of inspired oxygen (Fi_{O_2}) is often set lower in pediatric anesthesia, especially in infants, because of concerns for oxygen toxicity and retinopathy of prematurity. When FGF is also set low, the Fi_{O_2} may need to be set higher in order to compensate for oxygen extraction. Diligence to the inspired oxygen concentration is of utmost importance to avoid delivering a hypoxic mixture. In addition, side stream gas analyzers often remove 200 mL/min FGF from the circuit, which must be accounted for when using very low FGF, because not all systems return that volume to the circuit after analysis. Low-flow techniques result in more rapid exhaustion of CO_2 absorbent. Contrary to how many anesthesiologists practice, the most efficient use of absorbent results from changing it based on consistently increased inspired CO_2 concentration rather than after a predetermined period of time or with the appearance of an indicator.[13]

The carbon footprint of an anesthetic that uses any volatile agent is dramatically higher than an anesthetic that uses only neuraxial, regional, or intravenous agents[14] (**Fig. 1**). The GHG emissions that result from using desflurane without N_2O (discussed later) are approximately 2600 times the emissions that result from an anesthetic using propofol; roughly 32,000 g of CO_2 equivalents (gCO_2e) versus roughly 12 gCO_2e. Sevoflurane is far less detrimental to the atmosphere than desflurane, but its use still results in approximately 135 times greater emissions as using propofol (roughly 1600 gCO_2e versus roughly 12 gCO_2e). Although the environmental impact of pharmaceuticals is also concerning, it is drastically less than the environmental impact of volatiles, making total intravenous anesthesia the superior choice.

Box 3
Choice of volatile anesthetic agent and the rate of FGF are the most important determinants of the carbon footprint of a gas-based anesthetic.

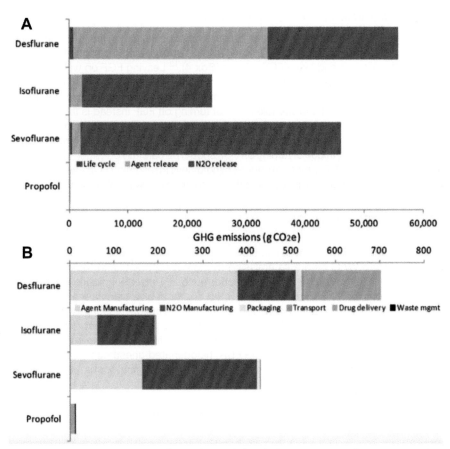

Fig. 1. Life cycle GHG emissions of anesthetics, (A) including waste anesthetic gas emissions of volatile agents and N_2O, and (B) excluding waste anesthetic gas emissions to show the lesser impact of manufacturing, transport, packaging, and drug delivery. Note the differing scales. gCO_2e, grams of CO2 equivalents; mgmt, management. (*From*: Sherman J et al. Life Cycle Greenhouse Gas Emissions of Anesthetic Drugs. Anesth Analg 2012;114:1086 –90; Used with permission from Wolters Kluwer Health, Inc.)

Mask Induction of Anesthesia

Mask induction of anesthesia is unique to pediatrics and presents an additional challenge to minimizing the venting of volatile anesthetic to the atmosphere. In addition, N_2O is often used during mask induction; this is discussed later. High flows are generally used to facilitate rapid changes in inspired sevoflurane during mask induction, and the resulting wasted anesthesia gas is considerable. Flows need not be higher than 5 to 8 L/min initially during mask induction and should be decreased when uptake by the patient has slowed. This slowed uptake is indicated by the expired agent concentration approaching the inspired concentration until nearly balanced and approximating the desired MAC value. Rebreathing increases when FGF decreases, which may decrease the delivered anesthetic concentration, so vigilance is important during this period.[12] Setting alarm limits for low inspired agent concentration is an easy way to ensure that adequate depth of anesthesia is maintained when FGF is reduced.

Fresh Gas Flow Management During Intubation

When a volatile agent has been initiated before intubation (ie, during induction), it is preferable during intubation to turn off FGF and leave the vaporizer at its set point rather than turn off the vaporizer and leave FGF flowing (**Box 4**).[12] Leaving FGF on with the circuit disconnected allows washout of volatile agent from the internal volume of the circuit into the room and requires the reestablishment of a volatile agent in the circuit once the circuit is reconnected. The preferable result of turning off FGF instead is the avoidance of environmental contamination during intubation and the ability to use a lower FGF to maintain circuit concentration after intubation. Although the circuit can be refilled quickly with high FGF, the technique of turning off FGF should be carefully considered in high-risk intubation scenarios. This practice requires mindfulness in resuming FGF after intubation, and individual practitioners must decide their comfort levels with this practice.

Waste Anesthesia Gas Recapture

As mentioned earlier, scavenged waste anesthesia gas (WAG) is typically vented directly out the roof of the hospital. However, several technologies are being developed to capture WAG before its emission to the environment, with the end goals of destruction, warehousing, or purification and reuse.[15] These techniques use adsorption of the volatile WAG onto either activated charcoal or a selective adsorbent, or condensation of the volatile agent to a liquid. A reversible adsorbent process is used by BlueZone Delta (Toronto) to collect WAG and allow for either destruction or reprocessing. Although no pharmaceutical originating from reprocessed or recycled product has yet to be approved by the FDA, halogenated anesthetics are good candidates for recycling in that they are recovered in their original forms, without additives, and are easily purified.[13]

Clinics care points/suggestions to decrease environmental impact:

- Eliminate desflurane

- Use low flow (<2 L/min) during maintenance

- Turn off FGF during intubation while leaving the vaporizer set to preserve volatile agent concentration in the circuit and avoid washout of volatile agent into the room

- Use total intravenous anesthesia to eliminate volatile anesthetic emissions whenever possible

---

NITROUS OXIDE

N_2O is not only a GHG like the volatile anesthetics but it also depletes ozone and persists in the atmosphere for more than 100 years. As a GHG, it has a global warming potential 298 times that of CO_2.[16] N_2O has a long tradition of use in pediatric anesthesia both to facilitate mask induction and as a maintenance anesthetic carrier gas. However, mask induction without N_2O is not only possible but also advantageous for multiple reasons. Most importantly, use of N_2O during induction decreases inspired oxygen concentration, eliminating preoxygenation, which decreases the time from

---

Box 4

Turn off FGF during intubation, leaving the vaporizer at its set point, to avoid washout of volatile agent from the circuit and contamination of the operating room (OR) environment.

apnea to desaturation, especially in young children.[17] Because young children are more prone to laryngospasm during induction, and by definition of receiving mask induction usually do not have intravenous access in place, preoxygenation is of utmost importance for safety.

As pediatric anesthesiologists can readily attest, placement of a mask on a child's face (even before a volatile agent is in the circuit) is often distressing to the child, and N_2O offers no benefit for at least 30 seconds after placement of the mask. However, distraction techniques are often effective to help children tolerate both mask placement and delivery of a gradually increasing concentration of sevoflurane. The second gas effect has been mostly studied in adults and with halothane, making application of the principle questionable for pediatric patients who have a larger ratio of alveolar ventilation compared with functional residual capacity and a larger fraction of their cardiac output delivered to the vessel-rich group, both of which serve to speed induction independent of a second gas effect compared with adults.[17] In clinical practice, mask induction with sevoflurane is not faster with N_2O than with 100% oxygen in children.

As an alternative to using N_2O during induction, consider using distraction to help the child tolerate mask placement and initiation of volatile anesthetic in the circuit. Screen technology is a powerful distraction tool for children, but storytelling, jokes, or casual conversation are also effective for different age groups. The advantages and disadvantages of N_2O during induction are summarized in **Table 3**.

N_2O is frequently used during maintenance of anesthesia. Although this allows for a decreased concentration of volatile agent, the overall carbon footprint of the anesthetic is increased when N_2O is used for maintenance compared with using volatile anesthetic in air and oxygen.[14]

Clinics care points/suggestions to decrease environmental impact:

• Avoid N_2O

MEDICATION WASTE

Medication waste is an unavoidable consequence of administering medications during anesthesia care. In anesthesia practice, propofol is the most wasted medication by volume, whereas emergency medications (succinylcholine, atropine, epinephrine, ephedrine, phenylephrine) have the highest waste fractions (percentage of opened medication that is not used and must be wasted).[18] Virtually all medications drawn up from vials end up in the environment in some form, and thus limiting preparation

Table 3
Nitrous oxide for mask induction: pros and cons

Advantages	Disadvantages
Euphoria and ambivalence to presence of volatile anesthetic	Prohibits preoxygenation, predisposing to rapid desaturation in the event of laryngospasm, bronchospasm, or apnea
Stable hemodynamics overall (but potential risk of increased pulmonary pressure)	Significant delay to onset of clinical effect of euphoria
	Dysphoria common with high inspiratory fraction
	Does not speed mask induction
	Increases risk of postoperative nausea and vomiting
	Increases carbon footprint of the anesthetic

Box 5

Virtually all medications drawn up from vials end up in the environment in some form.

---

to only medications that are planned to be used is the best way to decrease medication waste (**Box 5**).

Disposal of unused medications varies according to hospital policies as well as state and federal regulations. Controlled substances (all narcotics, benzodiazepines, barbiturates, ketamine, and in some states propofol) are considered hazardous waste pharmaceuticals; their disposal is regulated primarily by the Drug Enforcement Administration (DEA) and the Environmental Protection Agency (EPA) (**Boxes 6** and **7**). DEA regulations state that controlled substances must be "irretrievable and unusable after disposal."[19] The EPA dictates the manner in which controlled substances may be disposed and, in January 2020, banned the sewer system as an acceptable method of hazardous waste pharmaceutical disposal for all but personal and residential purposes.[20] Thus, controlled substances must be disposed of in appropriate containers, in full compliance with both DEA and EPA regulations, which generally requires incineration.

Uncontrolled medications are also preferably disposed of by incineration, thus preventing the eventual release into groundwater that occurs when medications leak through landfills. Neither landfills nor wastewater treatment facilities are designed to prevent pharmaceuticals from entering the environment. This finding is shown by well-documented pharmaceutical contamination of groundwater and surface water.[21] Because the environmental burden of a pharmaceutical generally correlates with the amount that is dispensed, the most commonly used medications (oral contraceptives, antihypertensives, antibiotics, antiepileptics, mood stabilizers, and over-the-counter analgesics) are those most frequently found in the environment.[22] Thus, although anesthesia-related medications are a small fraction of overall medication waste, the ubiquitous presence of pharmaceuticals in groundwater is cause for significant concern and serves as an entreaty to avoid unnecessary medication wastage.

Strategies to decrease medication waste include use of prefilled syringes, splitting of vials (especially in pediatric anesthesia) to accommodate smaller dose volumes, and avoiding drawing up medications that may not be used. Third-party vendors' prefilled syringes of emergency medications decrease waste because, unlike medication drawn up from a vial, an unused prefilled syringe can be returned to stock and has a long shelf life.[23] In addition, prefilled syringes are usually cost neutral or cost saving and their use has been found to decrease medication errors.[24] Another type of prefilled syringe is one created by splitting larger vials of medication under a pharmacy's sterile hood.[25] These syringes have a much shorter shelf life than commercially available ones but, for frequently used expensive medications (sugammadex, dexmedetomidine), they are preferable to wasting large fractions of a medication vial's contents. Proper disposal of pharmaceutical waste is expensive, and it is far less expensive to avoid generating pharmaceutical waste than to pay to dispose of it.

Clinics care points/suggestions to decrease environmental impact:

- Use prefilled syringes for emergency medications
- Request that pharmacy split vials under a sterile hood to decrease waste, which is also beneficial during drug shortages
- Maintain medications readily available but not opened when possible
- Use smaller vials for pediatrics (eg, propofol 10 mL vs 20 mL)
- Follow the controlled substances waste stream to ensure that these medications are not being disposed of by sewer, because this practice is prohibited by law

---
Box 6

DEA regulations require controlled substances to be irretrievable and unusable after disposal.

SINGLE-USE DEVICES

Health care in the United States uses a mind-boggling number of single-use devices. Anesthesia is no exception, and, with the recent trend of switching to single-use laryngoscopes, there are only a handful of reusable devices used in many practices currently. The switch to single-use devices has resulted from preference for convenience and concern for cross-contamination. However, the environmental impacts have been disastrous. United States hospitals generate approximately 6 million tons of waste annually (**Box 8**).[26] Plastic is the mainstay of single-use devices and containers, and, as a result, microplastics have become ubiquitous in the environment.[27] Infection control concerns must be addressed in any proposal to decrease use of single-use devices, and the Centers for Disease Control and Prevention (CDC) risk classification and guidelines for disinfection are useful to reference.[28]

Life-cycle analysis (LCA) is a scientific method used to quantify the environmental emissions of a process or product, including natural resource extraction, manufacturing, packaging, transportation, use/reuse, and waste management strategies.[29] A robust LCA represents the gold standard of a given product's environmental impact. Although only recently applied to health care, several LCAs are available for anesthesia equipment, including disposable and reusable laryngoscopes,[30] laryngeal mask airways,[31] and central line kits.[32] As more LCAs are published and demands mount on device manufacturers to disclose the environmental impacts of their products, it will become much easier to compare the environmental impacts of reusable and single-use devices.

Many hospitals utilize single-use device reprocessing through third-party vendors. Reprocessing refers to the process of sterilizing, tracking, and repackaging items originally manufactured for single use. The quality standards for this industry are the same as those applied to the original device manufacturers[33] and additionally require tracking of the number of reprocessing cycles for each individual device to ensure its removal before quality is compromised.

Clinics care points/suggestions to decrease environmental impact:

- Use supply chain data to determine costs of single-use devices used in a practice and the cost savings associated with switching to reusable devices
- Implement a reprocessing program to decrease waste, decrease carbon footprint of the operating room (OR), and reduce costs for OR equipment

---

HEATING, VENTILATION, AND AIR CONDITIONING

Hospitals use an immense amount of energy. The United States Energy Information Administration last quantified hospital energy use in 2007 and found that large

---
Box 7

EPA regulations specifically prohibit disposing of controlled substances into the sewer system (eg, wasting medications into the sink or toilet is illegal).

Box 8

Six million tons is equivalent to 25 of the world's largest cruise ships. US hospitals generate that much waste annually.

---

hospitals account for less than 1% of all commercial buildings but consume 5.5% of the total delivered energy used by the commercial sector.[34] In a detailed study, the HVAC system accounted for 65% of hospital energy use.[35] The OR uses 3 to 6 times more energy per square meter than any other area in the hospital,[36] and much of that impact is caused by strict requirements for the provision of suitably clean air during surgical procedures. These requirements are set by ANSI/ASHE/ASRAE standard 170-2017[37] and include requirements for air changes per hour (ACH). ORs are required to maintain 20 ACH (although this rate is also governed by state regulations) during surgical procedures, but only 6 ACH when the OR is not being used, provided that a positive-pressure relationship is maintained between the OR and its adjoining spaces. By setting back the ACH in an OR during off hours, many hospitals have significantly decreased their energy use, carbon footprint, and costs (**Box 9**).

HVAC controls are outside the realm of expertise of most anesthesiologists, and therefore adjustments of OR HVAC controls are a multidisciplinary undertaking. The building infrastructure must allow for computer-controlled adjustments to the HVAC system and real-time monitoring of the pressure relationships of the ORs. Synchronizing the OR setback schedule with the real-time surgery schedule is helpful, and a manual override must be in place to ensure OR ACH are appropriate in unforeseen circumstances. These strict protocols and planning may seem to make OR setbacks too cumbersome a project to initiate, but the cost savings realized by institutions that have successfully implemented setbacks speak to the incentive. Data from Practice Greenhealth (the largest networking organization for sustainable health care in the United States) indicate that member hospitals report a median saving of $2585 per OR per year, and median hospital savings of $33,600 per year attributable to OR setbacks.[38]

Clinics care points/suggestions to decrease environmental impact:

- Inquire about the HVAC system controls for your OR. If your hospital has a sustainability initiative in place, use that infrastructure to mobilize the relevant stakeholders needed for OR setbacks

---

SUMMARY

The challenges to human health are many. As of this writing, Sars-CoV-19 has established itself in the forefront of everyone's mind but climate change, although more insidious and more debated, remains the larger threat. There is high-level buy-in from the global community to minimize the spread of the novel coronavirus, protect those most vulnerable to infection, and to find treatments and vaccines. Humanity has faced the threat of infectious disease before, and, although the end of this

---

Box 9

Decreasing the ACH in the OR during unoccupied times results in a significant decrease in carbon footprint and energy costs for the hospital.

---

pandemic may be years away, the way forward is fairly clear. Climate change presents a much more difficult problem in that it has been created over several decades by humanity's choices, and, as a result, it will be impossible to effectively mitigate without global cooperation. Ultimately, climate change will affect every person on Earth. A problem of this magnitude must be addressed on every level and from every sector if any headway is to be made on turning the tide before irreversible changes occur. Everyone must each do their part, in both their personal and professional lives, to bring about global change. A desirable side effect of many sustainability efforts is significant cost savings, and this provides the leverage needed to convince departments and larger organizations to pursue sustainability projects.

Sustainability work in hospitals, specifically in ORs, has more impact than the same efforts in other settings because of the hospitals' and ORs' significant uses of energy, medications, and supplies. Anesthesia providers can decrease the environmental impact of their clinical care. They can choose to avoid desflurane and N_2O because of their high GWP_{100} status. They can minimize medication waste by only drawing up medications that are needed and by using prefilled syringes. They can use LCA studies to advocate for supplies with lower environmental impact and lower cost instead of submitting to the lure of convenience at the expense of the environment. They can collaborate with other experts in their hospitals to tackle larger projects, such as reducing unnecessary energy use, especially in ORs. As everyone makes changes in their own practices, they positively influence those around them to do the same and, slowly, the collective planetary benefit increases. It took considerable time to get the planet into the dangerous situation it is in, and it is going to take time to "right the ship." By learning about the carbon footprint of daily choices in anesthesia and adjusting clinical practice to minimize impact, clinicians are playing a part in healing the damage already done to the planet and setting the example for the future of anesthesia care.

DISCLOSURE

The author has nothing to disclose.

REFERENCES

1. Watts N, Amann N, Arnell N, et al. The 2018 report of the Lancet Countdown on health and climate change: shaping the health of nations for centuries to come. Lancet 2018;392(10163):2479–514.
2. National Health System Sustainable Development Unit. NHS Carbon Footprint. 2016. Available at: https://www.sduhealth.org.uk/policy-strategy/reporting/nhs-carbon-footprint.aspx. Accessed April 7, 2020.
3. United Kingdom National Statistics. 2015 UK Greenhouse Gas Emissions, Final Figures. Department for Business, Energy and Industrial Strategy. 2017. Available at: https://assets.publishing.service.gov.uk/government/uploads/system/uploads/attachment_data/file/604350/2015_Final_Emissions_statistics.pdf. Accessed April 7, 2020.
4. Pichler PP. International comparison of health care carbon footprints. Environ Res Lett 2019;14:064004. Available at: https://iopscience.iop.org/article/10.1088/1748-9326/ab19e1. Accessed April 1, 2020.
5. Boden TA, Andres RJ. National CO2 emissions from Fossil-Fuel Burning, Cement manufacture, and Gas Flaring: 1751-2014. Carbon Dioxide Information Analysis Center, Oak ridge national Laboratory, U.S. Department of energy 2017. https://

doi.org/10.3334/CDIAC/00001_V2017. Available at: https://cdiac.ess-dive.lbl. gov/trends/emis/overview_2014.html. Accessed April 7, 2020.

6. Eckelman MJ, Sherman J. Environmental Impacts of the U.S. Health Care System and Effects on Public Health. PLoS One 2016;11(6):e0157014. Available at: https://journals.plos.org/plosone/article?id=10.1371/journal.pone.0157014. Accessed April 7, 2020.

7. United Nations Environment Programme. Kigali Amendment: Nine Parties to the Montreal Protocol Have Ratified. 2018. Available at: https://ozone.unep.org/kigali-amendment-nine-parties-montreal-protocol-have-ratified. Accessed January 6, 2020.

8. National Health System Sustainable Development Unit. Carbon footprint update for NHS in England 2012 2013. Available at: https://www.sduhealth.org.uk/ policy-strategy/reporting/nhs-carbon-footprint.aspx. Accessed April 7, 2020.

9. Branche R, Feldman J, Hendrickx J. Low flow and CO2 absorbents. APSF Newsletter 2017;32(2):49–50. Available at: https://www.apsf.org/article/low-flow-and-co2-absorbents/. Accessed March 28, 2020.

10. Sevoflurane package insert. Available at: http://baxtersevo.com/downloads/ Sevoflurane%20PI%20460-220-13%20-%202011.pdf. Accessed April 3, 2020.

11. Keijzer C, Perez RS, de Lange JJ, et al. Compound A and carbon monoxide production from sevoflurane and seven different types of carbon dioxide absorbent in a patient model. Acta Anaesthesiol Scand 2007;51:31–7.

12. Feldman J. Managing fresh gas flow to reduce environmental contamination. Anesth Analg 2012;114(5):1093–101.

13. Sherman JS, Feldman J, Berry JM. Reducing Inhaled Anesthetic Waste and Pollution. Anesthesiology News 2017. Available at: https://www.anesthesiologynews. com/Commentary/Article/04-17/Reducing-Inhaled-Anesthetic-Waste-and-Pollution/ 40910. Accessed February 1, 2020.

14. Sherman J, Le C, Lamers V, et al. Life cycle greenhouse gas emissions of anesthetic drugs. Anesth Analg 2012;114:1086–90.

15. Eisenkraft JB, McGregor DG. Waste anesthetic gases and scavenging systems. In: Ehrenwerth J, Eisenkraft JB, Berry JM, editors. Anesthesia equipment: principles and applications. 2nd edition. Philadelphia: Saunders; 2013. p. 139–45.

16. Sulbaek Andersen MP, Nielsen OJ, Wallington TJ, et al. Assessing the impact on global climate from general anesthetic gases. Anesth Analg 2012;14(5):1081–5.

17. Banchs R, Lerman J, Wald SH. The use of nitrous oxide as an adjuvant for inhalation inductions with sevoflurane: a pro–con debate. Pediatr Anesth 2013;23: 557–64.

18. Mankes RF. Propofol wastage in anesthesia. Anesth Analg 2012;114(5):1091–2.

19. US DEA Final Rule for Disposal of Controlled Substances, 79 Fed Reg 53519 (Sep 9, 2014) (to be codified at 21 C.F.R. pts 1300, 1301, 1304, 1305, 1307, & 1317). Available at: https://www.federalregister.gov/documents/2014/09/09/ 2014-20926/disposal-of-controlled-substances. Accessed February 17, 2020.

20. US EPA Final Rule for Management Standards for Hazardous Waste Pharmaceuticals and Amendment to the P075 Listing for Nicotine, 84 Fed Reg 5816 (Aug 21, 2019) (to be codified at 40 C.F.R. pts 261-265, 268, 270, 273 & 266). Available at: https://www.federalregister.gov/documents/2019/02/22/2019-01298/managemen t-standards-for-hazardous-waste-pharmaceuticals-and-amendment-to-the-p075-listing-for. Accessed February 20, 2020.

21. World Health Organization. Pharmaceuticals in drinking-water. 2011. Available at: https://www.who.int/water_sanitation_health/publications/2011/pharmaceuticals_ 20110601.pdf. Accessed April 8, 2020.

22. Corcoran J, Winter MJ, Tyler CR. Pharmaceuticals in the aquatic environment: a critical review of the evidence for health effects in fish. Crit Rev Toxicol 2010; 40(4):287–304.
23. McCook A. Prefilled syringes cut waste—and bottom line on drugs. Anesthesiology News 2011. Available at: https://www.anesthesiologynews.com/Policy-Management/Article/10-11/Prefilled-Syringes-Cut-Waste-and-Bottom-Line-on-Drugs/19192. Accessed April 1, 2020.
24. Litman RS. How to prevent medication errors in the operating room? Take away the human factor. Br J Anaesth 2018;(120):440e442.
25. Buck D, Subramanyam R, Varughese A. A quality improvement project to reduce the intraoperative use of single-dose fentanyl vials across multiple patients in a pediatric institution. Pediatr Anesth 2016;26(1):92–101.
26. Practice GreenHealth: Waste. Available at: https://practicegreenhealth.org/topics/waste/waste-0. Accessed April 6, 2020.
27. Sherman J. Reusable vs. disposable laryngoscopes. APSF Newsletter 2019;33: 91. Available at: https://www.apsf.org/article/reusable-vs-disposable-laryngoscopes/. Accessed April 3, 2020.
28. Rutala WA, Weber D. The healthcare infection control practices Advisory Committee (HIPAC): guideline for disinfection and sterilization in healthcare facilities. Centers for Disease Control; 2008.
29. International Organization for Standardization, ISO 14040:2006, Environmental management, Life cycle assessment, Principles and framework. 2006. reviewed and confirmed 2016. Available at: https://www.iso.org/standard/37456.html. Accessed January 31, 2020.
30. Sherman JD, Raibley LA, Eckelman MJ. Life cycle assessment and costing methods for device procurement: comparing reusable and single-use disposable laryngoscopes. Anesth Analg 2018;127(2):434–43.
31. Eckelman M, Mosher M, Gonzales A, et al. Comparative life cycle assessment of disposable and reusable laryngeal mask airways. Anesth Analg 2012;114: 1067–72.
32. McGain F, McAlister S, McGavin A, et al. A life cycle assessment of reusable and single-use central venous catheter insertion kits. Anesth Analg 2012;114(5): 1073–80.
33. US FDA Reprocessing of single use devices. CPG Sec 300.500, CPG 7124.16 (Mar 18. 2005. Available at: https://www.fda.gov/media/71769/download. Accessed April 7, 2020.
34. US EIA: energy Characteristics and energy consumed in large hospital buildings in the United States in. Available at: https://www.eia.gov/consumption/commercial/reports/2007/large-hospital.php. Accessed April 3, 2020.
35. Sheppy M, Pless S, Kung F. Healthcare energy end-use monitoring. National Renewable Energy Laboratory; 2014. Available at: https://www.nrel.gov/docs/fy14osti/61064.pdf. Accessed March 25, 2020.
36. MacNeill AJ, Lillywhite R, Brown CJ. The impact of surgery on global climate: a carbon footprinting study of operating theatres in three health systems. Lancet 2017;1(9):PE381–8.
37. American National Standards Institute/American Society for Healthcare Engineering/American Society of Heating, Refrigeration, and Air Conditioning Engineers Standard 170-2017. Available at: https://www.ashrae.org/technical-resources/standards-and-guidelines/standards-interpretations/interpretations-for-standard-170-2017. Accessed April 5, 2020.

38. Practice GreenHealth 2019 Sustainability Benchmark Data. Available at: https://practicegreenhealth.org/sites/default/files/2019-11/2019_sustainability_benchmark_data.pdf. Accessed March 25, 2020.
39. United States Environmental Protection Agency. Understanding Global Warming Potentials. Available at: https://www.epa.gov/ghgemissions/understanding-global-warming-potentials. Accessed April 7, 2020.
40. The Intergovernmental Panel on Climate Change (IPCC) Working Group 1: The Carbon Cycle and Atmospheric Carbon Dioxide Content. Available at: https://archive.ipcc.ch/ipccreports/tar/wg1/016.htm. Accessed April 2, 2020.

Pediatric Obstructive Sleep Apnea and Neurocognition

Arvind Chandrakantan, MD, MBA*, Adam C. Adler, MS, MD

KEYWORDS

- Pediatric • Obstructive sleep apnea • Neurocognition • ADHD
- Memory and learning • Adenotonsillectomy • Sleep

KEY POINTS

- Pediatric obstructive sleep apnea affects up to 7.5% of children and has significant, long-lasting effects on memory, learning, and other executive functions.
- Adenotonsillectomy, which is first-line therapy, has equivocal results on neurocognitive function.
- There are certain subgroups, including low socioeconomic status and disadvantaged minorities, who seem to carry a higher morbidity from the illness and surgery.

INTRODUCTION

Pediatric obstructive sleep-disordered breathing (oSDB) affects up to 7.5% of the pediatric population.[1–4] Pediatric obstructive sleep apnea (OSA) is characterized by intermittent hypoxia and hypercapnia, sleep fragmentations, frequent arousals, and circadian rhythm disturbances. Pediatric OSA can have a variety of end-organ manifestations with effects on the heart, lungs, brain, gut microbiome, and genitourinary systems (**Fig. 1**). Clinical manifestations of pediatric oSDB are on a continuum with symptoms ranging from nasal turbulence, to snoring, to obstructive apnea. The population typically affected are children between 2 and 14 years of age. Adolescent OSA is considered a separate phenotype and has variable progression into adult OSA.[5] A main feature of pediatric OSA is the difference in both risk factors and disease expression and response to treatment when compared with adult OSA, often resulting in missed or delayed diagnosis (**Tables 1–3**).

Although obesity has clearly been identified as a causative factor in pediatric OSA,[6,7] 2 parts of the clinical phenotype exist, with a significant number of children being normal or even underweight.[8] Emerging data suggest that weight may be used to stratify pediatric OSA severity, as patient weight has been found to correlate with

Department of Anesthesiology, Perioperative and Pain Medicine, Texas Children's Hospital, Baylor College of Medicine, 6621 Fannin Street, A330, Houston, TX 77030, USA
* Corresponding author.
E-mail address: chandrak@bcm.edu

Anesthesiology Clin 38 (2020) 693–707
https://doi.org/10.1016/j.anclin.2020.05.004   anesthesiology.theclinics.com
1932-2275/20/© 2020 Elsevier Inc. All rights reserved.

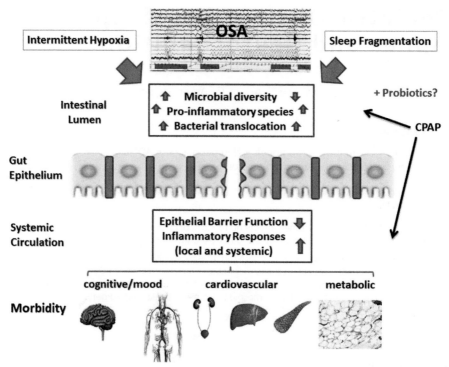

Fig. 1. End-organ sequelae of OSA. (*From* Farre N, et al. Sleep Apnea Morbidity: A Consequence of Microbial-Immune Cross-Talk? Chest. 2018 Oct;154(4):754-759 with permissions.)

Table 1
Characteristic differences between adult and pediatric patients with obstructive sleep apnea

	Adult	Pediatric
Gender predilection	Male >> Female	Male = Female
History	• Daytime somnolence • Fatigue • Memory impairment • Frequent headache	• Hyperactivity, • Emotional difficulties • Concertation difficulties • Impulsivity • Decreased academic performance
Physical examination	• Thick neck • Obesity • Symptoms of right heart failure	• Often of normal appearance • Syndromic facies • Midfacial hypoplasia • Micrognathic or retrognathic • Adenotonsillar hypertrophy
Treatment	• Lifestyle modifications • Continuous or bi-level positive airway pressure during sleep	• Surgical intervention with adenotonsillectomy is first-line treatment
Impact on growth	• Obesity	• Failure to thrive

Table 2
Polysomnographic differences between adult and pediatric patients with obstructive sleep apnea

	Adult	Pediatric
OSA Severity by AHI		
No OSA	0–5	0
Mild	6–20	1–5
Moderate	21–39	6–9
Severe	>40	>10

Abbreviations: AHI, apnea hypopnea index; OSA, obstructive sleep apnea.

the number of sites of airway obstruction.[9] This finding may, in part, explain the lack of resolution of OSA symptomatology following adenotonsillectomy surgery in a number of symptomatic children.[10] More critically, 2 recent large multicenter studies demonstrated the persistence of neurocognitive deficits following surgery.[11,12] Thus, early identification and treatment of oSDB is critical, as neurocognitive deficits at least in the short term may be irreversible once developed. The objective of this article was to summarize the neurocognitive expression of pediatric OSA, enumerate comorbid risk factors, discuss surgical timing/risk factors, and describe perioperative complications, all of which contribute to decision making with this common disorder.

NEUROCOGNITIVE EXPRESSION OF OBSTRUCTIVE SLEEP APNEA IN CHILDREN

There is a summative, temporal net effect of these physiologic perturbations on nearly every end-organ system, including the brain. Multiple areas of the brain are affected by persistent pediatric OSA. Because sleep is an essential piece of mammalian memory consolidation,[13,14] learning, memory, and attention deficits are seen in the clinical

Table 3
Polysomnographic differences between adult and pediatric patients with obstructive sleep apnea

	Adult	Pediatric
Apnea definition	Cessation of airflow for at least 2 respiratory cycles	Cessation of airflow for at least 10 s
Cortical arousal	Low frequency of cortical arousals (arousal following obstructive event)	Generally, apneic events are followed by a cortical arousal
Sleep state of OSA	Apnea and hypopnea events generally occur in REM phase	Apnea and hypopnea events Occur in both REM and non-REM phases
Sleep architecture	Normal sleep architecture	Fragmented sleep
Transcutaneous CO_2	$Paco_2$ often elevated	Often normal
Type of obstruction	Persistent and partial obstructions	Cyclical partial or complete obstruction of the upper airway
Severity scale of OSA	Vastly different between adult and pediatric	

Abbreviations: OSA, obstructive sleep apnea; REM, rapid eye movement.

phenotype of idiopathic sleep behavior disorders.[15] Learning, memory, and attention are largely hippocampally mediated in early life,[16–19] pointing to hippocampal damage as being seminal to the symptomatology seen from OSA in the developing brain.[20–23] One study demonstrated gray matter volume reductions in the left hippocampus/entorhinal cortex, left posterior parietal cortex, and left superior frontal gyrus in children with OSA.[24] These findings were similarly observed in adult patients with OSA, albeit with greater changes in the temporal gyri, insula, and posterior cingulate cortex.[25] All of these changes affect learning, memory, and other areas that govern critical thinking and outcomes processing. In addition, gray matter loss was noted within sites involving motor regulation of the upper airway as well as those responsible for cognitive function.[26,27] When taken together, effects on these brain structures result in a number of clinically observed changes.

CLINICAL MANIFESTATIONS OF OBSTRUCTIVE SLEEP APNEA

The neurocognitive effects from pediatric OSA can be broadly classified into those affecting executive function, learning and memory, or behavior. Extensive discussion on the effects of pediatric OSA on the brain can be found in our recent review article.[28]

CHANGES IN EXECUTIVE FUNCTIONING

Executive functioning encompasses a set of cognitive processes that includes a number of basic and higher-order functions.[29,30] Executive functioning is primarily measured by testing working memory, cognitive flexibility, and inhibitory control. Because arousal from sleep is the primary mechanism by which cognitive function is preserved in response to an obstructive event,[31] it seems logical that arousals from sleep would predict neurobehavioral morbidity. This has been demonstrated not to be the case.[32] Furthermore, adenotonsillectomy has not been shown to facilitate executive function recovery in children with mild-moderate sleep apnea.[33]

BEHAVIORAL CHANGES

Attention deficit/hyperactivity disorder (ADHD) has been reported at far higher rates in children with OSA.[34–36] Even very low apnea hypopnea index (AHI) rates have been correlated with ADHD.[37] There is also a significant increase in ADHD symptomatology with increased degree of hypoxia. However, to date there have been no large-scale trials to elucidate the link between ADHD and OSA, and therefore much remains unknown. However, this has led to multiple clinicians proposing to screen children with ADHD for sleep-disordered breathing phenotypes before initiating pharmacologic intervention.[38] Furthermore, early sleep deprivation is associated with a higher risk of developing ADHD later on.[39] MRI has demonstrated deficits in areas of the brain involved with emotional processing.[40] There have also been significant clinical functional deficits demonstrated within multiple domains, including compulsion, aggression, and somatization.[41] Adenotonsillectomy results in significant improvement in behavioral outcomes,[42,43] suggesting there is a strong link between pediatric OSA and ADHD. However, many of the issues related to pediatric OSA translate into academic difficulties for a number of children[44] compared with controls.[45] However, because of the behavioral and academic difficulties, a number of children with OSA are theorized to be incorrectly diagnosed with ADHD.

LEARNING AND MEMORY DEFICITS

Learning and memory deficits have been well characterized in pediatric OSA. These deficits are diverse and involve spatial memory, working memory, verbal comprehension, and reasoning. These deficits affect both acquisition and retention of newly learned material[46,47] and are worse in children with Trisomy 21.[48] The question that has eluded researchers for some time is the reversibility of these changes after therapy. Some measures of neuropsychological functioning seem to improve,[49] although specific improvements are difficult to demonstrate even with large cohorts.[50–53]

PRECLINICAL MODELS OF PEDIATRIC OBSTRUCTIVE SLEEP APNEA

There are 2 preclinical rodent models of OSA that have been used. One model is the intermittent hypoxia model, which uses 14 days of rapid cycling oxygen concentrations of between 10% and 21%. The neurobehavioral outcome was deficits in the Water Maze Task, which involves hippocampally based decision making.[54] The second model is the intermittent tracheal occlusion model which uses surgery for implantation of a silicone tube, which is intermittently inflated to occlude the trachea. This model has not been neurobehaviorally validated.[55] To date, however, there is no preclinical model for pediatric OSA.

COMORBID RISK FACTORS FOR PEDIATRIC OBSTRUCTIVE SLEEP APNEA

Obesity has been demonstrated to be a significant risk factor for the development of pediatric OSA.[56] Obesity also has a significant effect on worsening the neurocognitive profile of OSA,[57] which has been attributed to sleep fragmentation and poorer sleep quality.[58] Obesity also correlates with worse outcomes following adenotonsillectomy[59] and a higher risk of respiratory complications on the first postoperative night. Although most patients achieve a reduction in oSDB symptoms following adenotonsillectomy, obese patients are noted to have a significantly greater incidence of residual disease.[60–63] In addition, children with very high body mass index (z-scores >3) appear to benefit the least from adenotonsillectomy.[64] This subgroup may benefit from preoperative drug-induced sleep endoscopy to assess regions of obstruction, assess response to adenotonsillectomy, and identify additional areas of airway obstruction.[65,66]

RHINOSINUSITIS

A number of pediatric patients present to the ear, nose, and throat (ENT) surgeon with chronic rhinosinusitis concomitant with sleep-disordered breathing. The argument can be made in these children, that with a low impact on quality of life, an initial course of intranasal steroids can be used to assess symptomatology.[67] Intranasal steroids can also alleviate comorbid allergies and reduce mouth breathing.[68] African American children with rhinosinusitis seem to have an increased risk of OSA compared with white children.[69]

ASTHMA

A number of children with OSA also have coexisting asthma;[70,71] however, the presence of asthma seems to decrease the likelihood of concomitant OSA.[72] In children with both disorders, there are a number of other abnormalities in pulmonary and chemoreceptor function.[73] Given the overlap, it is important for the clinician to identify the presence of both conditions and focus therapies to address both.[74] In concomitant oSDB and asthma, there appears to be some improvement in asthma symptomatology[75] with adenoidectomy[76] and adenotonsillectomy.[77] However, comorbid asthma increases the likelihood of postoperative respiratory complications[78,79] as well as predicts a higher likelihood of postsurgical residual OSA disease.[80]

IMPACT OF RACE AND SOCIOECONOMIC STATUS ON PEDIATRIC OBSTRUCTIVE SLEEP APNEA

Several studies have characterized the relationship between demographics and pediatric OSA with regard to preoperative, intraoperative, and postoperative outcomes.[81] Parental education has been demonstrated to be a mitigating factor for the development of pediatric OSA, whereas lack of education represents a risk factor for the disease.[82] Furthermore, children with OSA are more likely to come from disadvantaged neighborhoods.[83] It is hypothesized that neighborhood distress may play a role in disease evolution.[84] A larger study looking at disease demographics demonstrated a higher incidence in African American children; when adjusting for poverty rate and single-female head of household factors, race was less of a factor.[85]

One smaller study[81] suggests that access to care is a significant determinant of health care outcomes, as distance from an urban center predicted loss to follow-up. However, even in an urban cohort, most of whom were on public insurance, almost 50% were lost to follow-up after initial ENT evaluation.[86] This finding was confirmed in a cohort of publicly insured patients in whom there was a significant delay in obtaining polysomnography (PSG) and definitive surgical intervention.[87] As far as school performance, only socioeconomic status (SES) is the common independent causative variable,[88] suggesting that other factors may be less important when studying the effects of OSA on academic indices alone.

Several studies have looked at disadvantaged minority children and the impact of pediatric OSA. African American race and environmental tobacco smoke exposure have both been demonstrated to increase disease severity.[89] These factors have similarly been demonstrated in Australia.[90] Despite these observations and the higher incidence of OSA in this population, these patients are less likely to present for ENT services[91] and are at higher risk of becoming lost to follow-up. Unfortunately, many patients with OSA in the at-risk populations (minorities, Medicaid recipients) often fail to seek care.[92] A recent meta-analysis identified low SES, uninsured or underinsured status, and nonwhite race as potential disparities for access to care.[93] Attempts to strictly define race as a standalone factor in pediatric studies has been obfuscated by the fact that race is largely self-supplied in most studies,[94] although African ancestry carries a genetic signature in an adult genome-wide association study analysis of OSA.[95]

Surgical Factors

There are multiple surgical techniques described for pediatric adenotonsillectomy in patients with oSDB.[96] However, bleeding rates may differ by surgical technique used.[97] A large Cochrane analysis found that existing data are insufficiently powered to demonstrate a difference in bleeding rates.[98] Over time, the pediatric ENT community is slowly shifting to monopolar electrocautery and coblation techniques and away from cold techniques.[99] Intracapsular tonsillectomy has been suggested to be superior in select patients with OSA with regard to complication rates.[100] However, one international study reviewed 1087 patients and found that monopolar techniques were associated with lower hemorrhage rates as compared with electrocautery.[101] Therefore, significant controversy remains in the literature surrounding the "optimal" surgical technique for pediatric adenotonsillectomy.[102–106]

Surgical Timing

Despite adenotonsillectomy being widely accepted as first-line treatment for pediatric OSA, there are limited data as to the optimal timing of surgery. Approximately 67% of all pediatric adenotonsillectomies are performed due to airway obstruction, which represents a shift away from the historical indication for this surgery, chronic tonsillitis.

However, in cases of mild OSA (AHI 1–5), nonsurgical management has been proposed as an option. Kohn and colleagues[107] retrospectively reported on 201 pediatric patients with mild OSA of whom 101 (52%) opted for nonsurgical management. Of the 91 patients completing a follow-up sleep study, 46% had a greater than 20% decrease in AHI and 41% had a greater than 20% increase in AHI. However, 11 patients had an increase in AHI greater than 5, and 6 of these patients were upgraded from mild to moderate OSA and 5 were upgraded to severe OSA. Twenty-four patients (26%) had resolution of OSA with AHI less than 1. Older children between the ages of 12 and 18 tended to have greater AHI means on repeat PSG testing. Kohn and colleagues[107] concluded that mild pediatric OSA had approximately equal chances of worsening or improving over time without surgical intervention.

Children with mild OSA often report poor quality of life (QOL) and can be very symptomatic. These children generally improve with surgical management. However, medical management is a possible option for children with mild OSA, particularly if the child is noted to have allergic rhinitis symptoms and a mild impact on QOL.

Therefore, in the absence of neurocognitive dysfunction, there are clearly subgroups with OSA for whom medical therapy may be of benefit. In the presence of neurocognitive sequelae, the optimal therapeutic path remains unclear. The CHAT study assessed children with mild-moderate OSA assigned to early intervention with adenotonsillectomy or symptomatic management. They found early adenotonsillectomy improves behavioral symptoms and QOL; however, these patients did not benefit from improvement in executive function.[11] This logically led to the hypothesis that the neurocognitive dysfunction could be mediated by time with disease burden, and therefore surgery earlier in life would allow for executive function recovery. This finding was the rationale behind the recently published POSTA study.[12] This study demonstrated that early adenotonsillectomy in young children was not beneficial in reversing changes in executive function.[53] At the minimum, these data suggest that the mechanism mediating neurocognitive recovery maybe different than purely the obstructive component of pediatric OSA. What remains unknown is the progression of neurocognitive dysfunction without therapy. The behavioral and QOL benefits, however, have to be weighed against the complications associated with adenotonsillectomy.

POSTSURGICAL COMPLICATIONS OF ADENOTONSILLECTOMY

The complications of adenotonsillectomy can be put into 2 major categories: respiratory and nonrespiratory.

Respiratory Complications

A major consideration for adenotonsillectomy is the risk of perioperative respiratory complications. One study retrospectively analyzed more than 3000 children younger than 6 and identified that children younger than 3 were at higher risk for respiratory complications.[108] Similarly, age-based risk stratification also demonstrated that children at or younger than 2 years of age were at higher risk than children between 2 and 3 years of age. Further, children weighing less than 14 kg also had a higher rate of post tonsillectomy respiratory complications and generally, children younger than 2 years of age weigh less than 14 kg.[109] In addition, obese children, as well as those with congenital/craniofacial syndromes, are also at higher risk of respiratory complications from OSA. Therefore, despite adenotonsillectomy on the whole being a safe procedure, there are certain subgroups for whom increased caution is warranted.[110,111]

Nonrespiratory Complications

The major nonrespiratory complications of this surgery include dehydration, hemorrhage, and postoperative fever.[112,113] Dehydration has typically been coupled with oropharyngeal pain, preventing adequate oral rehydration. Many patients are not compliant with postoperative pain regimens.[114] Furthermore, there is also an association with low SES and underprivileged minority status having a higher rate of urgent revisits not related to bleeding.[115] Younger children also have a higher risk of non–bleeding-related revisits.[116] This has led a push to focus on symptom control to help transition these patients in the postdischarge period.[117] In addition, societal guidelines have been projected to stratify patients by risk of complications.[118] There are some data to suggest that these guidelines have reduced the revisit rates for non–life-threatening complications.[119]

Post tonsillectomy hemorrhage (PTH) remains a major, and potentially life-threatening concern.[120,121] This complication is more common in young children, specifically those younger than 3,[122] although a recent meta-analysis also found children older than 8 to be at increased risk.[123] Obese children have also been found to be at greater risk.[124] Children with OSA are also known to have lower PTH rates than children with chronic tonsillitis.[125] Secondary PTH is more likely to be life threatening.[126] Further, there is a fair amount of debate within the ENT community about the contribution of surgical technique to postoperative PTH rates.[127] Last, the severity of OSA on presentation does not seem to influence the incidence of postoperative complications.[128]

SUMMARY

In summation, pediatric OSA is a common, heterogeneous disorder affecting many children. There are certain subgroups, including younger children, underprivileged minorities, and children with a low SES background, that have a higher morbidity of disease at presentation and a higher rate of complications with surgical therapy. These risks have to be balanced against the end-organ consequences of untreated disease, including neurocognitive morbidity in a vulnerable population. Although much is known about the disease, much remains to be elucidated, especially the reversibility of neurocognitive dysfunction after therapy.

Clinics Care Points

- Adenotonsillectomy is first-line therapy for pediatric obstructive sleep apnea (OSA). The effects of adenotonsillectomy on polysomnographic improvement in pediatric OSA is well documented. There are certain subgroups who are at higher risk for recurrent disease, including obese children and children with craniofacial syndromes.

- Children with mild OSA and minimal effect on quality of life and no neurocognitive dysfunction maybe medically managed.

- Postsurgical complications are higher in younger and underweight children who may also have a higher burden of disease. Therefore, the risk:benefit ratio needs to be calculated in these children before operative intervention.

REFERENCES

1. Bixler EO, Vgontzas AN, Lin HM, et al. Sleep disordered breathing in children in a general population sample: prevalence and risk factors. Sleep 2009;32(6): 731–6.
2. Li AM, So HK, Au CT, et al. Epidemiology of obstructive sleep apnoea syndrome in Chinese children: a two-phase community study. Thorax 2010;65(11):991–7.
3. O'Brien LM, Holbrook CR, Mervis CB, et al. Sleep and neurobehavioral characteristics of 5- to 7-year-old children with parentally reported symptoms of attention-deficit/hyperactivity disorder. Pediatrics 2003;111(3):554–63.
4. Lumeng JC, Chervin RD. Epidemiology of pediatric obstructive sleep apnea. Proc Am Thorac Soc 2008;5(2):242–52.
5. Chan KC, Au CT, Hui LL, et al. How OSA evolves from childhood to young adulthood: natural history from a 10-year follow-up study. Chest 2019;156(1):120–30.
6. Patinkin ZW, Feinn R, Santos M. Metabolic consequences of obstructive sleep apnea in adolescents with obesity: a systematic literature review and meta-analysis. Child Obes 2017;13(2):102–10.
7. Bin-Hasan S, Katz S, Nugent Z, et al. Prevalence of obstructive sleep apnea among obese toddlers and preschool children. Sleep Breath 2018;22(2):511–5.
8. Keefe KR, Patel PN, Levi JR. The shifting relationship between weight and pediatric obstructive sleep apnea: A historical review. Laryngoscope 2018.
9. Coutras SW, Limjuco A, Davis KE, et al. Sleep endoscopy findings in children with persistent obstructive sleep apnea after adenotonsillectomy. Int J Pediatr Otorhinolaryngol 2018;107:190–3.
10. Tan HL, Kheirandish-Gozal L, Gozal D. Obstructive sleep apnea in children: update on the recognition, treatment and management of persistent disease. Expert Rev Respir Med 2016;10(4):431–9.
11. Marcus CL, Moore RH, Rosen CL, et al. A randomized trial of adenotonsillectomy for childhood sleep apnea. N Engl J Med 2013;368(25):2366–76.
12. Waters KA, Chawla J, Harris MA, et al. Rationale for and design of the "POSTA" study: Evaluation of neurocognitive outcomes after immediate adenotonsillectomy compared to watchful waiting in preschool children. BMC Pediatr 2017; 17(1):47.
13. Boyce R, Glasgow SD, Williams S, et al. Causal evidence for the role of REM sleep theta rhythm in contextual memory consolidation. Science 2016; 352(6287):812–6.
14. Ravassard P, Hamieh AM, Joseph MA, et al. REM sleep-dependent bidirectional regulation of hippocampal-based emotional memory and LTP. Cereb Cortex 2016;26(4):1488–500.
15. Li X, Wang K, Jia S, et al. The prospective memory of patients with idiopathic REM sleep behavior disorder. Sleep Med 2018;47:19–24.
16. Krause AJ, Simon EB, Mander BA, et al. The sleep-deprived human brain. Nat Rev Neurosci 2017;18(7):404–18.
17. Rosero MA, Winkelmann T, Pohlack S, et al. Memory-guided attention: bilateral hippocampal volume positively predicts implicit contextual learning. Brain Struct Funct 2019;224(6):1999–2008.
18. Finn AS, Kharitonova M, Holtby N, et al. Prefrontal and hippocampal structure predict statistical learning ability in early childhood. J Cogn Neurosci 2018;1–12.
19. Goldfarb EV, Chun MM, Phelps EA. Memory-guided attention: independent contributions of the hippocampus and striatum. Neuron 2016;89(2):317–24.

20. Kheirandish-Gozal L, Sahib AK, Macey PM, et al. Regional brain tissue integrity in pediatric obstructive sleep apnea. Neurosci Lett 2018;682:118–23.
21. Kheirandish L, Gozal D. Neurocognitive dysfunction in children with sleep disorders. Dev Sci 2006;9(4):388–99.
22. Xu LH, Xie H, Shi ZH, et al. Critical role of endoplasmic reticulum stress in chronic intermittent hypoxia-induced deficits in synaptic plasticity and long-term memory. Antioxid Redox Signal 2015;23(9):695–710.
23. Feng J, Wu Q, Zhang D, et al. Hippocampal impairments are associated with intermittent hypoxia of obstructive sleep apnea. Chin Med J (Engl) 2012; 125(4):696–701.
24. Canessa N, Castronovo V, Cappa SF, et al. Obstructive sleep apnea: brain structural changes and neurocognitive function before and after treatment. Am J Respir Crit Care Med 2011;183(10):1419–26.
25. Song X, Roy B, Kang DW, et al. Altered resting-state hippocampal and caudate functional networks in patients with obstructive sleep apnea. Brain Behav 2018; 8(6):e00994.
26. Macey PM, Henderson LA, Macey KE, et al. Brain morphology associated with obstructive sleep apnea. Am J Respir Crit Care Med 2002;166(10):1382–7.
27. Morrell MJ, McRobbie DW, Quest RA, et al. Changes in brain morphology associated with obstructive sleep apnea. Sleep Med 2003;4(5):451–4.
28. Chandrakantan A, Adler AC. Pediatric obstructive sleep apnea: neurocognitive consequences. Curr Anesthesiol Rep 2019;9(2):110–5.
29. Diamond A. Executive functions. Annu Rev Psychol 2013;64:135–68.
30. Chan RC, Shum D, Toulopoulou T, et al. Assessment of executive functions: review of instruments and identification of critical issues. Arch Clin Neuropsychol 2008;23(2):201–16.
31. Malhotra RK, Kirsch DB, Kristo DA, et al. Polysomnography for obstructive sleep apnea should include arousal-based scoring: an American Academy of Sleep Medicine Position Statement. J Clin Sleep Med 2018;14(7):1245–7.
32. Chervin RD, Garetz SL, Ruzicka DL, et al. Do respiratory cycle-related EEG changes or arousals from sleep predict neurobehavioral deficits and response to adenotonsillectomy in children? J Clin Sleep Med 2014;10(8):903–11.
33. Venekamp RP, Hearne BJ, Chandrasekharan D, et al. Tonsillectomy or adenotonsillectomy versus non-surgical management for obstructive sleep-disordered breathing in children. Cochrane Database Syst Rev 2015;(10):CD011165.
34. Wu J, Gu M, Chen S, et al. Factors related to pediatric obstructive sleep apnea-hypopnea syndrome in children with attention deficit hyperactivity disorder in different age groups. Medicine (Baltimore) 2017;96(42):e8281.
35. Miano S, Amato N, Foderaro G, et al. Sleep phenotypes in attention deficit hyperactivity disorder. Sleep Med 2019;60:123–31.
36. Pagel JF, Snyder S, Dawson D. Obstructive sleep apnea in sleepy pediatric psychiatry clinic patients: polysomnographic and clinical correlates. Sleep Breath 2004;8(3):125–31.
37. Huang YS, Guilleminault C, Li HY, et al. Attention-deficit/hyperactivity disorder with obstructive sleep apnea: a treatment outcome study. Sleep Med 2007; 8(1):18–30.
38. Sedky K, Bennett DS, Carvalho KS. Attention deficit hyperactivity disorder and sleep disordered breathing in pediatric populations: a meta-analysis. Sleep Med Rev 2014;18(4):349–56.
39. Tso W, Chan M, Ho FK, et al. Early sleep deprivation and attention-deficit/hyperactivity disorder. Pediatr Res 2019;85(4):449–55.

40. Oznur T, Akarsu S, Karaahmetoglu B, et al. A rare symptom in posttraumatic stress disorder: spontaneous ejaculation. Am J Case Rep 2014;15:69–73.

41. Kaihua J, Yang Y, Fangqiao Z, et al. Event-related potentials and behavior performance scores in children with sleep-disordered breathing. Brain Dev 2019; 41(8):662–70.

42. Chervin RD, Ruzicka DL, Giordani BJ, et al. Sleep-disordered breathing, behavior, and cognition in children before and after adenotonsillectomy. Pediatrics 2006;117(4):e769–78.

43. Song IS, Hong SN, Joo JW, et al. Long-term results of sleep-related quality-of-life and behavioral problems after adenotonsillectomy. Laryngoscope 2020; 130(2):546–50.

44. Beebe DW, Ris MD, Kramer ME, et al. The association between sleep disordered breathing, academic grades, and cognitive and behavioral functioning among overweight subjects during middle to late childhood. Sleep 2010; 33(11):1447–56.

45. Gottlieb DJ, Chase C, Vezina RM, et al. Sleep-disordered breathing symptoms are associated with poorer cognitive function in 5-year-old children. J Pediatr 2004;145(4):458–64.

46. Kheirandish-Gozal L, De Jong MR, Spruyt K, et al. Obstructive sleep apnoea is associated with impaired pictorial memory task acquisition and retention in children. Eur Respir J 2010;36(1):164–9.

47. Spruyt K, Capdevila OS, Kheirandish-Gozal L, et al. Inefficient or insufficient encoding as potential primary deficit in neurodevelopmental performance among children with OSA. Dev Neuropsychol 2009;34(5):601–14.

48. Joyce A, Elphick H, Farquhar M, et al. Obstructive sleep apnoea contributes to executive function impairment in young children with down syndrome. Behav Sleep Med 2019;1–11.

49. Giordani B, Hodges EK, Guire KE, et al. Changes in neuropsychological and behavioral functioning in children with and without obstructive sleep apnea following Tonsillectomy. J Int Neuropsychol Soc 2012;18(2):212–22.

50. Giordani B, Hodges EK, Guire KE, et al. Neuropsychological and behavioral functioning in children with and without obstructive sleep apnea referred for tonsillectomy. J Int Neuropsychol Soc 2008;14(4):571–81.

51. Gozal D, Kheirandish-Gozal L, Bhattacharjee R, et al. Neurocognitive and endothelial dysfunction in children with obstructive sleep apnea. Pediatrics 2010; 126(5):e1161–7.

52. Rhodes SK, Shimoda KC, Waid LR, et al. Neurocognitive deficits in morbidly obese children with obstructive sleep apnea. J Pediatr 1995;127(5):741–4.

53. Waters KA, Chawla J, Harris MA, et al. Cognition after early tonsillectomy for mild OSA. Pediatrics 2020;145(2).

54. Gozal D, Daniel JM, Dohanich GP. Behavioral and anatomical correlates of chronic episodic hypoxia during sleep in the rat. J Neurosci 2001;21(7): 2442–50.

55. Crossland RF, Durgan DJ, Lloyd EE, et al. A new rodent model for obstructive sleep apnea: effects on ATP-mediated dilations in cerebral arteries. Am J Physiol Regul Integr Comp Physiol 2013;305(4):R334–42.

56. Krajewska Wojciechowska J, Krajewski W, Zatonski T. The association between ENT diseases and obesity in pediatric population: a systemic review of current knowledge. Ear Nose Throat J 2019;98(5):E32–43.

57. Shen YC, Kung SC, Chang ET, et al. The impact of obesity in cognitive and memory dysfunction in obstructive sleep apnea syndrome. Int J Obes (Lond) 2019;43(2):355–61.

58. Hannon TS, Rofey DL, Ryan CM, et al. Relationships among obstructive sleep apnea, anthropometric measures, and neurocognitive functioning in adolescents with severe obesity. J Pediatr 2012;160(5):732–5.

59. Lee CH, Hsu WC, Chang WH, et al. Polysomnographic findings after adenotonsillectomy for obstructive sleep apnoea in obese and non-obese children: a systematic review and meta-analysis. Clin Otolaryngol 2016;41(5):498–510.

60. Imanguli M, Ulualp SO. Risk factors for residual obstructive sleep apnea after adenotonsillectomy in children. Laryngoscope 2016;126(11):2624–9.

61. Mitchell RB, Kelly J. Outcome of adenotonsillectomy for obstructive sleep apnea in obese and normal-weight children. Otolaryngol Head Neck Surg 2007; 137(1):43–8.

62. O'Brien LM, Sitha S, Baur LA, et al. Obesity increases the risk for persisting obstructive sleep apnea after treatment in children. Int J Pediatr Otorhinolaryngol 2006;70(9):1555–60.

63. Com G, Carroll JL, Tang X, et al. Characteristics and surgical and clinical outcomes of severely obese children with obstructive sleep apnea. J Clin Sleep Med 2015;11(4):467–74.

64. Lennon CJ, Wang RY, Wallace A, et al. Risk of failure of adenotonsillectomy for obstructive sleep apnea in obese pediatric patients. Int J Pediatr Otorhinolaryngol 2017;92:7–10.

65. Kirkham E, Ma CC, Filipek N, et al. Polysomnography outcomes of sleep endoscopy-directed intervention in surgically naive children at risk for persistent obstructive sleep apnea. Sleep Breath 2020.

66. Adler AC, Musso MF, Mehta DK, et al. Pediatric drug induced sleep endoscopy: a simple sedation recipe. Ann Otol Rhinol Laryngol 2019. 3489419892292.

67. Jung YG, Kim HY, Min JY, et al. Role of intranasal topical steroid in pediatric sleep disordered breathing and influence of allergy, sinusitis, and obesity on treatment outcome. Clin Exp Otorhinolaryngol 2011;4(1):27–32.

68. Scadding G. Non-surgical treatment of adenoidal hypertrophy: the role of treating IgE-mediated inflammation. Pediatr Allergy Immunol 2010;21(8):1095–106.

69. Hui JW, Ong J, Herdegen JJ, et al. Risk of obstructive sleep apnea in African American patients with chronic rhinosinusitis. Ann Allergy Asthma Immunol 2017;118(6):685–688 e1.

70. Rogers VE, Bollinger ME, Tulapurkar ME, et al. Inflammation and asthma control in children with comorbid obstructive sleep apnea. Pediatr Pulmonol 2018;53(9): 1200–7.

71. Malakasioti G, Gourgoulianis K, Chrousos G, et al. Interactions of obstructive sleep-disordered breathing with recurrent wheezing or asthma and their effects on sleep quality. Pediatr Pulmonol 2011;46(11):1047–54.

72. Narayanan A, Yogesh A, Mitchell RB, et al. Asthma and obesity as predictors of severe obstructive sleep apnea in an adolescent pediatric population. Laryngoscope 2019.

73. He Z, Armoni Domany K, Nava-Guerra L, et al. Phenotype of ventilatory control in children with moderate to severe persistent asthma and obstructive sleep apnea. Sleep 2019.

74. Trivedi M, ElMallah M, Bailey E, et al. Pediatric obstructive sleep apnea and asthma: clinical implications. Pediatr Ann 2017;46(9):e332–5.

75. Sanchez T, Castro-Rodriguez JA, Brockmann PE. Sleep-disordered breathing in children with asthma: a systematic review on the impact of treatment. J Asthma Allergy 2016;9:83–91.
76. Goldstein NA, Thomas MS, Yu Y, et al. The impact of adenotonsillectomy on pediatric asthma. Pediatr Pulmonol 2019;54(1):20–6.
77. Kheirandish-Gozal L, Dayyat EA, Eid NS, et al. Obstructive sleep apnea in poorly controlled asthmatic children: effect of adenotonsillectomy. Pediatr Pulmonol 2011;46(9):913–8.
78. Lavin JM, Shah RK. Postoperative complications in obese children undergoing adenotonsillectomy. Int J Pediatr Otorhinolaryngol 2015;79(10):1732–5.
79. Kalra M, Buncher R, Amin RS. Asthma as a risk factor for respiratory complications after adenotonsillectomy in children with obstructive breathing during sleep. Ann Allergy Asthma Immunol 2005;94(5):549–52.
80. Bhattacharjee R, Kheirandish-Gozal L, Spruyt K, et al. Adenotonsillectomy outcomes in treatment of obstructive sleep apnea in children: a multicenter retrospective study. Am J Respir Crit Care Med 2010;182(5):676–83.
81. Xie DX, Wang RY, Penn EB, et al. Understanding sociodemographic factors related to health outcomes in pediatric obstructive sleep apnea. Int J Pediatr Otorhinolaryngol 2018;111:138–41.
82. Friberg D, Lundkvist K, Li X, et al. Parental poverty and occupation as risk factors for pediatric sleep-disordered breathing. Sleep Med 2015;16(9):1169–75.
83. Brouillette RT, Horwood L, Constantin E, et al. Childhood sleep apnea and neighborhood disadvantage. J Pediatr 2011;158(5):789–795 e1.
84. Spilsbury JC, Storfer-Isser A, Kirchner HL, et al. Neighborhood disadvantage as a risk factor for pediatric obstructive sleep apnea. J Pediatr 2006;149(3):342–7.
85. Wang R, Dong Y, Weng J, et al. Associations among neighborhood, race, and sleep apnea severity in children. A six-city analysis. Ann Am Thorac Soc 2017;14(1):76–84.
86. Harris VC, Links AR, Kim JM, et al. Follow-up and time to treatment in an urban cohort of children with sleep-disordered breathing. Otolaryngol Head Neck Surg 2018;159(2):371–8.
87. Boss EF, Benke JR, Tunkel DE, et al. Public insurance and timing of polysomnography and surgical care for children with sleep-disordered breathing. JAMA Otolaryngol Head Neck Surg 2015;141(2):106–11.
88. Chervin RD, Clarke DF, Huffman JL, et al. School performance, race, and other correlates of sleep-disordered breathing in children. Sleep Med 2003;4(1):21–7.
89. Weinstock TG, Rosen CL, Marcus CL, et al. Predictors of obstructive sleep apnea severity in adenotonsillectomy candidates. Sleep 2014;37(2):261–9.
90. Tamanyan K, Walter LM, Davey MJ, et al. Risk factors for obstructive sleep apnoea in Australian children. J Paediatr Child Health 2016;52(5):512–7.
91. Walker B Jr. Social and economic determinants of occupational health policies and services. Am J Ind Med 1989;16(3):321–8.
92. Penn EB Jr, French A, Bhushan B, et al. Access to care for children with symptoms of sleep disordered breathing. Int J Pediatr Otorhinolaryngol 2012;76(11):1671–3.
93. Jabbour J, Robey T, Cunningham MJ. Healthcare disparities in pediatric otolaryngology: a systematic review. Laryngoscope 2018;128(7):1699–713.
94. Grossman NL, Ortega VE, King TS, et al. Exacerbation-prone asthma in the context of race and ancestry in asthma clinical research network trials. J Allergy Clin Immunol 2019;144(6):1524–33.

95. Wang H, Cade BE, Sofer T, et al. Admixture mapping identifies novel loci for obstructive sleep apnea in Hispanic/Latino Americans. Hum Mol Genet 2019; 28(4):675–87.

96. Cassano M, Bayar Muluk N, Di Taranto F, et al. A comparison of intraoperative haemostatic techniques during tonsillectomy: Suture vs electrocautery-A study to assess postoperative pain scores and duration to resumption of normal diet. Clin Otolaryngol 2018;43(5):1219–25.

97. Lane JC, Dworkin-Valenti J, Chiodo L, et al. Postoperative tonsillectomy bleeding complications in children: a comparison of three surgical techniques. Int J Pediatr Otorhinolaryngol 2016;88:184–8.

98. Pynnonen M, Brinkmeier JV, Thorne MC, et al. Coblation versus other surgical techniques for tonsillectomy. Cochrane Database Syst Rev 2017;(8):CD004619.

99. Walner DL, Mularczyk C, Sweis A. Utilization and trends in surgical instrument use in pediatric adenotonsillectomy. Int J Pediatr Otorhinolaryngol 2017; 100:8–13.

100. Chang DT, Zemek A, Koltai PJ. Comparison of treatment outcomes between intracapsular and total tonsillectomy for pediatric obstructive sleep apnea. Int J Pediatr Otorhinolaryngol 2016;91:15–8.

101. Brkic F, Mujic M, Umihanic S, et al. Haemorrhage rates after two commonly used tonsillectomy methods: a multicenter study. Med Arch 2017;71(2):119–21.

102. Mitchell RM, Parikh SR. Hemostasis in tonsillectomy. Otolaryngol Clin North Am 2016;49(3):615–26.

103. Baik G, Brietzke SE. Comparison of pediatric intracapsular tonsillectomy and extracapsular tonsillectomy: a cost and utility decision analysis. Otolaryngol Head Neck Surg 2018;158(6):1113–8.

104. Bagwell K, Wu X, Baum ED, et al. Cost-effectiveness analysis of intracapsular tonsillectomy and total tonsillectomy for pediatric obstructive sleep apnea. Appl Health Econ Health Policy 2018;16(4):527–35.

105. Guest JF, Rana K, Hopkins C. Cost-effectiveness of Coblation compared with cold steel tonsillectomies in the UK. J Laryngol Otol 2018;132(12):1119–27.

106. Hoey AW, Foden NM, Hadjisymeou Andreou S, et al. Coblation((R)) intracapsular tonsillectomy (tonsillotomy) in children: A prospective study of 500 consecutive cases with long-term follow-up. Clin Otolaryngol 2017;42(6):1211–7.

107. Kohn JL, Cohen MB, Patel P, et al. Outcomes of children with mild obstructive sleep apnea treated nonsurgically: a retrospective review. Otolaryngol Head Neck Surg 2019;160(6):1101–5.

108. Statham MM, Elluru RG, Buncher R, et al. Adenotonsillectomy for obstructive sleep apnea syndrome in young children: prevalence of pulmonary complications. Arch Otolaryngol Head Neck Surg 2006;132(5):476–80.

109. Baijal RG, Bidani SA, Minard CG, et al. Perioperative respiratory complications following awake and deep extubation in children undergoing adenotonsillectomy. Paediatr Anaesth 2015;25(4):392–9.

110. Yumusakhuylu AC, Binnetoglu A, Demir B, et al. Is it safe to perform adenotonsillectomy in children with Down syndrome? Eur Arch Otorhinolaryngol 2016; 273(9):2819–23.

111. Isaiah A, Hamdan H, Johnson RF, et al. Very severe obstructive sleep apnea in children: outcomes of adenotonsillectomy and risk factors for persistence. Otolaryngol Head Neck Surg 2017;157(1):128–34.

112. Konstantinopoulou S, Gallagher P, Elden L, et al. Complications of adenotonsillectomy for obstructive sleep apnea in school-aged children. Int J Pediatr Otorhinolaryngol 2015;79(2):240–5.

113. Curtis JL, Harvey DB, Willie S, et al. Causes and costs for ED visits after pediatric adenotonsillectomy. Otolaryngol Head Neck Surg 2015;152(4):691–6.
114. Lavin J, Lehmann D, Silva AL, et al. Variables associated with pediatric emergency department visits for uncontrolled pain in postoperative adenotonsillectomy patients. Int J Pediatr Otorhinolaryngol 2019;123:10–4.
115. Bhattacharyya N, Shapiro NL. Associations between socioeconomic status and race with complications after tonsillectomy in children. Otolaryngol Head Neck Surg 2014;151(6):1055–60.
116. Chang IS, Kang KT, Tseng CC, et al. Revisits after adenotonsillectomy in children with sleep-disordered breathing: a retrospective single-institution study. Clin Otolaryngol 2018;43(1):39–46.
117. Shay S, Shapiro NL, Bhattacharyya N. Revisit rates and diagnoses following pediatric tonsillectomy in a large multistate population. Laryngoscope 2015; 125(2):457–61.
118. Roland PS, Rosenfeld RM, Brooks LJ, et al. Clinical practice guideline: polysomnography for sleep-disordered breathing prior to tonsillectomy in children. Otolaryngol Head Neck Surg 2011;145(1 Suppl):S1–15.
119. Lee HH, Dalesio NM, Lo Sasso AT, et al. Impact of clinical guidelines on revisits after ambulatory pediatric adenotonsillectomy. Anesth Analg 2018;127(2): 478–84.
120. De Luca Canto G, Pacheco-Pereira C, Aydinoz S, et al. Adenotonsillectomy complications: a meta-analysis. Pediatrics 2015;136(4):702–18.
121. Subramanyam R, Varughese A, Willging JP, et al. Future of pediatric tonsillectomy and perioperative outcomes. Int J Pediatr Otorhinolaryngol 2013;77(2): 194–9.
122. Lawlor CM, Riley CA, Carter JM, et al. Association between age and weight as risk factors for complication after tonsillectomy in healthy children. JAMA Otolaryngol Head Neck Surg 2018;144(5):399–405.
123. Burckardt E, Rebholz W, Allen S, et al. Predictors for hemorrhage following pediatric adenotonsillectomy. Int J Pediatr Otorhinolaryngol 2019;117:143–7.
124. Kshirsagar R, Mahboubi H, Moriyama D, et al. Increased immediate postoperative hemorrhage in older and obese children after outpatient tonsillectomy. Int J Pediatr Otorhinolaryngol 2016;84:119–23.
125. Perkins JN, Liang C, Gao D, et al. Risk of post-tonsillectomy hemorrhage by clinical diagnosis. Laryngoscope 2012;122(10):2311–5.
126. Windfuhr JP, Schloendorff G, Baburi D, et al. Serious post-tonsillectomy hemorrhage with and without lethal outcome in children and adolescents. Int J Pediatr Otorhinolaryngol 2008;72(7):1029–40.
127. Reusser NM, Bender RW, Agrawal NA, et al. Post-tonsillectomy hemorrhage rates in children compared by surgical technique. Ear Nose Throat J 2017; 96(7):E7–11.
128. Kang KT, Chang IS, Tseng CC, et al. Impacts of disease severity on postoperative complications in children with sleep-disordered breathing. Laryngoscope 2017;127(11):2646–52.

Using Electroencephalography (EEG) to Guide Propofol and Sevoflurane Dosing in Pediatric Anesthesia

Ian Yuan, MD[a,*], Ting Xu, MD[b,c], Charles Dean Kurth, MD[a,d]

KEYWORDS

• EEG • Electroencephalogram • Sevoflurane • Propofol • Anesthesia

KEY POINTS

• The dose of sevoflurane and propofol that produces unconsciousness varies by age group (neonates, infants, and children) as well as between patients within the same age group, potentially creating risk for underdose and overdose in pediatric patients.

• Intraoperative electroencephalography (EEG) can be used as a biomarker of hypnotic depth in neonates, infants, and children to guide the dose of propofol and sevoflurane to the individual patient.

• Numeric proprietary indices on intraoperative EEG monitors do not reliably correlate with anesthetic dose in neonates and young infants. EEG waveforms and other nonproprietary EEG parameters, however, change reliably with increased doses of sevoflurane and propofol across all ages and can be utilized in pediatric anesthesia.

INTRODUCTION

Inhaled sevoflurane and intravenous (IV) propofol are 2 of the primary drugs used to anesthetize children. Dosing for these agents is guided by monitoring expired concentration for sevoflurane or infusion pump rate for propofol total IV anesthetic (TIVA);

[a] Department of Anesthesiology and Critical Care Medicine, The Children's Hospital of Philadelphia, University of Pennsylvania, Perelman School of Medicine, 3401 Civic Center Boulevard, Philadelphia, PA 19104, USA; [b] Department of Anesthesiology, Laboratory of anesthesia and Critical Care Medicine, Translational Neuroscience Center, West China Hospital, Sichuan University and The Research Units of West China, Chinese Academy of Medical Sciences, Chengdu 610041, Sichuan, China; [c] Department of Anesthesiology, Sichuan Academy of Medical Sciences & Sichuan Provincial People's Hospital, 32#, 2nd Section (West), 1st Ring Road, Chengdu 610072, China; [d] Department of Pediatrics, The Children's Hospital of Philadelphia, University of Pennsylvania, Perelman School of Medicine, Philadelphia, PA, USA
* Corresponding author.
E-mail address: YUANI@EMAIL.CHOP.EDU

Anesthesiology Clin 38 (2020) 709–725
https://doi.org/10.1016/j.anclin.2020.06.007
1932-2275/20/© 2020 Elsevier Inc. All rights reserved.
anesthesiology.theclinics.com

additional considerations include changes in heart rate, blood pressure, and movement in response to stimulation. None of these factors directly assesses the anesthetic state of the brain. EEG allows measurement of cortical electrical activity and can be used to assess hypnotic depth to adjust dosing of anesthetic agents to the individual patient.[1–5] EEG monitoring recently has been recommended as one of the vital organ monitors used to guide anesthetic management.[6] Potential benefits of intraoperative EEG monitoring include less incidence of hypotension and awareness under anesthesia, faster wakeup and recovery times, and less amount of drugs administered.[2,6,7] Intraoperative EEG monitoring might be particularly beneficial in neonates and young infants undergoing major surgery and pediatric patients with cardiovascular disease, as they have greater risk of respiratory and cardiovascular events during anesthesia.[8,9] Intraoperative EEG monitoring might also be suited for propofol TIVA to assess propofol effect site concentration, which cannot be assessed otherwise, unlike sevoflurane anesthesia in which the expired concentration can be used to assess sevoflurane effect site concentration.[6,10–12]

This article describes the rationale and application of EEG to guide sevoflurane and propofol TIVA dosing in children aged 0-12 years and specifically discusses the fundamentals necessary to interpret EEG, changes in EEG with age and anesthetic state, the interaction between anesthetic state and pharmacology, and how EEG can be used to guide dosing of sevoflurane and propofol.

EEG FUNDAMENTALS
Intraoperative EEG Monitors

EEG measures the electrical activity in the neocortex, which is generated by the summation of excitatory and inhibitory postsynaptic activities from pyramidal neurons.[3] Although it has been known for many years that EEG changes with increasing doses of volatile and IV anesthetics, intraoperative EEG monitoring was uncommon until recently. The increased use of intraoperative EEG monitoring has been driven by clinical and media reports of intraoperative awareness and advances in EEG technology that make it more accessible to anesthesiologists.[10] These advances include creation of a numeric proprietary index that provides an overview of hypnotic depth and improvements in sensor and signal processing technology to enable rapid application and noise-filtering.

Smaller and more practical than EEG machines utilized by neurologists, intraoperative EEG monitors typically combine 4 to 8 electrodes into a disposable sensor placed on the forehead. Intraoperative EEG monitors approved for pediatric use include BIS (Medtronic, Minnesota, Minnesota), Narcotrend (MonitorTechnik, Bad Bramstedt, Germany), and SedLine (Masimo, Irvine, California).[10] These monitors display both unprocessed (EEG waveforms) and processed EEG (numeric proprietary indices and nonproprietary parameters). Because many anesthesiologists have some experience using numeric proprietary indices (eg, BIS), the emphasis of this article is on using EEG waveforms and nonproprietary EEG parameters to guide anesthetic dosing, since numeric proprietary indices are not always reliable in the pediatric population.[13]

EEG Waveforms

EEG waveforms can be described using frequency and amplitude/power. Frequency (hertz) is the number of times the EEG waveform crosses 0 within a second and is grouped into frequency bands, from lowest to highest frequencies: slow (<1 Hz), delta (1–4 Hz), theta (5–8 Hz), alpha (9–12 Hz), beta (13–25 Hz), and gamma (26–80 Hz).[5]

Amplitude (microvolts) is the height of the EEG waveform and indicates the synchrony of the underlying neuronal discharges; the larger the EEG amplitude, the more synchronized the neuronal discharges, indicating a deeper state of unconsciousness. Slow and delta waves with large amplitudes are seen in deep sleep or coma, whereas theta waves are present in light sleep. Alpha waves are seen in an awake state with eyes closed or when meditating, whereas beta waves are present in a state of active thinking.[3] EEG power (decibels) is the quantity of EEG activity at a given frequency; with increased depth of unconsciousness, EEG power typically decreases in higher frequencies and increases in lower frequencies. Amplitude and power are related mathematically but in processed EEG, power is used instead of amplitude because it is easier to display graphically.

EEG Artifacts

EEG amplitude is 100 times less than electrocardiography and 10 times less than electromyography (EMG), thereby making intraoperative EEG highly susceptible to electrical interference (eg, electrocautery), motion artifact, and contamination from electrocardiography and EMG.[3] Intraoperative EEG is able to overcome many of these limitations using filters and signal processing to remove or identify artifacts. Although the patient usually is immobile during anesthesia, motion artifact often is unavoidable in head and neck surgery, rendering EEG interpretation problematic. The sterile field in craniofacial surgery may also preclude EEG monitoring. The EEG module should not be located next to warming devices or the table controller as both can generate electrical noise.

Processed EEG Parameters

Using signal processing, a complex EEG waveform can be broken down into multiple waveforms of discrete frequencies; a mathematical process known as Fourier transformation.[5] **Fig. 1** shows an example of a complex waveform that contains three underlying waveforms of frequencies 4, 8, and 32 Hz which are decomposed into three simple waveforms of those three frequencies. The decomposition of an EEG

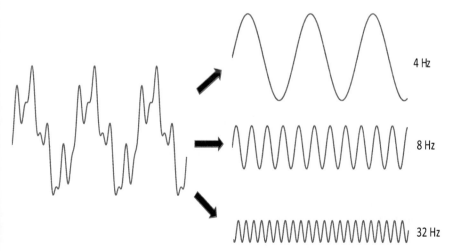

4 Hz

8 Hz

32 Hz

Fig. 1. Decomposition of complex waveform into 3 simple waveforms of distinct frequencies.

waveform into discrete frequency bands (e.g. slow, delta, theta, alpha, beta, and gamma) over time allows creation of a spectrogram also known as a density spectral array (DSA), a type of processed non-proprietary EEG parameter.[5]

The DSA displays the relationship between EEG power and frequency over time. In the DSA, the x-axis represents time and y-axis represents frequency. To display EEG power at a certain frequency and time, a colored or grey scale is used to represent power intensity, with dark-brilliant colors representing higher power and light-dull colors denoting lower power.[5] **Fig. 2** illustrates an example of DSA during 30 minutes of a propofol anesthetic. At minutes 0-5 (see **Fig. 2**), the majority of EEG power is concentrated in lower frequencies, denoted by the intense red color at frequencies < 3 Hz (lower left in **Fig. 2**), while a minority of EEG power exists in higher frequencies, denoted by blue color at frequencies > 15 Hz. At minutes 8-27 (see **Fig. 2**), there is an increase in power at frequencies 10-12 Hz as indicated by the appearance of yellow/orange colors, along with a decrease in power at frequencies < 5 Hz as indicated by the change from red to yellow. The DSA shows that the level of hypnosis was greater at minutes 0-5 than at 8-27, as indicated by the majority of power existing in lower frequencies in minutes 0-5. Because propofol and sevoflurane exert dose-dependent effects on frequency and power, the DSA can visually display hypnotic level during the course of the anesthetic. Purdon and colleagues[5] provides an excellent tutorial on interpreting DSA for the clinical anesthesiologist.

Many intraoperative EEG monitors display their proprietary index along with EEG waveforms, DSA, and nonproprietary processed parameters (**Fig. 3**). These nonproprietary processed EEG parameters include spectral edge frequency (SEF), burst suppression ratio (BSR), and relative beta ratio (RBR). SEF95 is the frequency below which 95% of EEG power is located.[5] A lower SEF95 represents a deeper state of hypnosis.

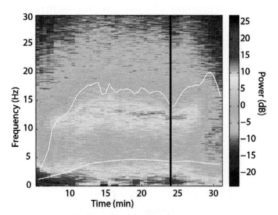

Fig. 2. DSA (EEG spectrogram) displays the power spectrum over time. X axis denotes time and Y axis denotes frequency on left axis, while power is on right axis, denoted using color (red for increased and blue for decreased power). The top white line indicates SEF95 (Spectral Edge Frequency), where 95% of power lies below that frequency. The bottom white line indicates SEF50 or median frequency, where 50% of power lies below that frequency. Note that negative power on DSA represents very low EEG waveform amplitude and not negative amplitude. (*From* Purdon PL, Sampson A, Pavone KJ, Brown EN. Clinical electroencephalography for anesthesiologists. Part I: background and basic signatures. Anesthesiology: The Journal of the American Society of Anesthesiologists. 2015 Oct 1;123(4):937-60; with permission.)

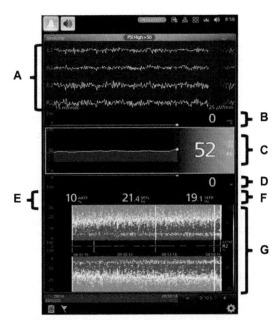

Fig. 3. SedLine EEG monitor. EEG parameters are indicated by letters. A, EEG waveforms shows graphic 4-channel recordings from left and right forehead; B, percentage of EMG interference as number and graphic recording; C, PSI, a numeric proprietary index; D, percentage of BSR; E, percentage of artifact; F, SEF95 from left and right forehead; G, DSA: top graph is from left forehead and bottom graph is from right forehead; white line going across shows the spectral edge frequency encompassing SEF95.

In the DSA in **Fig. 2**, SEF95 is shown by the top white line and is less than 5 Hz at minute 0, steadily increasing to 12 Hz by minute 10, indicating decreased hypnotic depth over time. DSA and SEF95 often are used together to assess hypnotic depth: SEF95 provides a numeric index of EEG frequency and power at a moment in time, whereas DSA provides a graphical representation of EEG frequency and power over time. BSR shows the percentage of time that EEG is isoelectric, which indicates an electrically inactive cortex and very deep hypnosis.[14,15] RBR is the ratio of power in theta versus beta frequency bands; a higher ratio indicates more power in the slower frequencies and a deeper state of hypnosis.[5,10]

A non-EEG parameter is EMG, which shows the amount of temporalis muscle activity. EMG represents an alert for artifact and potentially erroneous calculation of the EEG parameters; muscle relaxants can decrease EMG artifact. EMG activity also can indicate increased muscle tone consistent with light anesthesia.

Proprietary indices (eg, BIS, Narcotrend index, and Patient State Index [PSI]) are calculated from an algorithm that uses a combination of EEG and non-EEG parameters to construct the numeric index ranging from 0 to 100; a lower value represents a deeper state of hypnosis. In general, hypnotic states representing sedation, surgical anesthesia, and burst suppression/isoelectricity correspond to proprietary indices of 60-80, 40-60, and 0-20, respectively, which in turn correspond to SEF95 ranges of 15-20 Hz, 6-14 Hz, and <5 Hz.[5,10]

Traditionally, pediatric anesthesiologists have relied primarily on the numeric proprietary index to determine anesthetic depth.[10] This practice has several issues: (1) the index may be inaccurate for certain age groups and anesthetic drugs; (2) the index is subject to artifact and noise, which may not be properly accounted for; and (3) the index does not measure the nonhypnotic components of the anesthetic state (eg, muscle tone–immobility, awareness, and analgesia), which are important in assessing overall anesthetic depth. Therefore, proper use of EEG requires (1) knowledge of age and drug effects on EEG, which are discussed later; (2) basic understanding of the EEG waveform and commonly used nonproprietary EEG parameters (eg, DSA and SEF95) to aid interpretation of the index; and (3) understanding the limitations of EEG in assessing the overall anesthetic state. To understand these limitations, the components of the anesthetic state and involvement of the neocortex are described next.

ANESTHETIC STATE

The anesthetic state includes components of hypnosis (unconsciousness), analgesia, areflexia (immobility), and amnesia (awareness). The anesthetic state is induced by drugs interfering with synaptic transmission within or between several brain regions. γ-Aminobutyric acid (GABA) and α-adrenergic neurotransmitter-receptor systems in the neocortex, thalamus, and brainstem strongly influence the level of consciousness.[5,16,17] Opioid and glutamate neurotransmitter-receptors in the amygdala, thalamus, brainstem, and spinal cord strongly affect analgesia.[18,19] Memory formation, which is key to awareness, involves several neurotransmitter-receptor systems in many areas of the neocortex as well as the hippocampus.[20] As a monitor of neocortical activity, EEG is able to assess the level of hypnosis and, in theory, also can assess the risk of awareness.[3–5,16,21] EEG does not assess the analgesia or areflexia components of the anesthetic state.[3]

PEDIATRIC EEG CHANGES WITH AGE

For anesthesiologists taking care of young children, understanding normal EEG changes with age is important because it can affect the interpretation of intraoperative EEG. By ages 10 to 14 years, the EEG resembles that of an adult. In children older than age 3 years, all EEG frequency bands are present.

The neonatal and infant EEG is characterized by low frequency and power compared with older children.[15] In preterm neonates 28 weeks to 34 weeks postmenstrual age, periods of isoelectric EEG are common, occurring during both awake and sleep. Thus, a normal EEG in a non-anesthetized neonate or infant could be similar to the EEG in an anesthetized child or adult. Accordingly, proprietary indices that were developed in adults are not reliable in neonates and infants.[13] EEG waveform and some nonproprietary processed EEG parameters, however, can be used to assess the level of hypnosis for all ages, as described later.

EEG TO GUIDE ANESTHETIC DOSE

Using EEG to guide sevoflurane and propofol TIVA dosing requires knowledge of each drug's pharmacokinetics and pharmacodynamics. Therefore, each section starts with an introduction to the pharmacokinetics-pharmacodynamics of each drug, followed by a description of the EEG parameters that can be used to adjust dosing across all age groups; the sections end with sample cases demonstrating EEG-guided dosing.

Sevoflurane

Pharmacokinetics-pharmacodynamics
The effect of sevoflurane on synaptic neurotransmission is related to its partial pressure in the brain and spinal cord, represented at equilibrium by the alveolar

concentration. The rate constant between brain and lung is 6 minutes, indicating rapid equilibration between brain and alveolar concentrations.[22] Sevoflurane alveolar concentration is related directly to the inhaled concentration and minute ventilation, and indirectly to its solubility and cardiac output. Sevoflurane solubility is similar in neonates, infants, and children.[23] Because the ratio of alveolar ventilation and cardiac output per body weight is similar from neonates through childhood, sevoflurane pharmacokinetics behaves similarly in the pediatric population regardless of age.[24]

Sevoflurane pharmacodynamics are described in terms of the minimum alveolar concentration (MAC) of sevoflurane required to suppress movement to a surgical incision in 50% of the patients.[22,25] MAC of sevoflurane varies by age, ranging from 2.4% in premature infants, 3.2% in infants, and 2.1% in young adults. Individual differences also exist within the same age group.[22,25] For example, even though the MAC of sevoflurane is 3.2% for age 0-6 months, the dose of sevoflurane for 95% of young infants in that age group to not move during surgical incision could range from 2.5% to 3.8%.[22,24] Because of these inherent variabilities in MAC, there is a potential risk of underdose/overdose in an individual pediatric patient when using population-based MAC and expired sevoflurane concentration as a dosing guide. EEG permits titration of hypnotic dose to the individual patient, often at a lower dose than that based on MAC and cardiovascular parameters. This is useful particularly for neonates and infants undergoing major surgery as well as neonates, infants, and children with cardiovascular disease, because these patients are at greater risk of hypotension during anesthesia.[8,9,14,26]

EEG parameters for sevoflurane dosing

Proprietary EEG indices are unreliable in neonates and young infants ages less than 6 months but are generally reliable in children ages greater than 1 year.[13,27–29] Unreliability in infants is due to the proprietary EEG indices being developed in adults without consideration for the normal age-related EEG changes in infants.[10,13,30] Even in older infants and children, proprietary EEG indices do not always correlate with sevoflurane concentration.[3,12,13] For example, in children ages 6 months to 12 years, BIS index decreased from sevoflurane 1% to 3%, as expected, and then paradoxically increased from sevoflurane 3% to 5%. This is due to the proprietary index misinterpreting high frequency epileptiform EEG activity during high-dose sevoflurane as a lighter state of hypnosis.[12,31,32]

By comparison, nonproprietary EEG parameters have been shown to reflect sevoflurane concentration in infants ages greater than 3 months but not in infants ages less than 1 month. For example, in infants ages less than 1 month, SEF95, BSR, and RBR do not reliably indicate changes in sevoflurane concentration, whereas they do by ages 3 months to 5 months.[29] In infants ages greater than 3 months, Koch and colleagues[33] have identified SEF95 values (cutoffs) of less than 7 Hz (deep anesthesia), less than 13 Hz (surgical anesthesia), and greater than 20 Hz (sedation/consciousness) that can be utilized to indicate time to intubate, start surgery, and emerge/extubate, respectively. Accordingly, SEF95 at 15 Hz to 20 Hz, 10 Hz to 15 Hz, and 6 Hz to 14 Hz are targets for sedation, surgical maintenance, and laryngoscopy/surgical incision, respectively.

Given the unreliability of proprietary indices for infants ages less than 1 year and nonproprietary processed EEG parameters for infants ages less than 3 months, anesthesiologists can use the EEG waveform to identify isoelectricity as an indicator of cortical inactivity and excess sevoflurane dose. Isoelectricity is common during sevoflurane anesthesia in neonates and infants when the dose is guided by MAC and hemodynamic parameters, and is associated with low arterial pressure.[14,34] When an infant demonstrates isoelectricity on the EEG, sevoflurane dose should be decreased until activity returns on EEG waveform. Case 1 demonstrates how to use EEG waveform to titrate sevoflurane dose in a young infant.

Case 1

A 2-month-old term infant was scheduled for laparoscopic inguinal hernia repair. Sevoflurane anesthesia with endotracheal tube and local anesthetic infiltration were planned. During sevoflurane induction, SedLine EEG sensors were applied on the forehead. EEG waveform revealed EMG artifact (23%), consistent with patient movement during induction (**Fig. 4**A). After inserting an IV catheter, 1 mg/kg of propofol, was given for intubation. In **Fig. 4**B, EEG waveform revealed isoelectricity and SEF95 was 3 Hz; DSA showed stronger power (green) in lower frequencies and weaker power (blue) in higher frequencies, all consistent with deep hypnosis. The numeric proprietary index, however, was inaccurately high (PSI 82). At incision, expired sevoflurane was 1.5% (0.47 MAC); EEG continued to display isoelectricity, indicating unnecessarily deep anesthesia, yet PSI still was inaccurately high (not shown in screenshot). Inspired sevoflurane was decreased to 1.2% (0.35 MAC) and shortly afterward, EEG activity resumed (**Fig. 4**C). SEF95 increased to 6.8 Hz, and DSA showed red in lower frequencies and green in higher frequencies (see **Fig. 4**C), a preferred level of anesthetic depth. At the end of surgery, the patient was extubated after demonstration of purposeful, spontaneous movement, and expired sevoflurane was less than 0.2%. EEG waveforms after extubation (**Fig. 4**D) showed increased activity (increased EEG frequency and amplitude) compared with earlier (see **Fig. 4**C); both PSI and SEF95 were similar between the 2 screenshots, suggesting that EEG waveforms can more reliably differentiate between anesthetic states than processed EEG parameters in this patient.

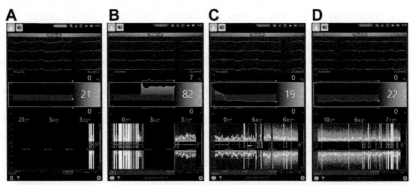

Fig. 4. SedLine EEG in a 2-month full-term infant, American Society of Anesthesiologist physical status class I, for inguinal hernia repair using sevoflurane anesthesia. (*A*) During sevoflurane induction, EEG waveform revealed EEG activity with EMG artifact 23%, consistent with patient movement during induction. (*B*) After intubation and before incision, EEG waveform displayed isoelectricity, indicating that the patient was "way too deep" and PSI was 82 and erroneously high. (*C*) During surgery, inspired sevoflurane was decreased to 0.5 MAC to regain EEG activity, upon which frequency bands delta (*red*) and theta (*green*) appeared, although SEF95 was only 6.8 Hz, indicating that the infant was still too deep. Inspired sevoflurane was subsequently decreased further (0.35 MAC) (*D*) At extubation, EEG waveforms, DSA, and indices were similar to (*C*), yet the patient was moving with expired sevoflurane concentration less than 0.2%. Possible explanations include measured sevoflurane was erroneously low due to not sampling alveolar concentration and/or brain concentration actually was higher from the 6-minute time delay from brain to alveolus.

This case illustrates that (1) the initial sevoflurane dose after intubation was higher than necessary based on isoelectric EEG, despite the dose being well below 1 MAC; (2) numeric proprietary index is unreliable as an indicator of hypnotic depth in young infants; and (3) nonproprietary parameters, such as SEF95, are not always reliable in infants less than 3 months, and use of the EEG waveform is recommended.

Propofol Total Intravenous Anesthetic

Pharmacokinetics-pharmacodynamics

Propofol acts at the $GABA_A$ receptor to disrupt the thalamocortical and corticocortical neurotransmitter systems, resulting in unconsciousness.[5,16,17] The effect of propofol is related to its effect-site concentration (Ce) in the brain, which is influenced by pharmacokinetics, a function of (1) the 3 volume compartments—central (eg, brain and heart), fast-peripheral (eg, liver and kidneys), and slow-peripheral (eg, skin and muscle); (2) drug distribution between the 3 compartments; and (3) drug clearance from the body.[35] The distribution half-life from the blood to the central compartment is 2 minutes to 4 minutes, indicating rapid equilibration between the blood and brain.[36] To achieve a target Ce, propofol is administered as a loading dose (bolus) followed by a maintenance infusion. Without the loading dose, Ce increases slowly and may take longer than desired to reach the target Ce.[7]

Propofol pharmacokinetics change with age as a result of developmental changes in the compartment volumes and clearances.[35] Neonates and young infants have higher central and fast-peripheral volumes and lower slow-peripheral volumes. Consequently, to achieve equivalent Ce, the loading dose bolus of propofol is higher in neonates and young infants than in older infants and children.[35] Drug clearance increases during the first year of life due to increases in liver cytochrome P450 enzyme function and glomerular filtration rate. As a result, to maintain equivalent Ce, the maintenance infusion dose of propofol is lowest in neonates and increases throughout infancy and childhood.[35]

Propofol pharmacodynamics are described in terms of propofol Ce, which is the same as blood propofol concentration at equilibrium. Brain Ce levels corresponding to different clinical endpoints (eg, unconscious and intubation) have been determined from blood Ce drawn at steady state from healthy adult volunteers.[37] Analogous to MAC, there is Ce-awake and Ce-immobility to stimuli. The propofol Ce-awake is 2 µg/mL, Ce-immobility to tactile pressure is 4 µg/mL, and Ce-immobility to laryngoscopy is 6 µg/mL.[38–40] For procedures with painful stimuli, remifentanil commonly is combined with propofol for synergistic effects. Remifentanil at 0.1 µg/kg/min to 0.8 µg/kg/min decreases the propofol Ce-awake and Ce-immobility by 30% to 70%.[40–42]

Propofol dosing

Many anesthesiologists dose propofol based on hemodynamic parameters and patient movement, which often delivers more propofol than necessary to achieve hypnosis.[3,14] Propofol also can be dosed according to an established pharmacokinetic equation, or model, that calculates the infusion dose needed to achieve a targeted Ce corresponding to the desired hypnotic level.[35] Because of pharmacokinetic variability by age group, propofol models or dosing regimens exist for adults,[43] children (ages 3–12 year),[44] infants (1–36 months),[45,46] and neonates (32–44 weeks postmenstrual age).[47]

Propofol TIVA according to the dosing model can be delivered by an infusion pump, with the dose adjusted manually based on a patient's age and duration of infusion (**Table 1**). The table can be entered into an anesthesia workstation computer or a smartphone for easy reference. Alternatively, in countries where targeted controlled

Table 1
Dosing regimens for propofol in neonates, infants, and children

Age Group	0–1 mo	1–3 mo	3–6 mo	6–12 mo	12–36 mo	3–12 y
Propofol bolus mg/kg	3.5	3	3	3	3	2.5
Propofol 0–15 min (µg/kg/min)	183	200	200	208	217	250
Propofol 16–30 min (µg/kg/min)	167	183	192	200	200	217
Propofol 31–60 min (µg/kg/min)	150	167	175	183	192	183
Propofol 61–120 min (µg/kg/min)	133	158	167	175	183	167
Propofol 121–180 min (µg/kg/min)	117	150	158	167	175	150
Propofol 181–300 min (µg/kg/min)	100	133	150	158	167	142

The dose regimens for ages 0 to 36 mo and 3 to 12 y based on pharmacokinetic models.[44,45,47] Doses targeted to yield propofol level in brain (Ce) 3 µg/mL to produce hypnosis.

For mild noxious stimulation, add remifentanil 0.1 to 0.2 µg/kg/min (procedural analgesia). For severe noxious stimulation, add remifentanil 0.2 to 0.4 µg/kg/min (surgical analgesia).

infusion (TCI) devices are available, the TCI device automatically adjusts the infusion dose over time according to the inputted target Ce (usually 3 μg/mL, as in **Table 1**). TCI is not available in the United States but is available and widely used in Canada, Mexico, and many countries in Europe and Asia.

Fig. 5 and **Table 1** illustrate the application of pharmacokinetics-pharmacodynamic models to the dosing of propofol in neonates, infants, and children. **Fig. 5** displays Ce during a hypothetical anesthetic from induction through emergence. To rapidly achieve the target Ce for surgery (3–5 μg/mL), propofol is dosed as a rapid bolus followed by a maintenance infusion (see **Fig. 5**). The propofol bolus and maintenance dose are selected from **Table 1** according to the age group. If regional analgesia or remifentanil are coadministered, propofol Ce is targeted to 3 μg/mL, the most common technique for propofol TIVA. For major noxious stimulation (incision and intubation), concomitant administration of remifentanil, 0.3 μg/kg/min to 0.4 μg/kg/min, is recommended. For minor noxious stimulation (preparation and wound closure), administration of remifentanil, 0.1 μg/kg/min to 0.2 μg/kg/min, is recommended. The remifentanil infusion dose is adjusted during surgery according to the severity of surgical stimulation, varying from 0.1 μg/kg/min to 0.4 μg/kg/min. Note that according to **Table 1**, the propofol maintenance infusion dose must be decreased over time for all age groups; otherwise Ce steadily increases, resulting in a higher Ce than desired and the potential for hypotension and prolonged emergence and recovery. By comparison, remifentanil does not accumulate over time and, therefore, its dose can remain constant.[35,42] If TCI is available, the dosing table has been programmed into the device; the target Ce is entered into the device and the device automatically adjusts the maintenance infusion over time to achieve the target Ce. For emergence, the propofol infusion is stopped and propofol Ce decreases rapidly, with consciousness returning at Ce 1.8 μg/mL.

Because these dosing regimens are derived from age-matched cohorts, pharmacokinetic variability exists for individuals within the same age group. The absolute prediction error of these dosing models ranges from 50% to 200%.[43–47] In neonate and infant models using weight, age, and time as parameters, the actual Ce could range from 75% to 183% of the target Ce.[47] Thus, in a neonate or infant receiving propofol TIVA

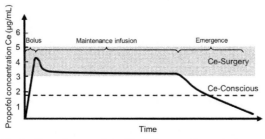

Fig. 5. Schematic illustration of propofol effect Ce over time during propofol TIVA. Solid line shows Ce over time during propofol administration as a bolus, maintenance infusion, and discontinuation of infusion (emergence). Clinical endpoints for Ce are indicated: dashed line is Ce-conscious (1.8 μg/mL); shaded area is Ce-surgery (3–5 μg/mL), with the range reflecting the intensity of noxious surgical stimulation and whether remifentanil is coadministered or regional analgesia is employed. After propofol bolus, there is a rapid rise in Ce, followed by a sharp decrease corresponding to redistribution. Steady state Ce for surgery (in this example, Ce target is 3 μg/mL) is achieved by a continuous infusion of propofol. After discontinuing propofol infusion (emergence), the Ce decreases over time, with consciousness returning when Ce less than 1.8 μg/mL.

according to **Table 1** or TCI, if the target Ce is 3 µg/mL, the actual Ce can range from approximately 2.3 to 5.4 µg/mL. Unlike sevoflurane, where expired concentration can be measured to infer brain sevoflurane concentration, blood propofol levels are not measured with propofol TIVA, which leaves uncertainty about brain Ce and raises concern about both overdose (hypotension) and underdose (intraoperative awareness). To overcome this, the dosing model can be used as a starting guide, while EEG can be used to further titrate dosing to the desired hypnotic level of the individual patient.

Electroencephalography parameters for propofol total intravenous anesthetic dosing

Numeric proprietary EEG indices may not be reliable in infants ages less than 1 year receiving propofol TIVA, whereas they generally are reliable in infants ages greater than 1 year. As with sevoflurane, this is due to the proprietary index being developed in adults and not accounting for the age-related differences in infant EEG.[11] In children greater than 1 year, processed EEG parameters can serve as a biomarker for propofol Ce and be used to adjust propofol dose, analogous to expired concentration serving as a biomarker for sevoflurane brain concentration. Several studies have observed that as propofol dose increases, BIS values decrease proportionately.[2,12,48,49] Compared with adults, however, children have relatively greater power in the high frequency bands, which may lead the proprietary EEG indices to be erroneously high; as a result, the anesthesiologist interprets the index to indicate light anesthesia and inappropriately administers more propofol.[5,11] The EEG waveforms and other EEG parameters should be evaluated to confirm the veracity of the index value.

In the authors' experience, EEG waveforms, DSA, and SEF95 can be used to assess hypnotic depth for propofol TIVA in all ages. For infants and children, the authors target SEF95 to 15 Hz to 20 Hz, 10 Hz to 15 Hz, and 6 Hz to 14 Hz for sedation, surgical maintenance, and laryngoscopy/surgical incision, respectively.[1] On raw EEG and DSA, increased power in beta and alpha bands indicate entry to deep sedation.[1,4] Decreased power in beta band along with increased power in theta and delta bands reflect an excellent depth of hypnosis.[1] Distinct power in the alpha band also demonstrates an excellent depth of hypnosis. Because these SEF95 and frequency band targets are not as reliable in neonates,[11] the authors also use EEG waveforms to identify isoelectricity as an indicator of cortical inactivity and excessively high propofol dose; when isoelectricity is encountered, the maintenance dose is decreased until EEG activity returns. As with sevoflurane, isoelectricity is common during propofol TIVA in neonates and infants when dose is guided by hemodynamic parameters.[14] Case 2 demonstrates how to use the dosing table and EEG to titrate a propofol infusion dose in a young child.

Case 2

A 13-month-old boy presented for robot-assisted laparoscopic excision of müllerian duct remnants, bilateral orchidopexy, and hypospadias repair. Propofol TIVA with remifentanil and continuous epidural anesthesia was planned. The authors followed the dosing regimen in **Table 1** (ages 12–36 months), selecting a remifentanil infusion dose of 0.2 µg/kg/min to cover minor noxious stimulation because the epidural was expected to provide significant analgesia. After induction with 3 mg/kg of propofol, SedLine EEG sensors were applied, and 0.2 mg/kg of cisatracurium and 1 µg/kg of fentanyl were administered. Propofol was infused using the Paedfusor TCI model, with a target Ce 3 µg/mL, which corresponded to 217 µg/kg/min (see **Table 1**) (0–30 minutes).

After intubation and placement of a low thoracic epidural catheter, 10 mL of 0.2% ropivacaine was injected and the propofol infusion was decreased to 192 µg/kg/min (see **Table 1**) (30–60 minutes). The EEG around the time of surgical incision is shown in **Fig. 6**A. The SEF95 was 12 Hz and the DSA showed strong power in < 4 Hz (red), weaker power in 8-10 Hz (yellow) and 12-15Hz (scattered yellow), corresponding to an anesthetic depth suitable for surgery. The target SEF95 for the anesthetic mainte-nance phase during surgery is 10-15Hz. **Fig. 6**B showed EEG at 90 minutes after inci-sion with propofol infusion at 183 μg/kg/min (see **Table 1**, 60-120 min). The SEF95 has now increased to 16 Hz and DSA showed decreased power (orange/red) in < 4 Hz and increased power (yellow) in 8-10 Hz and 12-15 Hz, indicating that the anesthetic depth needed to be increased to decrease the SEF95 back to the 10-15 Hz range. Therefore, TCI programmed Ce was increased to 4 μg/mL, corresponding to a 10% increase in propofol infusion to 200 μg/kg/min. At 200 minutes into surgery, surgical closure began. To prepare for emergence, TCI was decreased to Ce, 2 μg/mL, corresponding to a decrease in propofol from 167 μg/kg/min (see **Table 1**) (180 minutes–300 minutes) to 100 μg/kg/min. Shortly after the decrease, **Fig. 6**C shows SEF95 at 20 Hz and DSA showed increased power (yellow) at 12 Hz to 16 Hz, indicating decreased hypnotic depth. At the end of surgery, propofol and remifentanil were discontinued; 5 minutes later, the patient was extubated in the operating room. In the recovery area, **Fig. 6**D shows that SEF95 was low (2 Hz), DSA had increased power (red) in less than 4 Hz, and EEG waveforms showed large amplitude and low frequency, all consistent with natural sleep. This case demonstrates the use of the propofol dosing table and TCI-programmed Ce to dose propofol and then using EEG during surgery to adjust the pro-pofol dose for the individual patient.

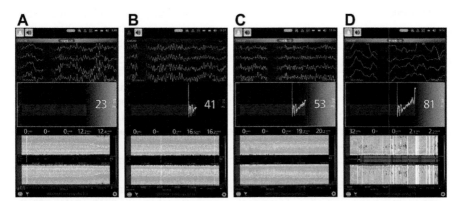

Fig. 6. SedLine EEG in a 13 month old, American Society of Anesthesiologist physical status class III, for urologic surgery using propofol and remifentanil TIVA with epidural analgesia. (*A*) Shortly before incision, propofol infusion 192 μg/kg/min corresponding to TCI program Ce 3 μg/mL. The EEG waveforms and DSA showed strong power in frequency bands theta-delta (*red band*) and alpha (*yellow band in middle of green band*), SEF95 12.4/12.2 Hz, indi-cating a good surgical level. (*B*) During surgery, EEG waveforms and DSA display increased power in bands alpha (*wider yellow band*) and beta (*brighter green band above alpha band*), SEF95 16.5/16.2 Hz, indicating that the patient was too light. Propofol infusion dose was increased by 10%, corresponding to TCI program Ce increase to 4 μg/mL. (*C*) Dur-ing surgical closure, propofol infusion dose was decreased from 167 μg/kg/min to 100 μg/kg/min in preparation for emergence, corresponding to TCI program Ce decrease to 2 μg/mL. EEG waveforms and DSA showed power in alpha (*broad yellow band*) and beta (*green band above yellow band*), SEF95 19.7/20.2 Hz, indicating ready for emergence. (*D*) At the end of surgery, propofol and remifentanil were discontinued and the patient was extubated in the operating room. EEG in the recovery room showed patterns that mimicked natural sleep: SEF95 less than 5 Hz and DSA showed power in theta bands.

SUMMARY

The dose of sevoflurane and propofol that produces unconsciousness varies by age group as well as between patients within the same age group, potentially creating risk for underdose and overdose in pediatric patients. Intraoperative EEG can be used as a biomarker of hypnotic depth in neonates, infants, and children to guide the dosing of propofol and sevoflurane to the individual patient. Although EEG proprietary numeric indices are unreliable as biomarkers of hypnosis in neonates and young infants, and more reliable in older children, EEG waveforms and nonproprietary processed EEG parameters are reliable biomarkers of propofol and sevoflurane levels across all ages. This article describes how to use EEG waveforms and nonproprietary processed parameters to guide dosing in pediatric anesthesia.

Clinics Care Points

- Electroencephalography (EEG) parameters, such as EEG waveforms, density spectral array, spectral edge frequency, and proprietary indices (eg, Bispectral Index-BIS), can be combined to help guide anesthetic dosing in pediatric patients.

- EEG can guide sevoflurane dosing to the individual patient, often resulting in a lower dose than suggested by standard minimum alveolar concentration (MAC) formulas.

- Pharmacokinetic models and EEG can guide propofol and remifentanil dosing in neonates, infants, and children. EEG can serve as a biomarker of propofol effect site concentration.

DISCLOSURE

The authors have nothing to disclose.

REFERENCES

1. Xu T, Kurth CD, Yuan I, et al. An approach to using pharmacokinetics and electroencephalography for propofol anesthesia for surgery in infants. Pediatr Anesth, in press.
2. Louvet N, Rigouzzo A, Sabourdin N, et al. Bispectral index under propofol anesthesia in children: a comparative randomized study between TIVA and TCI. Pediatr Anesth 2016;26(9):899–908.
3. Constant I, Sabourdin N. The EEG signal: a window on the cortical brain activity. Pediatr Anesth 2012;22(6):539–52.
4. Brown E, Purdon PL, Akeju O, et al. Using EEG markers to make inferences about anaesthetic-induced altered states of arousal. Br J Anaesth 2018;121(1):325–7.
5. Purdon PL, Sampson A, Pavone KJ, et al. Clinical electroencephalography for anesthesiologists: part I: background and basic signatures. Anesthesiology 2015; 123(4):937–60.
6. Chan MT, Hedrick TL, Egan TD, et al. American Society for Enhanced Recovery and Perioperative Quality Initiative Joint Consensus Statement on the role of neuromonitoring in perioperative outcomes: electroencephalography. Anesth Analg 2020;130(5):1278–91.
7. Nimmo A, Absalom A, Bagshaw O, et al. Guidelines for the safe practice of total intravenous anaesthesia (TIVA) Joint Guidelines from the Association of Anaesthetists and the Society for Intravenous Anaesthesia. Anaesthesia 2019;74(2): 211–24.
8. Habre W, Disma N, Virag K, et al. Incidence of severe critical events in paediatric anaesthesia (APRICOT): a prospective multicentre observational study in 261 hospitals in Europe. Lancet Respir Med 2017;5(5):412–25.

9. Kurth CD, Tyler D, Heitmiller E, et al. National pediatric anesthesia safety quality improvement program in the United States. Anesth Analg 2014;119(1):112–21.

10. Fahy BG, Chau DF. The technology of processed electroencephalogram monitoring devices for assessment of depth of anesthesia. Anesth Analg 2018; 126(1):111–7.

11. Lee JM, Akeju O, Terzakis K, et al. A prospective study of age-dependent changes in propofol-induced electroencephalogram oscillations in children. Anesthesiology 2017;127(2):293–306.

12. Rigouzzo A, Khoy-Ear L, Laude D, et al. EEG profiles during general anesthesia in children: a comparative study between sevoflurane and propofol. Pediatr Anesth 2019;29(3):250–7.

13. Davidson A, Skowno J. Neuromonitoring in paediatric anaesthesia. Curr Opin Anaesthesiol 2019;32(3):370–6.

14. Yuan I, Landis WP, Topjian AA, et al. Prevalence of isoelectric electroencephalography events in infants and young children undergoing general anesthesia. Anesth Analg 2020;130(2):462–71.

15. Tsuchida TN, Wusthoff CJ, Shellhaas RA, et al. American clinical neurophysiology society standardized EEG terminology and categorization for the description of continuous EEG monitoring in neonates: report of the American Clinical Neurophysiology Society critical care monitoring committee. J Clin Neurophysiol 2013;30(2):161–73.

16. Lee U, Mashour GA, Kim S, et al. Propofol induction reduces the capacity for neural information integration: implications for the mechanism of consciousness and general anesthesia. Conscious Cogn 2009;18(1):56–64.

17. Speigel I, Bichler EK, García PS. The influence of regional distribution and pharmacologic specificity of GABAAR subtype expression on anesthesia and emergence. Front Syst Neurosci 2017;11:58.

18. Pathan H, Williams J. Basic opioid pharmacology: an update. Br J Pain 2012; 6(1):11–6.

19. Pereira V, Goudet C. Emerging trends in pain modulation by metabotropic glutamate receptors. Front Mol Neurosci 2019;11:464.

20. Camina E, Güell F. The neuroanatomical, neurophysiological and psychological basis of memory: current models and their origins. Front Pharmacol 2017;8:438.

21. Avidan MS, Mashour GA. Prevention of intraoperative awareness with explicit recallmaking sense of the evidence. Anesthesiology 2013;118(2):449–56.

22. Behne M, Wilke H-J, Harder S. Clinical pharmacokinetics of sevoflurane. Clin Pharmacokinet 1999;36(1):13–26.

23. Malviya S, Lerman J. The blood/gas solubilities of sevoflurane, isoflurane, halothane, and serum constituent concentrations in neonates and adults. Anesthesiology 1990;72(5):793–6.

24. Goa KL, Noble S, Spencer CM. Sevoflurane in paediatric anaesthesia. Paediatr Drugs 1999;1(2):127–53.

25. Patel SS, Goa KL. Sevoflurane. Drugs 1996;51(4):658–700.

26. Olbrecht VA, Skowno J, Marchesini V, et al. An international, multicenter, observational study of cerebral oxygenation during infant and neonatal anesthesia. Anesthesiology 2018;128(1):85–96.

27. McKeever S, Johnston L, Davidson AJ. Sevoflurane-induced changes in infants' quantifiable electroencephalogram parameters. Pediatr Anesth 2014;24(7): 766–73.

28. Dennhardt N, Arndt S, Beck C, et al. Effect of age on Narcotrend index monitoring during sevoflurane anesthesia in children below 2 years of age. Pediatr Anesth 2018;28(2):112–9.

29. Hayashi K, Shigemi K, Sawa T. Neonatal electroencephalography shows low sensitivity to anesthesia. Neurosci Lett 2012;517(2):87–91.

30. Cornelissen L, Kim S-E, Purdon PL, et al. Age-dependent electroencephalogram (EEG) patterns during sevoflurane general anesthesia in infants. Elife 2015;4: e06513.

31. Kim H, Oh AY, Kim C, et al. Correlation of bispectral index with end-tidal sevoflurane concentration and age in infants and children. Br J Anaesth 2005;95(3): 362–6.

32. Kreuzer I, Osthaus WA, Schultz A, et al. Influence of the sevoflurane concentration on the occurrence of epileptiform EEG patterns. PLoS One 2014;9(2): e89191.

33. Koch S, Stegherr A, Mörgeli R, et al. Electroencephalogram dynamics in children during different levels of anaesthetic depth. Clin Neurophysiol 2017;128(10): 2014–21.

34. Cornelissen L, Bergin AM, Lobo K, et al. Electroencephalographic discontinuity during sevoflurane anesthesia in infants and children. Pediatr Anesth 2017; 27(3):251–62.

35. Anderson BJ, Bagshaw O. Practicalities of total intravenous anesthesia and target-controlled infusion in children. Anesthesiology 2019;131(1):164–85.

36. Kataria BK, Ved SA, Nicodemus HF, et al. The pharmacokinetics of propofol in children using three different data analysis approaches. Anesthesiology 1994; 80(1):104–22.

37. Absalom A, Mani V, De Smet T, et al. Pharmacokinetic models for propofol— defining and illuminating the devil in the detail. Br J Anaesth 2009;103(1):26–37.

38. Iwakiri H, Nishihara N, Nagata O, et al. Individual effect-site concentrations of propofol are similar at loss of consciousness and at awakening. Anesth Analg 2005;100(1):107.

39. Fuentes R, Cortínez I, Ibacache M, et al. Propofol concentration to induce general anesthesia in children aged 3–11 years with the Kataria effect-site model. Pediatr Anesth 2015;25(6):554–9.

40. Kuizenga MH, Colin PJ, Reyntjens KM, et al. Population pharmacodynamics of propofol and sevoflurane in healthy volunteers using a clinical score and the patient state index a crossover study. Anesthesiology 2019;131(6):1223–38.

41. Johnson KB, Syroid ND, Gupta DK, et al. An evaluation of remifentanil propofol response surfaces for loss of responsiveness, loss of response to surrogates of painful stimuli and laryngoscopy in patients undergoing elective surgery. Anesth Analg 2008;106(2):471–9.

42. Minto CF, Schnider TW, Egan TD, et al. Influence of age and gender on the pharmacokinetics and pharmacodynamics of remifentanil. I. Model development. Anesthesiology 1997;86(1):10–23.

43. Eleveld D, Colin P, Absalom A, et al. Pharmacokinetic–pharmacodynamic model for propofol for broad application in anaesthesia and sedation. Br J Anaesth 2018;120(5):942–59.

44. McFarlan CS, Anderson BJ, Short TG. The use of propofol infusions in paediatric anaesthesia: a practical guide. Pediatr Anesth 1999;9(3):209–16.

45. Steur R, Perez R, De Lange J. Dosage scheme for propofol in children under 3 years of age. Pediatr Anesth 2004;14(6):462–7.

46. Absalom A, Kenny G. 'Paedfusor'pharmacokinetic data set. Br J Anaesth 2005; 95(1):110.

47. Morse J, Hannam JA, Cortinez LI, et al. A manual propofol infusion regimen for neonates and infants. Pediatr Anesth 2019;29(9):907–14.

48. Park HJ, Kim YL, Kim CS, et al. Changes of bispectral index during recovery from general anesthesia with 2% propofol and remifentanil in children. Pediatr Anesth 2007;17(4):353–7.

49. Akeju O, Pavone KJ, Westover MB, et al. A comparison of propofol-and dexmedetomidine-induced electroencephalogram dynamics using spectral and coherence analysis. Anesthesiology 2014;121(5):978.

Moving?

Make sure your subscription moves with you!

To notify us of your new address, find your **Clinics Account Number** (located on your mailing label above your name), and contact customer service at:

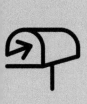

Email: journalscustomerservice-usa@elsevier.com

800-654-2452 (subscribers in the U.S. & Canada)
314-447-8871 (subscribers outside of the U.S. & Canada)

Fax number: 314-447-8029

Elsevier Health Sciences Division
Subscription Customer Service
3251 Riverport Lane
Maryland Heights, MO 63043

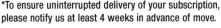

*To ensure uninterrupted delivery of your subscription, please notify us at least 4 weeks in advance of move.

ELSEVIER

Printed and bound by CPI Group (UK) Ltd, Croydon, CR0 4YY

08/05/2025

01864694-0005